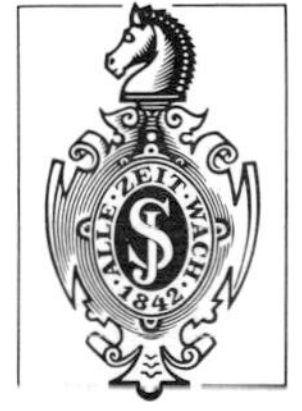
ALLE · ZEIT · WACH
1842

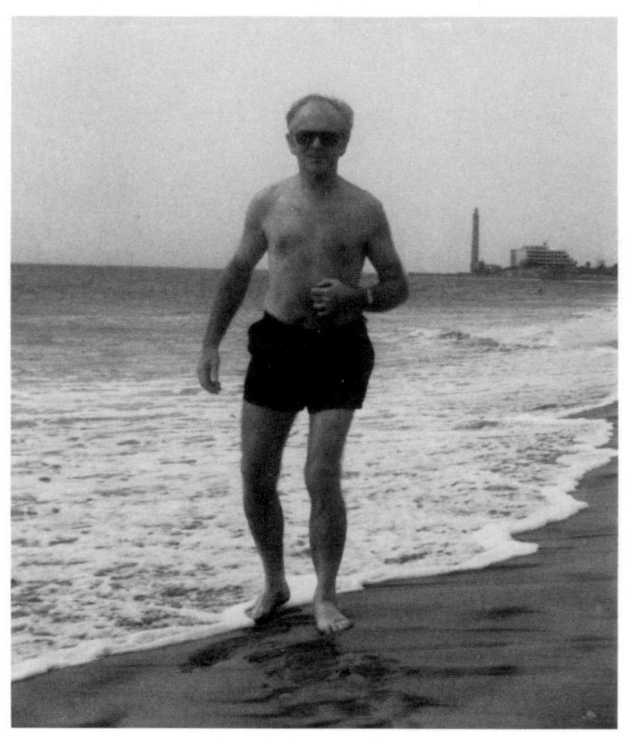

Free to choose where, when and with whom he would like to be, or even to be on his own

(Chapter 10)

Patricia M. Davies

Steps To Follow

A Guide to the Treatment of Adult Hemiplegia

Based on the Concept of K. and B. Bobath

With a Foreword by W. M. Zinn

With 326 Figures in 492 Separate Illustrations

Springer-Verlag
Berlin Heidelberg New York Tokyo

Patricia M. Davies, MCSP Dip. Phys. Ed.
Loc. Capannaccia
I-07020 Palau (SS)
Sardegna

Photographs:
David J. Brühwiller
CH-7310 Bad Ragaz

1st edition 1985, 8th printing 1993

ISBN 3-540-13436-0 Springer-Verlag Berlin Heidelberg New York Tokyo
ISBN 0-387-13436-0 Springer-Verlag New York Heidelberg Berlin Tokyo

Library of Congress Cataloging in Publication Data
Davies, Patricia M.
Steps to follow.
Bibliography: p. Includes index. l. Hemiplegics – Rehabilitation. I. Title. RC406.H45D38
1985 616.8'1 84-14066 ISBN 0-387-13436-0 (U. S.)

Typesetting and printing: Appl, Wemding
Binding: Schäffer, Grünstadt
21/3145 - 10 9 8 - Printed on acid-free paper

Foreword

The treatment and reintegration of adults with brain damage sustained as a result of illness or accident is one of the most important and challenging tasks in the field of rehabilitation. This is not only due to the complexity of the lost functions, but also because stroke is the most frequent cause of severe disability in our society. Approximately 25% of all severely disabled persons are hemiplegics (Nichols 1976). Brain damage caused by vascular disease is a tremendous problem for any population and civilization. Causes and effects, with the resulting symptoms, vary so widely that the problems are only gradually being recognized, and then perhaps not fully, even by the most committed research workers, doctors and therapists. The functional disturbances that arise as a result of cerebro-vascular accident, that is following stroke, in young and old do not differ fundamentally for the different age groups. Treatment and rehabilitation do however become more difficult with increasing age due mainly to the frequent presence of multiple disease, multiple sites, the diffuse spread of the vascular disease and the brain damage itself, the decreasing plasticity of the central nervous system and the frequent absence of a partner, of relatives and friends in later years.

Deep down inside everyone knows that a stroke is one of the most devastating traumas to the whole personality, that it is a dreadful blow to the person directly affected and to his family and friends as well.

In recent years the frequency of cerebro-vascular accident has finally started to decline slightly, as more is now known about the causative factors and their early detection, and certain measures of prophylaxis are therefore possible. The medical statistics in various countries document the effectiveness of such prophylactic measures and that doctors currently in practice are making increasing efforts to fulfil their obligations in this respect.

Size of the Problem

According to Dutch (Herman et al. 1980), American (Robins and Baum 1981), Finnish (Kallio 1980) and Swiss (Zinn 1978) studies, in western countries an average of about 320–400 people per year out of every 100,000 can be expected to suffer a first stroke. In Switzerland this would mean a total of over 20,000 people newly affected by stroke every year (Zinn 1981). There is a fairly linear increase in frequency rising from 5 per 100,000 of the population under the age of 20, to 1800 per 100,000 by the age of 85. About 25% of the patients are under 50 and just under 70% are over 60 years old. Men are more frequently affected than women, the male/female ratio being 144 : 100 within any age group (Robins and Baum 1981). Because many newly affected stroke patients will not survive the insult, and on the other hand many will be only slightly affected, it can be expected that in any one year there will be approximately 6000 new hemiplegic patients in Switzerland who would be able to benefit substantially from specific therapy and rehabilitation programs.

Neurophysiological Aspects

According to Bobath (1970) the central nervous system is an organ of re-action rather than of action, and reacts to stimuli converging on it from outside and within the body. Certainly only a small proportion of our actions are the result of a completely free decision, which in fact is hard to picture neurophysiologically. We are only able to select a course of action or a function from pe-existing, learned and well controlled circuits within the brain. Everything else that we do occurs automatically.

In most cases, of course, even the choice of action is governed by reflexes or determined by the strength and nature of the approaching stimuli and whether in-put exceeds the threshold of stimulation. We do not normally remember turning off the alarm clock in the morning, getting out of bed, washing, dressing and having breakfast, or how we drove the car and reached work at more or less the right time, not to mention the many mistakes we make even in decisive situations.

The power of habit is the result of acquired control circuits in the central nervous system, which have been facilitated by repetition and in this way stored or been assimilated, becoming second nature to us so that we continually fall back on them in our daily life.

The central nervous system is an organ of perception with prompt serial and intermodal integration and virtually instant programming and coordination of the corresponding reactions to the overall sensory stimulation or information. The capacity for perceiving is much greater than that for production. We are, then, dependent upon redundant sensory stimulation, and even small defects in perception have substantial results in terms of impaired performance. If problems of perception go unrecognized they can therefore quickly lead to overstrain and frustration or neglect, depression or neurosis. These in turn impede many opportunities for further communication and development.

The activity of the cells in our central nervous system can be excitatory or inhibitory. The most important function of the central nervous system is its ability to inhibit unco-ordinated or unwanted activity and to facilitate usable functions and so make possible the storing of information, in other words our capacity for learning. In physiological terms this is called plasticity. The plasticity of our central nervous system is at the very crux of our existence and development. Every learning process, and thus also the practical work of rehabilitation depends upon the preconditions of stimulability, inhibition and facilitation. The greater the patient's residual learning capacity, in other words the plasticity of his central nervous system, the more successful will his rehabilitation be.

Rehabilitation medicine, like every other branch of medicine is based on successful communication, and on learning from one another. We must aim to recognize all the patient's problems and to find the channels of communication best suited to him or her as an individual. More than anything else, therefore, the treatment poses problems of teaching, learning and instruction. Doctor, nurse, occupational therapist, physiotherapist, social worker and neuropsychologist should all recognize the necessity for a sound knowledge of modern educational theory and modern developmental psychology for teaching and learning, and have such knowledge at their finger tips.

The human being develops millions of nerve cells and nerve fibres and an inconceivable number of synapses between them, with parallel fibres and cross connections for possible by-passes. We also have more primitive functions from an earlier stage in development which are normally blocked and not evident, but may be used again as substitutes. Every function of the central nervous system, every sensation, every act of recognition, every movement, requires its own control circuit, and the action potentials needed for these circuits sometimes pass a great many contact points (synapses), which means that they have to be connected to umpteen different circuits. If an activity is repeated the resistance drops at the synapses through which the electrical potentials required for the activity pass. The conduction at the synapses from one nerve cell to another therefore becomes easier or is facilitated. Those nerve fibres not needed for that particular task gradually become blocked or inhibited. When this inhibition or facilitation has taken place, the function has been learned or stored. From then on it is available for recalling and using on the basis of an automatic or, occasionally, also of a voluntary process of selection or decision-making.

Piaget and Morf (1958), Piaget (1961), Affolter (1966, 1967) and Affolter et al. (1974a, b) have shown that of the many sensory modalities, three main channels of perception are important and must be intact for normal child development: the tactile/kinesthetic, the visual and the auditory channels. That is to say, feeling, seeing and hearing. To learn and develop normally, we need not only a qualitative sensory or modality specific capacity for perceiving, but must also be in a position to follow up, integrate and store impressions and sequences from a sensory modality even when they follow each other in rapid succession. I refer here to the serial integration of signals following each other in time very quickly, and also, of course to the integration of sequences of actions, movements and thought processes. The intramodal, or channel-specific serial capacity for integration must also be accompanied by the intermodal linkage of sensory impressions, that is, intermodal integration, if normal development is to take place.

Various stages of perception can be observed during normal development, giving the child the ability to choose, make decisions and to plan. Affolter (1976) refers to transitional stages of planning which follow one after the other as we develop.

Affolter and co-workers (1974a) have confirmed in various controlled studies that for the learning of functions needed in our daily life the most important is an intact tactile/kinesthetic channel and also the capacity for serial and intermodal integration. During a course held in the Hermitage, which is the post-graduate school attached to our clinic, Dr. Affolter conducted a controlled study using the course participants as subjects. The results showed that information about three-dimensional physical activities was substantially better received and remembered when it was felt (up to 80%), than when it was only seen or heard (20–40%). Since in the case of restoration of function after a brain lesion, the greatest emphasis is on three-dimensional recognition and movement patterns, it is obvious that in rehabilitation generally, in the fascinating process of teaching and learning between patient and therapist, it is not auditory and visual communication that plays the major part, but communication by way of the tactile/kinesthetic channel, that is by feeling. But, our development also depends on the intensity and variety of the stimulation to which we are exposed. The more intensive and varied the stimulation, the thicker our nerve fibres become, and the more synapses and connections are formed by our nerve cells (Eccles 1975; Rosenzweig 1980). We need, therefore to present children, pupils and adults with impressions to challenge and encourage them, to help them to train their personalities, their ethical natures, their minds and their bodies, in order to give them the opportunity of a fulfilled life. The maximum learning effect is reached if we manage to hold their full attention and maintain it at the peak performance level for a certain period during the learning process. The degree of attention can only be monitored by constant and precise observation. Motivation is increased by wide and frequent variation in the training program.

If we also give the central nervous system the rest periods it needs, it will eventually build up a maximum of assimilated circuits for comparing and recalling.

As modern developmental psychology and gerontology have confirmed, however, the process of development by no means comes to an end at a certain age, but continues throughout life until shortly before death (Agruso 1977; Baltes 1979). The learning capacity admittedly declines somewhat in later life (Zinn 1981), but this is mainly because the adult gradually forgets how to make use of the learning strategies which he used during school years or training, and also does not acquire any of the new learning techniques which have been developed since then. However, because of his or her experience and better judgement as to the value of the information to be learned, the adult can be in a better position to learn more rationally and effectively than children or young people (Weinert 1981).

The function of our central nervous system, our learning capacity, and our overall development are therefore dependent upon what we have received in the way of genetically determined factors, and also what we have facilitated, stored and learned through experience as a result of stimulation from our environment. This means that we learn and develop by way of our sensory system and all that we perceive.

Design for Therapy

How can a therapy, a re-education, personal relationships, a whole new life be instructed when perception has been impaired as a result of brain damage during adult life? How can we best help such patients day by day?

Close collaboration with several research groups and the rapidly increasing knowledge on the neurophysiology of restoration of function after brain damage have encouraged us to adopt a more energetic and enthusiastic approach in the treatment of patients with brain lesions. In this way we have been able to make a much better assessment of the patient's potential for functional gains in the rehabilitation process and to realize this potential in the restoration of function far more successfully than before (Zinn 1981). The main emphasis is on determining perceptual impairment by observation, and the subsequent training of perceptual performances (Affolter 1977).

In the brain-damaged patient the control circuits of the enormous store of habits and experience which he or she has accumulated, have been interrupted – either definitely destroyed or merely functionally blocked, in any event they cannot be recalled. In the treatment of severely affected patients in particular, the first priority is to find function circuits that are still intact though at the time not able to be used, and to unblock them by confrontation with suitable material. The activities and objects used are those with which the patient was familiar in his daily life before his illness, because the chance of recognition and recall will then be facilitated during the stage of post-stroke or post-traumatic amnesia. The transference to his new day-to-day life will also be easier. The exercise situation must be taken from the patient's own reality and include the problems confronting him in daily life. We do not work with individual stimuli, but with complete events taken from his own experience. The regained circuits serve as a support for the recovery of further functions. From the beginning the patient, his trunk and extremities, need support and must be guided along natural patterns of movement to provide him with natural perceptive stimuli, i.e. the resistance of the objects of our environment. The therapist quickly feels the patient perceiving a resistance, recognizing it more readily, taking over and then learning the practised movement. Finally he will reach a point where integration takes place. If we work in natural, physiologically appropriate movement patterns the patient will learn through repetition and will make constant progress.

Results

Steinmann (1977) advocated the incorporation of the Bobath concept into the treatment immediately after onset of stroke. He showed that nursing care, physiotherapy and occupational therapy for patients with vascular hemiplegia in acute hospitals, or early transfer to a rehabilitation centre with an appropriate treatment concept could bring about a marked reduction in the occurrence of secondary complications, and make it possible for a much larger proportion of the patients to become completely or almost independent in daily life. Garraway et al. (1980) later provided unequivocal evidence of this. We ourselves have been able to achieve at least equivalent results in our intercantonal hospital in Valens (Zinn 1981). Expanding and intensifying the treatment design, and incorporating and evaluating the ideas put forward by the quoted and many other authors will undoubtedly allow further progress in the treatment and rehabilitation of brain-damaged adults. Our work is still in its early stages, and it has not yet been possible to evaluate any comparative, statistically controlled studies. Nonetheless, on the basis of our experience, extending over several years, it seems clear to us that many severely affected patients with vascular and traumatic brain damage can now be helped and rehabilitated, where previously neither we nor other practicing doctors and therapists had much to offer them. Finally it should not be forgotten that the commitment of those involved in treatment, rehabilitation and social net-work around the patient can contribute substantially to its success. Joyce (1982) and Joyce and Swallow (1964) have shown that whole-hearted commitment can increase the success rate of a therapy by up to 40%!

About the Author

Patricia Davies, the author of this book, has a background that makes her particularly qualified in the field of physiotherapy for neurological patients. Her own natural talent and her training in this specialized field as well as in education have combined to equip her for the work. Her book is the product of many years of practical experience and study in several countries.

Ms. Davies is certainly exceptionally well suited to integrate the rapidly accumulating results of empirical, clinical and experimental neurophysiological observation and research into an ordered treatment system for physiotherapy for adult patients with hemiplegia, and to present it extremely clearly.

She refers modestly and gives credit to the concepts of great creative thinkers, whom we also hold in high esteem, but this should not prevent us from pointing out the substantial nature of the author's own contribution and her many interesting suggestions. I refer here to "the problems we cannot see", "re-educating functional walking", the chapter shedding some more light on the shoulder problems and to the "pusher syndrome" which as far as I know is included and described here for the first time.

By confining herself to those aspects that are essential for physiotherapy, Ms. Davies has documented her critically scientific attitude and work. On the other hand, large parts of her book also provide indispensable bases for medical and nursing care, occupational therapy, speech therapy, neuropsychology and social work.

Many years of close collaboration with K. and B. Bobath, Kay Coombes, Felicie Affolter and her group have given her the opportunity to further develop the rehabilitation of brain-damaged patients. It has been a privilege for me to be allowed to observe and encourage the author as she progressively linked and integrated the ideas offered by the various concepts in physical therapy. Her work has met with great and increasing interest from therapists in this field as is evident from the growing numbers applying to attend her courses. It is particularly pleasing that gradually doctors too, especially neurologists and rehabilitation specialists with a particular interest in therapy, are also starting to come for information. By reading this book and by constant close co-operation doctors can inspire and enhance the contribution of the physiotherapist. Close cooperation of this kind will certainly stimulate research in neurophysiology, which in recent years has confirmed some of the processes involved in recovery as observed in clinical practice, and clarified their mechanisms.

Wilhelm M. Zinn

References

Affolter F (1976) Auditive Wahrnehmungsstörungen und Lernschwierigkeiten. Monatsschr Kinderheilkd 124: 612

Affolter F (1977) Neue Aspekte der Wahrnehmungsleistungen und ihrer Störungen. Merkblatt der Medizinischen Abteilung Bad Ragaz, No 126

Affolter F, Stricker E (eds) (1980) Perceptual progresses as prerequisites for complex human behavior. Hans Huber, Bern

Affolter F, Brubaker R, Bischofberger W (1974a) Comparative studies between normal and language-disturbed children. Acta Otolaryngol [Suppl 323]

Affolter F, Brubaker R, Stockman IJ, Constam AG, Bischofberger W (1974b) Prerequisites for speech development: Visual, auditory and tactile patterns discrimination. Med Progr Technol 2: 93

Agruso VM, Jr (1977) Learning in the later years. Academic, New York

Baltes PB (ed) (1979) Entwicklungspsychologie der Lebensspanne. Klett-Cotta, Stuttgart

Bobath B (1970) Adult Hemiplegia: Evaluation and treatment. Heinemann Medical, London

Bobath K (1964–1978) Oral presentations during courses in the Medical Department Bad Ragaz and at the intercantonclinic at Valens

Eccles JC (1975) Wahrheit und Wirklichkeit. Springer, Berlin

Garraway WM, Akthar AJ, Prescott RJ, Hockey L (1980) Management of acute stroke in the elderly: Preliminary results of a controlled trial. Br Med J 1: 1040

Hermann B, Schulte BPM, Luijk JH, Leyten ACM, Frenken CWGM (1980) Epidemiology of stroke in Tilburg/NL. The population-based stroke incidence register. I. Introduction and preliminary results. Stroke 11: 162

Joyce CRB (1982) How to improve clinical judgment? Merkblatt der Medizinischen Abteilung Bad Ragaz, No 238

Joyce CRB, Swallow JN (1964) The controlled trial in dental surgery. Premedication of handicapped children with carisoprodol. Dent Pract 15: 44–47

Kallio V (1980) Ergebnisse der Mini-Finnland-Studie. (Oral presentation) 1980

Nichols PJR (1976) Rehabilitation medicine. Butterworths, London

Piaget J (1961) Les mecanismes perceptifs: Modèles, probabilistes, analyse génétique, relations avec l'intelligence. Presses Universitaires de France, Paris

Piaget J, Morf A (1958) Les préinférences perceptives et leurs relations avec les schèmes sensorimoteurs et opératoires. In: Bruner J, Bresson F, Morf A, Piaget J (eds) Logique et perception. Bibliotheque scientifique internationale, études d'épistémologie génétique. Presses Universitaires de France, Paris

Robins M, Baum HM (1981) Incidence. In: Weinfeld FD (ed) The national survey of stroke. Stroke 12: [suppl 1, chap IV]

Rosenzweig MR (1980) Animal models for effects of brain lesions and for rehabilitation. In: Bach-y-Rita P (ed) Recovery of function: Theoretical considerations for brain injury rehabilitation. Huber, Bern

Steinmann B (1977) Behandlung und Management von Patienten mit Hemiplegie. Vortrag an der gemeinsamen Fortbildungstagung der Schweizerischen Arbeitsgemeinschaft für Prothetik und Orthotik und der Schweizerischen Arbeitsgemeinschaft für Rehabilitation, Bern

Weinert FE (1981) Entwicklungspsychologie des Erwachsenenalters. Merkblatt der Medizinischen Abteilung Bad Ragaz No 231

Zinn WM (1978) Assessment, treatment and rehabilitation of adult patients with brain damage. Int Rehab Med 1: 3–9

Zinn WM (1981a) Vaskuläre Hirnschäden im Alter, Analyse und Lösung der Probleme. Bericht über die wissenschaftlichen Verhandlungen an der Jahrestagung der Schweizerischen Gesellschaft für Gerontologie, St. Gallen, 12.–14. 11. 1981

Zinn WM (1981b) Möglichkeiten, Grenzen und Finanzierung der Rehabilitation von Apoplektikern (inkl. Hilfsmittel). Ther Umsch 38: 776–790

Preface

> People need hope,
> People need loving,
> People need trust from a fellow man,
> People need love to make a good living,
> People need faith in a helping hand.
>
> Abba

For the last 7 years my professional time has been divided roughly in half, between treating patients and giving courses on the treatment of neurological disorders, mainly adult hemiplegia, for members of the medical and paramedical professions. Both the patients and course members alike frequently ask me if there is not a book which contains all that they have learnt, so that they can read more to deepen and stabilise their knowledge. I have found it difficult to advise them what to select from the enormous amount of rather theoretical literature, which often fails to give practical guide-lines on just how to cope with the manifold problems which confront them.

I hope that this book will fill the gap, and in writing it I have tried to be practical and at the same time as scientific as possible. But essentially it is a book about people, the patients and those who care for them, and people are not made up of facts and figures as the literature tends to imply. Furthermore, I hope that all the many therapists, nurses and relatives of patients who do not have the opportunity to attend special courses will also find the book useful. As Sagan (1977) writes, it has been possible to learn from a book since the invention of writing and not be entirely dependent on the "lucky accident" that there is someone nearby to teach us in person.

Apart from caring for or treating the patient in the hospital or rehabilitation centre, it is important to see how he manages in the world outside, with all its variety and challenge. It is part of rehabilitation to observe the patient in as many and as various situations as possible. Many judgements as to the success of the rehabilitation programme are made solely on the patient's performance in a very sheltered environment. Because of the pleasant custom in Switzerland, where by the patient at the end of a period of treatment invites his therapists and his doctor to a meal, I personally have learnt a great deal and have been forced to alter many preconceived ideas. There is an enormous difference between "can walk 45 m unaided" and walking to a table in a crowded restaurant. Eating together also provides a valuable time for listening to what the patient says, time which is often missing in a busy department.

For the therapists and others who read this book I should like to offer a few thoughts which could be of help, especially for those who may have had little experience in treating patients with hemiplegia before, or in using the concept described.

1. Because it is a concept rather than a technique, there is no absolute prescription which would suit every patient. Anything which results in a new ability for the patient, or enables him to move in a more normal way, can be used without hesitation.

2. The treatment of hemiplegia is not a series of isolated exercises performed in a set order, but is a sequence of activities in preparation for an actual function.
3. Rehabilitation starts on the day when the patient suffers a stroke, and not only when he is fit enough to attend a rehabilitation centre.
4. All who work with the patient must be very convinced of the importance of each position or activity used, because if we are not convinced he certainly will not be.
5. Not all hemiplegic patients are old and decrepit, and they will have expectations from their rehabilitation which extend way beyond just independence in self-care in the home, or managing to walk 45 m slowly even if unaided. It is important to try to achieve far higher goals for each patient. And even if the patient is old, his age should not exclude him from a full and active treatment programme. Age has been shown to be no deterrent to rehabilitation or recovery (Andrews et al. 1982, Adler et al. 1980).
6. The patient should be spoken to in a normal adult way and care must be taken to avoid a singsong voice and the use of the "we" form when he alone is being asked to do something. Much can be asked of him as long as we talk and discuss matters with him seriously. Hemiplegia is, after all, a very serious event in his life, and he has a right to be involved in decisions concerning his future. Particular care must be taken when addressing the patient who has aphasia. Being able to watch the speaker's face and the use of short, concise sentences will help him to understand what is being said.
7. When ever possible, negative feedback should be avoided, as the patient's day can otherwise be filled with "nos" and "don'ts". Merely by changing a few words the same correction can be given in a positive form.

Patients of all ages and at different stages of their rehabilitation have been used for the illustrations in the following chapters, to try to give an idea of the great diversity of people suffering from the effects of a stroke. The ages of the patients shown in the book range from 30 to 80 years.

For purposes of clarity, the masculine pronoun has been used in the entire text to refer to the patient, and the feminine form for the therapist or assistant. In the legends the correct form of the pronoun is used according to the sex of the person in the photograph.

Bad Ragaz, November 1984 *Pat Davies*

Acknowledgements

On completing this book I have the urge to express my gratitude to so many people who have contributed to its publication, perhaps without realising how much they have inspired or taught me along the way. Such a list would be far too long, so I must try to reduce it to those who have been directly connected with the actual material presented and the preparation of the manuscript. I hope that all those friends and colleagues not mentioned by name will accept my thanks indirectly.

First and foremost, I should like to express my sincere thanks to Karel and Bertie Bobath for developing their concept of inhibition of spasticity and facilitation of normal movement which has brought so much to patients and therapists all over the world. Without their teaching this book could never have been written.

I should also like to express my gratitude to my employers, *Thermalbäder und Grand Hotels,* Medical Department Bad Ragaz, for allowing me the time to undertake the writing of the book. Without their generosity the task would not have been accomplished. For his support and encouragement in all my work in Switzerland I wish to thank Dr. Wilhelm Zinn. His open-mindedness and faith in my abilities have provided a constant stimulation and allowed me the freedom to develop my ideas.

I owe my understanding of the problems which we cannot see directly to Dr. Felicie Affolter, and I am so very grateful to her for opening my eyes to them.

Learning from Kay Coombes how to deal with the problems of the face and oral tract has been a great joy, and I thank her not only for enabling me to write Chapt. 13 but also on behalf of the many patients who have difficulties in this area. I should like to thank Jennifer Todd, who developed many of the ideas used in the treatment during the acute phase and who originally helped me to organise other activities into sequences for teaching.

I should like to thank Dr. Eric Hamilton and Margaret Stewart for their encouragement and support when I was developing my approach at Kings College Hospital, London. I am grateful to the many, many course members who by their enthusiasm and interest have been partly responsible for my putting pen to paper. Their questions and difficulties in treatment have guided me in the planning of the book.

I should like to say a very big "thank you" to all the patients who so willingly agreed to be photographed, making the information in the book much clearer than words alone could ever have been. I am very sad that some of them did not live to see the book completed.

To the team in Valens I should like to express my gratitude for putting the concept into practice and proving that it really does work. It was a joy to see it happening in the Lucas-Stichting Rehabilitation Centre in Hoensbroek as well.

Until preparing the manuscript for publication, I had never fully understood why authors always thanked so fervently those who had typed for them. I understand now, and would like to express a multitude of thanks to Mrs. Gisela Jäger, Mrs. Margit Bischofberger, Ms. Jeannette Bauder and Ms. Astrid Wälti for deciphering my handwriting, bringing order to the chaos and typing and retyping the manuscript. To Karl and Jill Sprogis, I should like to express my sincere thanks for reading and correcting the different chapters so carefully, despite the pressure of time.

I am deeply grateful to Gisela Rolf, who has supported me both professionally and privately throughout the whole time of writing this book. She has given me courage when mine has failed, and in so many practical ways has helped me to complete the manuscript. I should like to thank her for her tolerance, understanding and never-failing support.

Finally, to my mother and father, who enabled me to study first physical education and then physiotherapy, I should like to say a big "thank you", for that was the beginning of it all.

Contents

1 The Problems We Cannot See

There is a widespread tendency in the rehabilitation of patients who have suffered a stroke to focus attention on problems which can actually be seen. The therapist observes the patient and immediately notices the position of his spastic arm, his inability to move his fingers or use his hand. She can see at a glance that he walks with his leg extended and is unable to dorsiflex his foot to clear the ground. Most treatment concepts in present day use concentrate on reducing spasticity and stimulating activity in the paralysed muscles. The word "hemiplegia" itself emphasises these problems with its original meaning – a paralysis of half (of the body).

Unfortunately, for many patients with hemiplegia the problems are far more complex. Failure to recognise the problems which we cannot see directly will lead to disappointment and frustration for therapist and patient in the rehabilitation programme. Success is dependent on the recognition of the problems and the inclusion of specific therapy to overcome the difficulties arising from them. In a survey of the long-term outcome for patients and their families, Coughlan and Humphrey (1982) found persisting problems of self-care in two-thirds of 170 surviving stroke patients who had been treated during an 8-year period.

Jimenez and Morgan (1979) give a figure of only 59% of patients with a stroke who were able to care for themselves at time of discharge from hospital. Satterfield (1982), in a survey of over 2000 patients, describes only 46% as having been taught independence in dressing. Lehmann et al. (1975) show a figure of approximately 78% who could dress independently at time of discharge.

The reasons which are generally given for stopping active treatment before complete independence has been achieved vary. Adams and Hurwitz (1963) write:

> Some patients are said to have been confused or unco-operative; others to have had no drive or initiative; and yet others to have had inadequate mentation or lack of motivation. These terms, however expressive or elegant, imply only that the patient was getting nowhere. They do not say why, and sometimes they attach a misleading label of impending dementia to a patient whose true disability is a focal cerebral lesion causing impaired comprehension, loss of recent memory, postural imbalance, apraxia, or loss of body awareness with neglect, anosognosia, or denial of ownership of the affected limbs.

All such problems can be said to arise from disturbances of perception and are the problems which we cannot see. They can only be observed indirectly by observing many different performances, making inferences about their prerequisite perceptual processes and then comparing them (Affolter and Stricker 1980).

It may help to understand the nature and effects of such problems by using a concrete example. Patients with hemiplegia often have considerable difficulty in learning to dress themselves. If a patient is observed as he struggles unsuccessfully to get dressed, an insight can be gained as to the complexity of the problems. The movements do not flow, he cannot put on his clothes in the correct order, he may not find the armhole and sometimes ends up with the garment on back to front. The activity is slow and laborious, and very often the patient will be unable to complete the task at all, and resign after a few unsuccessful attempts.

By comparison, a normal subject simulating a total paralysis on one side of the body can dress himself with one hand easily and efficiently in less than 5 min. The activity proceeds effortlessly, and the model adjusts quickly to the new experience. After a few practice runs he will have no difficulty in carrying out the task. The same applies to a patient whose disability is primarily a motor one. Even without specific training he will learn to dress himself with one hand in a very short time, as many indeed do.

1.1 Perception and Perceptual Problems

Our ability to learn and to adapt continually to our ever-changing environment is dependent on intact perceptual processes. The concept of perception is very complex, and as Affolter and Stricker (1980) state: "Perception includes all mechanisms used in processing the stimuli of an actual situation, including the different sensory modalities, supramodal organisation levels, respective storage systems, and recognition performances." In a similar way, Carterette and Friedman (1973) have defined perception as "understanding the way in which the organism transforms, organises and structures information arising from the world in sense data or memory."

In normal life, from the time we wake up till the time we go to sleep we are constantly solving problems and making decisions for the necessary adaptation – to movement, to happenings and to other people around us. Adaptation is dependent on intact perceptual processing, so that the hemiplegic patient who has a disturbance of the perceptual processes due to the lesion will fail to behave and adapt adequately in his daily life as a result. If, as Pitt (1976) has shown, problem-solving by normal adults entails up to 24 subroutines consisting of heuristic subprocesses and strategies, it is easy to understand that even a small lesion could interfere with the complex process and limit the patient's ability to solve the problems which confront him.

The tactile-kinaesthetic sensory system is the perceptual process which is essential for adaptation and the development of more complex performances. Visual and auditory information are secondary. It can be postulated, therefore, that patients who fail in complex human behaviour receive inadequate or distorted tactile-kinaesthetic information from their environment (Affolter and Stricker 1980).

Many terms, such as "apraxia", "agnosia" and "psycho-organic syndrome", have been attached to the perceptual problems experienced by hemiplegic patients, but such words only describe a group of symptoms. They do not explain the underlying cause of the difficulty, which the therapist would need to know in order to treat the patient appropriately.

It is important to realise that the patient who has difficulty in performing one task will also fail to perform other tasks of a similar complexity. For example, the patient's unsuccessful attempt to dress himself will not be an isolated failure but only a visible symptom of the whole problem. No area of the brain is so specialised as to control only one function. As Mountcastle (1978) writes, "... one can localise a lesion but not a function". Ruskin (1982) describes how "the simplest of activities such as taking an apple from a bowl requires the participation of a near totality of the central nervous system as well as the entire musculoskeletal system." He describes most clearly the importance of the dynamic interaction of the brain as a whole, and writes:

> The largest amount of the central nervous system white matter is utilized not by direct pathways, as was previously thought, but by internuncial neurons participating in feedback and feed-forward types of communication, interrelating all of the cells in a highly integrated whole and uniting the two sides of the central nervous system at every level of the neuraxis.
>
> When damage occurs in any portion of the brain, not only are those functions which might be the primary concern of that region disturbed, but the entire brain suffers from the loss of communication with the injured portion. The remaining normal portions of the brain are deprived of input from the damaged area, and they are also subject to abnormal messages and misinformation generated as a result of a lesion.
>
> From this basic understanding of the neuron, it is seen that there is no such thing as a simple stroke with only hemiplegia. The victim of the stroke will have significant difficulties with both sides of the body, and these difficulties will extend in some degree to all functions of the brain. Motor function will be impaired on both sides. Balance and coordination will not be the same. Sensory perception and spatial orientation will be impaired with far-reaching and often disastrous effects. Memory, cognition, and behaviour will all be altered, often presenting the most formidable challenges of rehabilitation.

Bach-y-Rita (1981) also emphasises the dynamic characteristics of the brain:

> Traditionally neurology has emphasised the correlation between the localisation of the lesion and the deficit of function. While certainly essential to an understanding of neurological symptoms and syndromes, this approach has frequently been accompanied by therapeutic nihilism. Greater emphasis on this plasticity of the brain (specifically on its capacity to mediate recovery of function) should lead to increased efforts to obtain the maximum recovery and reorganization of function that the damaged nervous system is capable of sustaining.

1.2 Implications for Therapy

The aim of therapy is that the patient should learn maximally, and learning takes place through repeated experience with the environment. Affolter and Stricker (1980) maintain that "interaction between the environment and the individual requires contact. Contact means to be 'in touch with'. To be in touch or in contact with can be realised only through the tactile kinesthetic sensory system."

As Moore (1980) says:

> The nervous system learns by doing. Active involvement has repeatedly been shown to be superior to passive participation in order for the nervous system to learn, mature and remain viable. Granted one can learn by observation but this has never been as effective as learning actively. The organism needs to 'get into the act' so to speak, and go through the process of an activity before permanent memory engrams are laid down.

It is easier for patients to learn in real life situations where they can draw on past experience to assist them. "And of course, it should be realized that the mechanism of forming a new memory must be inherently more complex than recalling an old one . . ." (Russell and Dewar, 1975). "Learning occurs only from successful performance. Attempts resulting in non-performance or inaccurate performance do not train the sensorimotor system to perform the desired task. Repeated erroneous responses only train the performance of that erroneous task" (Kottke 1978). Kottke also believes that optimal learning takes place when the patient is practising just below the peak of his best performance. "It is only when practising near the peak of performance that the level of performance increases."

The therapist may have difficulty in deciding what the patients best level of performance is. Patients who have suffered a brain lesion may often be functioning on a far lower level of planning as described by Affolter (1981) than before their stroke. Because some of the patients have such a high level of speech performance, the actual planning and performance level may be over estimated. A patient may be able to speak in detail about Beethoven or Picasso, where he is merely drawing on previously stored information. Retrieving such verbal information from memory requires no new planning or decision-making. It could be likened to a computer programme. He may, however, be unable to find his way to his own room. The therapist can estimate the patient's actual performance level by observing his attentiveness while carrying out tasks during therapy.

Attention is judged by:

The silence while the patient is working.
The intent expression on his face.
The appropriate eye contact for the task: i.e. he does not look around vaguely, but will either be looking at what he is doing or tensing the muscles around his eyes intently, to the point of closing them, as we do when we are thinking deeply.

Patients react in characteristic ways when the task confronting them is too complex or too easy, just as we all do. The patient with a brain lesion only reacts more strongly!

When too much is demanded of him:

The patient shows panic or fear. He cries out or clutches desperately on to someone or something.
He may talk exaggeratedly about irrelevant matters, e.g. old family history, or tell repetitive jokes.
He may make constant requests to visit the toilet.
He complains of other symptoms which could account for his lack of success, e.g. backache, old war wounds or lack of sleep.
He may even show signs of aggression directed towards the therapist or nurse.

When too little is demanded of him:

The patient appears bored and disappointed.
He chatters inconsequentially, and makes repetitive jokes.
He is inattentive and keeps looking at other stimuli, e.g. at fellow patients or out of the window.

When working at his individual peak performance level the patient recognises his successful performance and is motivated to continue to work at the task. "It does not help the patient to tell him a given step has been performed (well or not well) as long as he cannot experience the success of that step of the event himself" (Affolter 1981). "When we are working intensively we feel keenly the progress of our work; we are elated when our progress is rapid, we are depressed when it is slow" (Polya 1973). "And the typical consequence of prolonged or frequent failure is a general feeling of apathy. In the world of children, the concept is expressed as an I-don't-want-to-play-any-more attitude. The game is too hard. The rewards, while attractive, are too far removed to be a strong motivating force" (Jeffrey 1981).

1.3 Application to Therapy

"Animal experiments have shown that enriched experience promotes overall recovery of function. Even damaged brains can benefit from experience and their full capacity cannot be determined without training and/or enriched experience" (Rosenzweig 1980).

Bach-y-Rita (1981) writes that "it is now clear that neuronal dendritic growth results from functional demands. Furthermore, extensive growth of dendritic arborizations occurs in man even in old age. This growth is evidentally accompanied by new synapse formation."

It would seem obvious, therefore, that in the treatment of the hemiplegic patient sensory stimulation is essential if he is to achieve his maximal potential. As Affolter (1981) so rightly says:

> There is only one sensory modality which one can activate directly and that is the tactile-kinaesthetic system. By taking the hands or the body of the patient, and by guiding them to explore stimuli of the situation, some input can be assured. In addition to allowing input, the tactile-kinaesthetic system is unique among the sensory systems because it is the only sensory system that relates directly to reality. Looking at the world, nothing will be changed. Listening to the world, again the world will not be changed. However, the world cannot be touched without some changes. The tactile-kinaesthetic system combines receiving and exploratory functions, perceptual and motor processes. Developmentally, processing of tactile-kinaesthetic cause-effect information can be considered to be fundamental for building up cognitive and emotional experience.

1.4 Guiding

The therapist places her hand over that of the patient and guides the correct manipulation of the objects as he carries out a task. Only the patient's hands, not the therapist's, are in contact with the objects, so that he obtains the normal input or experience of the movement. By skilled guiding the therapist allows the activity to continue at a normal speed and in a harmonious rhythm. When the therapist feels that the patient is taking over the movement himself she reduces her assistance imperceptibly while he continues adequately. The moment she realises that a breakdown in the performance is imminent, she immediately guides his hands further to maintain the smooth continuity of the activity in a normal pattern.

Following the same principles, the therapist can assist the patient as he rises from the chair to perform an appropriate activity in a standing position, only now her hands may be assisting other parts of his body as well. e.g. she may hold his iliac crests as he walks to carry a tray to another room or to brush his teeth, so that she guides the correct gait pattern.

By guiding the patient the therapist can enable him to work at his correct level of planning irrespective of his motor ability. She can also ensure that he completes the task successfully and does not experience repeated failure as he might otherwise do. In order to guide the patient the therapist must know exactly how the movements would normally take place. When guiding the patient the therapist does not give him verbal instructions or feedback. Her voice would only distract him from the activity, or provide a clue to the next step, a clue which he would then need when attempting to carry out a similar task on his own.

The following example illustrates how the principles can be applied in everyday situations in the rehabilitation centre. As frequently happens, a patient pushes his chair against a fixed object and cannot continue further. If the therapist reverses the chair for him and steers it away from the hindrance so that he can push the chair further she will have taken over and made the necessary plan for him. He will only have learned then that when the chair becomes wedged he must have someone to help him. And so he calls for help next time it happens, or waits expectantly for someone to come to his aid. In a similar way, if the therapist tells the patient what he must do each time, she is actually doing the planning for him. Her verbal instruction is the next step required before he can complete the task.

Instead, the therapist, finding the patient in the situation, should take his hand and guide it to the wheel of the wheelchair and then reverse the chair by guiding his hand on the wheel. In this way he learns the necessary sequence, through feeling and storing. Later he will be able to produce the steps on his own in any situation where his wheelchair becomes wedged against an object. The same principle should be applied, whatever the task confronting the patient, e.g. dressing himself, washing, standing up.

1.5 Considerations

The successful rehabilitation of patients with perceptual problems may be long and arduous, but the improved independence and quality of life justify the time and effort.

> It is often noted in the neurological and rehabilitation literature . . . that virtually all the recovery from stroke that will take place occurs during the first 6 months. Many laboratory and some clinical studies do not support this view, and the possibility exists that the cessation of recovery after 6 months may be a result of a self-fulfilling prophecy: the clinician's attitude in this regard may influence the outcome.
>
> Laboratory studies have demonstrated that recovery of function continues to occur more than 5 years after a stationary lesion. (Bach-y-Rita 1981)

Bach-y-Rita and other authors have reported several cases where continuing recovery of function occurred up to as long as 7 years after onset of stroke.

Many patients with comparatively slight hemiplegia also suffer from perceptual disorders which are often not recognised on routine clinical examination. As Sagan

(1977) writes: "For example, lesions in the right hemisphere of the cerebral cortex may lead to impairments in thought and action, but in the nonverbal realm, which is by definition difficult for the patient or the physician to describe."

Brodal (1973), reporting on his own experiences following an acute left-sided hemiparesis, notes:

> ... the patient has found that destruction of even a minor part of the brain causes changes in a number of functions, which are difficult to study objectively. They are, however, very obvious to him. They are what one might call general defects in the functions of the brain: loss of powers of concentration, reduced short-term memory, increased fatigue, reduced initiative, incontinence of movements of emotional expression and other phenomena.
>
> It has also been astonishing to note how long it takes for these symptoms to improve visibly. Even after ten months, if the patient seems to be as he was, apart from his slight remaining pareses, he is painfully aware himself that this is not so.

Even if it is not possible to overcome all the patient's difficulties, care must be taken to preserve his self-respect. The problems arise from the lesion and the patient should in no way be blamed for his failure to achieve the desired rehabilitation goals. Because of the constant problem-solving and decision-making which are necessary for adaptation in normal daily life, behaviour modification approaches do not equip the hemiplegic patient for his life outside the rehabilitation centre. Such approaches only train habits which the patient is not able to modify or use in other situations.

The principles of learning described in this chapter apply throughout the book. In the following chapters ways are described by which the therapist can improve the patient's sensory/motor abilities so that he is better able to meet the demands of his daily life and enjoy his leisure hours as well.

2 Normal Movement Sequences and Balance Reactions

The treatment of patients with hemiplegia is a process of teaching and learning. The therapist teaches, the patient learns. When teaching, it is important that the teacher should know her subject very well, and in this case, where it is movement and reactions that are being retaught, the therapist must know exactly what should take place, i.e. how people move and react normally. Despite individual variations, we all move in basically similar patterns, common to us all. These patterns start developing from earliest childhood and become automatic in adult life so that they occur throughout the day without our being aware of them. How we get out of bed in the morning, how we stand up, walk, sit down, drink a cup of coffee and even how we speak all are carried out in a certain pattern of movement. Each of these activities has been learned and we notice at once when someone else performs them in an unfamiliar or strange way. The background of automatic movement is such that we do not have to think consciously how we have to move – the movements occur spontaneously. For example, when writing we do not think how to form each letter but concentrate on the content. The same applies when we speak to someone. When we walk we do not consider the act of moving each leg but can admire the surroundings or concentrate on our destination, or even hold a conversation on the way (Fig. 2.1).

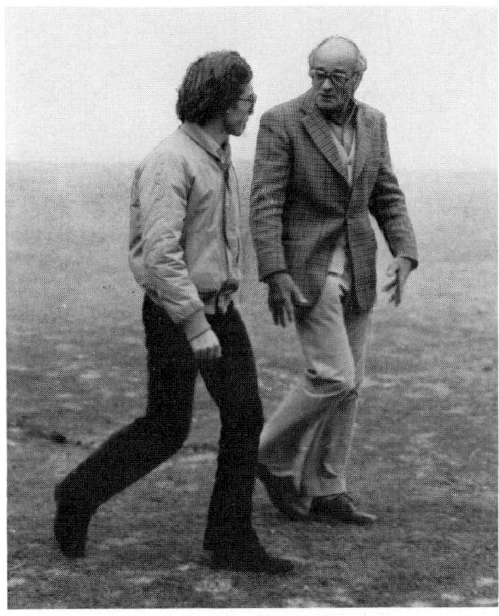

Fig. 2.1. Walking and talking

If we consider the action of walking, we see that every person walks in a similar way, one foot moving forwards and then the other, arms swinging and the body upright. Yet small individual differences enable us to recognize someone in the far distance, or even when we can only hear his footsteps approaching. Such individual variations can be observed whenever we move and are usually related to the following:

Our build – whether we are short or tall, fat or thin, long-legged or not
What we have learned by imitation from a very early age, from the customs or habits of those around us
Our personality, with its variety of inhibitions or lack of them, and the situation in which we find ourselves at the time
The presence of any stiffness or pain which causes us to move differently. Even a corn on the little toe changes someone's walking pattern considerably, as does a stiff neck or shoulder
Concentrated training for a particular sport, dance form or profession.

Despite these variations, so similar are our patterns of movement that they can be used diagnostically, if someone is seen to do something very differently from everyone else. For adults the repertoire of movement possibilities is enormous, but a few everyday examples have been selected which are very important in the treatment of hemiplegic patients. Normal people generally perform these activities in the same basic economic way. If a patient cannot perform one of the activities in this way, the therapist must discover why he cannot do so. The answer to the "why" will later become the basis of the treatment. She will try to enable the patient to carry out the movement normally and economically once again. To do so she will have to analyse very carefully which component of the movement is preventing him from carrying out the activity. Only as a result of such careful analysis can the treatment be appropriate and exact.

2.1 Analysis of Certain Everyday Movements

The analysis is not highly detailed. For each example, it is important to decide which observations led to the conclusion that a person was moving normally. The therapist needs to observe how these activities are usually performed so that she can facilitate or guide a patient correctly, enabling him to relearn the movement by feeling it.

2.1.1 Rolling over from Supine to Prone (Fig. 2.2)

We lift our head from the supporting surface and then turn our face to the side towards which we are rolling. The head never bangs against the floor, changing from being held in some flexion to held in some extension appropriately, a protection for the face or back of the head alternately. When the movement is completed, the head returns to rest gently on the supporting surface.

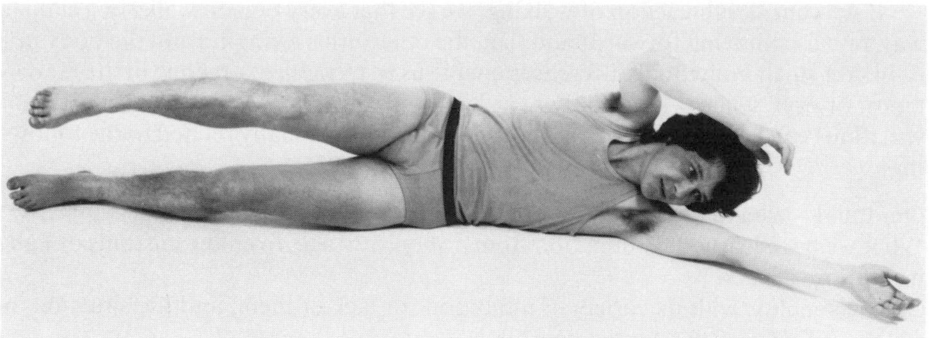

Fig. 2.2. Rolling over from supine to prone

The arms move out of the way so as not to impede the movement. They may do so in a variety of ways, either by being held above the head or by moving in front of the body, but never appearing to be in the way or remaining trapped beneath the body. Our arms sometimes swing to add momentum to the movement. During normal rolling we do not use our hands to pull ourselves over, nor do we push on the floor behind or in front of us to assist the movement, or to prevent ourselves from falling forwards or backwards.

Trunk rotation takes place so that the movement is smooth and harmonious, and the body does not jerk forwards in one piece, en bloc, while rolling forward or thud backwards when moving from the side to supine position.

Our legs move as if a step were being taken, the size of the step altering from person to person. The upper leg moves forward while the lower leg rolls into outward rotation, until it lies flat on the supporting surface. Rarely do we push off with one foot behind us or attempt to pull ourself forwards with the underneath leg. When we roll right over, our legs are extended before we reach the prone position, as flexion at the hips would impede the movement.

The activity of rolling is effortless, rhythmic and smooth, and we roll along a fairly straight line, even with our eyes closed.

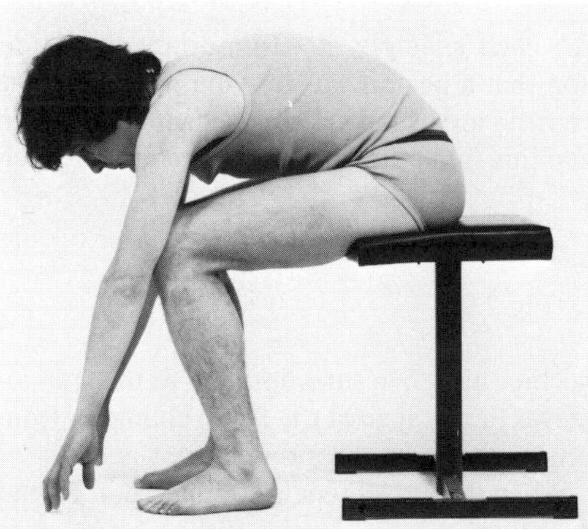

Fig. 2.3. Sitting, leaning forward. The feet remain flat on the floor and show no activity

2.1.2 Sitting, Leaning Forwards to Touch the Feet (Fig. 2.3)

When we sit, our feet rest on the floor without pushing actively against it. If we lean forward to touch our toes or to pick up something from the floor, our feet still do not participate by pushing against the floor or raising the heels. The same applies when we return to the upright position again. The head comes naturally forward as we lean forward or return to the starting position, without being held fixedly in extension. We can, however, hold it in different positions without interfering with the movement.

2.1.3 Standing from Sitting on a Chair

To stand up from a chair both feet are placed flat on the floor, either parallel to one another or with one in front of the other. The feet are drawn sufficiently far back toward the chair for the knees to be over the toes, if not further. We then lean forward by flexing the hips until our head is approximately over our toes. With back and neck held fairly straight we rise to our feet, with our arms either swinging forward or pushing off lightly to assist us (Fig. 2.4). If the seat is very low, or when we stand up very slowly, the arms come actively forward in extension. The knees move forwards over our feet as a result of increasing dorsal flexion at the ankle. Both thighs maintain the same angle relative to the mid-line (Fig. 2.5).

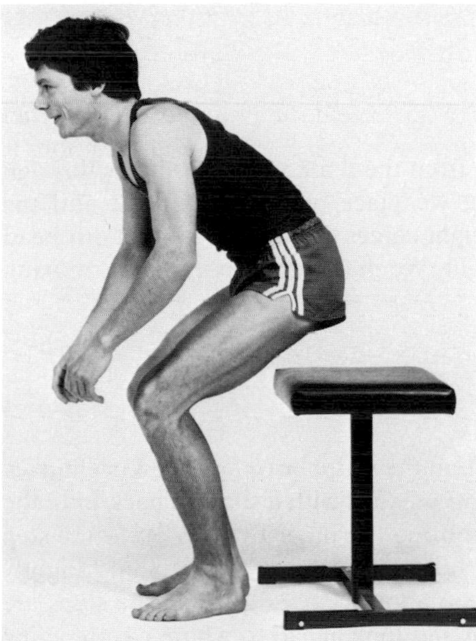

Fig. 2.4. Standing up from a sitting position, lateral view. The head leads the way, moving forwards over the feet and further

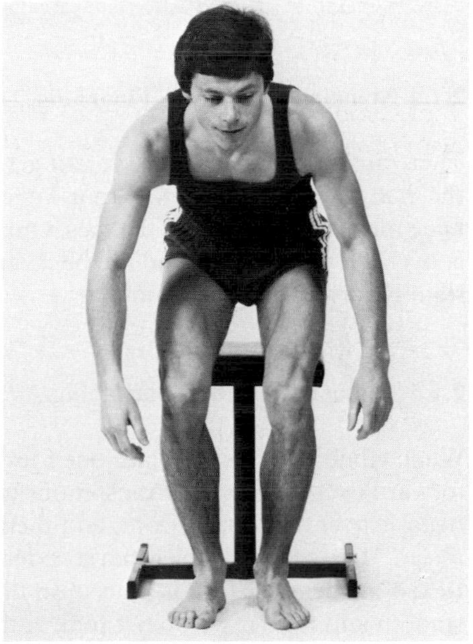

Fig. 2.5. Standing up from a sitting position, frontal view. The weight ist taken equally through both legs and the body shows an overall symmetry

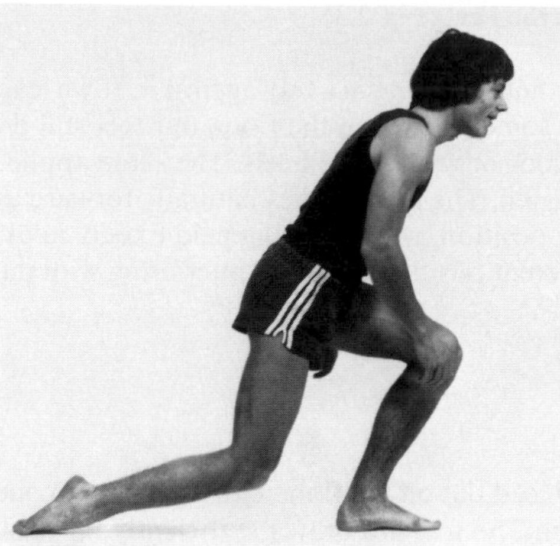

Fig. 2.6. Standing up through half-kneeling. Considerable dorsiflexion of the foot in front allows the knee to move forward

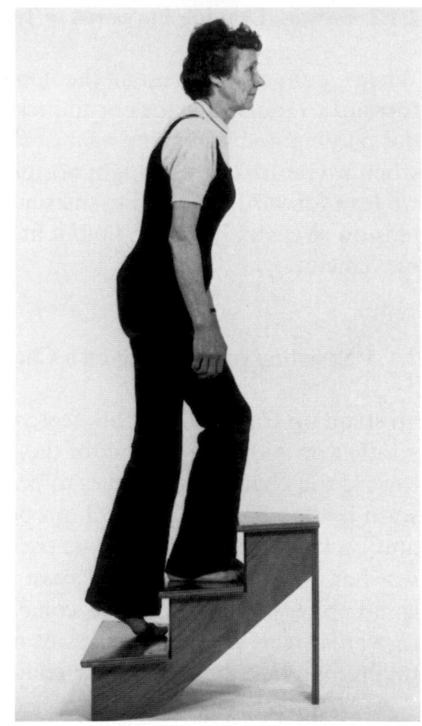

Fig. 2.7. Going upstairs

2.1.4 Standing up from the Floor (Fig. 2.6)

There are many ways which we can get up from the floor, one of which is through the half-kneeling position. From kneeling we place one foot in front and the knee moves forwards over the toes. Our weight comes forward so far that our head is over the foot in front and the back straight. We then stand up, the arms moving slightly forwards as we do so.

2.1.5 Going up and down Stairs (Fig. 2.7)

When climbing stairs we place one foot flat on the stair above and the knee moves forward over the toes. We transfer our weight forward with a straight back until the head is over the foot in front, and then we bring the other foot up on to the step ahead. The supporting leg never extends fully at the knee, but remains slightly flexed as the other foot is placed on the step above (Fig. 2.8). When the steps are smooth and regular we do not look at them, but look ahead to where we are going or to the steps ahead of us.

When we are going down stairs one foot moves forward and downward, and just before it reaches the step below we transfer our weight forward by lifting the heel of the supporting leg behind (Fig. 2.9). The heel must come off the step above,

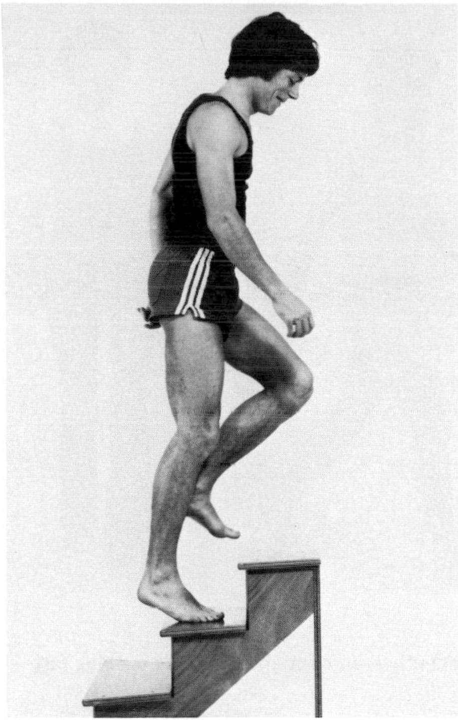

Fig. 2.8. Going upstairs the legs are in constant motion as in bicycle-riding and the knees are never fully extended

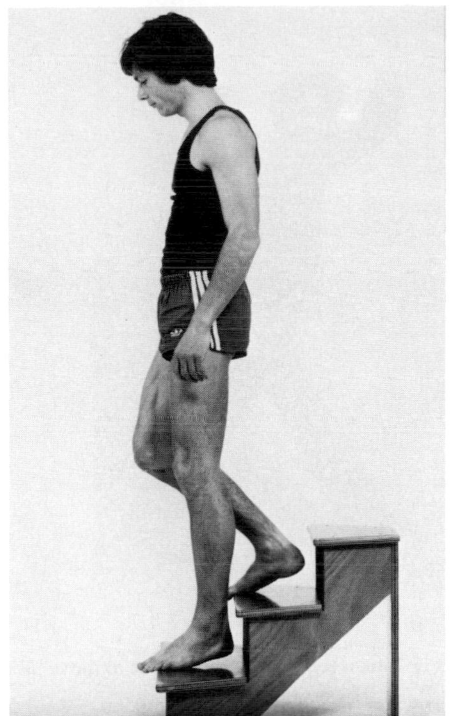

Fig. 2.9. Going downstairs. The weight keeps moving forward over the leg in front

as we would otherwise not have sufficient range of dorsal flexion at the ankle to allow the movement of the weight forward. Once the leg below has taken our weight with the foot flat on the step, the other leg swings forward with momentum and the sequence is repeated.

2.1.6 Walking

Walking has been often and most fully analysed by many authors. To gain an overall impression it is sufficient to consider the following points. The action of walking is rhythmic and apparently effortless. We can walk easily for an hour without being out of breath or exhausted. Walking is not dependent on a specific position of the head, so that we are able to look around freely while we walk and even wave to someone (Fig. 2.10). Our arms swing alternately forwards or backwards, due to the rotation between pelvis and shoulder girdle and also due to the transference of weight forwards. As one foot comes forward the arm on the opposite side swings forwards. The arm swing is dependent on the speed of the walking and will vary accordingly. We do not consciously move our arms. The strides are of the same

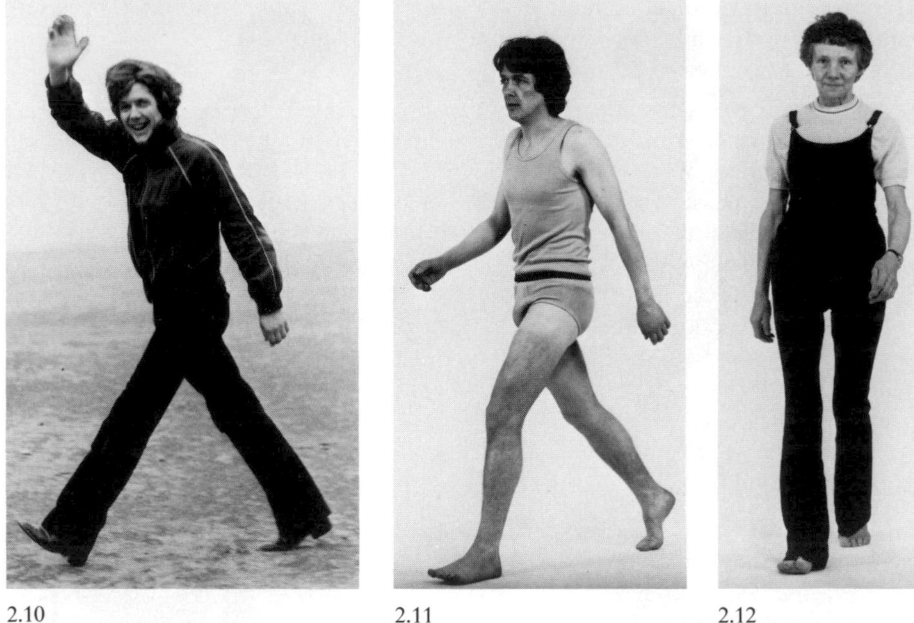

2.10 2.11 2.12

Fig. 2.10. Head and arms are free to move independently even when the subject is walking fast

Fig. 2.11. Normal economic walking

Fig. 2.12. Both feet assume the same position relative to the mid-line when they meet the ground in front. Their angle is determined by the rotation at the hip as the leg swings forwards

length and speed and the feet make the same noise when they make contact with the floor. We each have an individual rhythm when we walk. It is important to notice that the heel strikes the floor first in front and that the big toe behind leaves the floor last (Fig. 2.11), and for a short period both are in contact with the ground. We do not lift our leg actively from the hip to take a step; it swings forward as we push off with the supporting foot. We transfer our weight forwards before the heel makes contact with the ground in front. It is as if we are losing our balance and are only saved by the foot reaching the ground in time. The position which the foot assumes on the ground varies slightly from person to person, but it is important to notice that normally the angle from or toward the mid-line is the same for both feet (Fig. 2.12).

2.2 Balance, Righting and Equilibrium Reactions

Every activity we carry out requires that we react to gravity, and our body has to adjust accordingly in order to maintain balance. K. Bobath (1980) has described this ability as the "normal postural reflex mechanism". It is dependent on:

Normal tone in the musculature, which needs to be sufficiently high for us to support ourselves and move against gravity but not so high that it impedes movement

Reciprocal innervation or reciprocal inhibition, which enables us to stabilise certain parts of our body while we move other parts selectively
Patterns of movement common to us all.

The normal postural reflex mechanism presupposes an intact adult brain and provides the background for all skilled movement. In the upright posture, particularly when standing, we need very highly developed balance reactions. Equilibrium reactions make possible the maintenance of balance while sitting, standing and walking. As a result the upper limbs are released from their early function of support so that they may become the tools for skilled manipulative activities (Fiorentino 1981). These reactions are automatic, although we can control or modify them voluntarily for functional use. They range from tiny invisible tonus changes to gross movements of the trunk and limbs. When we consider that posture is arrested movement, that if we stop at any stage of any movement and hold the position we have adopted a posture, it becomes clear that the combinations and possibilities are infinite.

In our daily life we have to react to gravity in different situations where balance is required.

1. We move to perform an activity while the supporting surface remains stable and level. For example, while sitting in a chair we reach out for a required object or while standing we put on a shoe or step out of the way to avoid something. No matter how small the movement, there will be an adjustment in the tone and position of many other parts of the body. We see the need for this adjustment most clearly when working with patients with complete spinal cord lesions above the level of C5. With the help of the therapist, it is possible to find a position in which unsupported sitting is achieved, but even turning to look at something causes the patient to fall over because the necessary adjustment cannot take place.
2. The supporting surface moves and we react to maintain our balance, as when sitting in a moving motor car or standing in a crowded train.
3. We move on a stable but uneven supporting surface and the body reacts appropriately, as when we walk in a meadow of long grass, climb stairs or walk along a winding path.

The following examples of balance and equilibrium reactions require careful study because their re-education is an essential part of the treatment of hemiplegia.

2.2.1 Lying on a Surface Which Tilts Sideways

Although balance in lying is seldom required, it is interesting to note that the pattern of the reactions which develops in babyhood in this position will also occur in sitting and standing (Fig. 2.13).

The head flexes laterally to the upper side of the surface, i.e. the side working against the pull of gravity.
Almost simultaneously the trunk side flexes, concave towards the uppermost surface.
The arm and leg of the uppermost side abduct and extend.

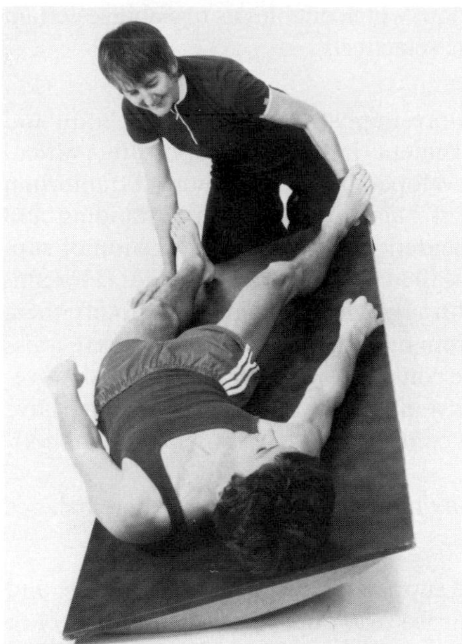

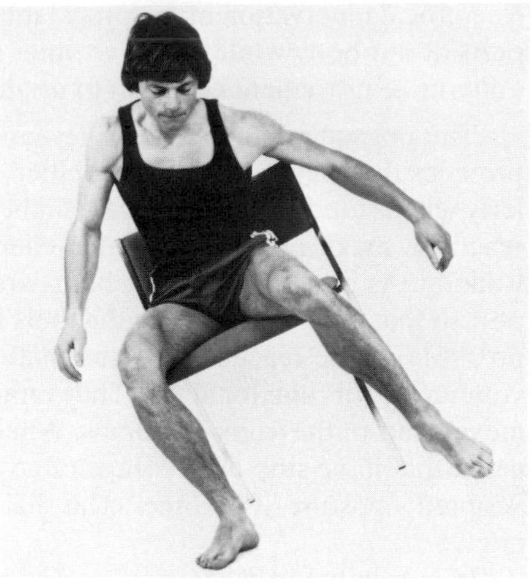

Fig. 2.14. Balance reactions in a sitting position when the supporting surface tilts

◁ **Fig. 2.13.** Balance reactions in a lying position when the surface tilts sideways

Trunk rotation takes place, the lower arm coming forwards across the body.
The lower leg also comes forwards and finally the person turns completely over into prone lying.

2.2.2 Sitting on a Surface Which Tilts Sideways (Fig. 2.14)

The same sequence of movement takes place as in lying. When the chair tips towards the right:

The head flexes to the left, so that the eyes are horizontal and facing forwards.
The right side of the trunk elongates as the weight comes over the right buttock.
The arms abduct in extension.
The lower leg rolls outwards from the hip.
The uppermost leg abducts in some extension and leaves the floor.

If the chair tips further, the right shoulder and arm move forwards across the body with trunk rotation, or the right leg makes a quick protective step sideways in abduction.

2.2.3 Sitting, Being Drawn Sideways by Another Person

Although the surface remains stationary, because the body is moving the pull of gravity changes. The sequence of the reactions is therefore the same as before (Fig. 2.15). The lower leg rolls outwards at the hip to allow the weight to be transferred, adjusting to the changed alignment of the trunk. The free upper leg, in relative extension, provides a counterweight by moving further and further into abduction. Shortly before the person loses his balance, the foot dorsiflexes with pronation.

2.2.4 Sitting with Both Legs Flexed and Turned to One Side

The head, trunk and arms react in the same pattern, but the movements are exaggerated, requiring more activity because the leg can no longer extend and abduct to act as a counterweight. The trunk rotation occurs earlier (Fig. 2.16).

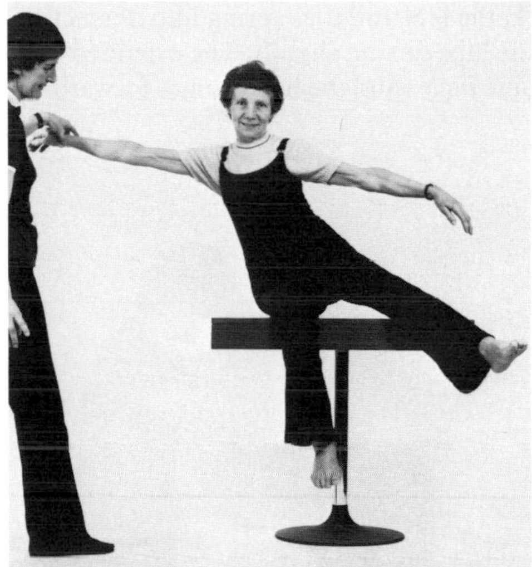

Fig. 2.15. Balance reactions in a sitting position when the supporting surface is stationary

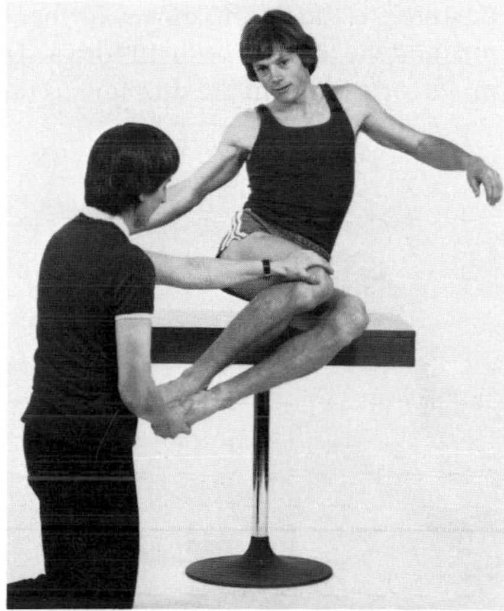

Fig. 2.16 Increased head and trunk reactions when the legs are not participating

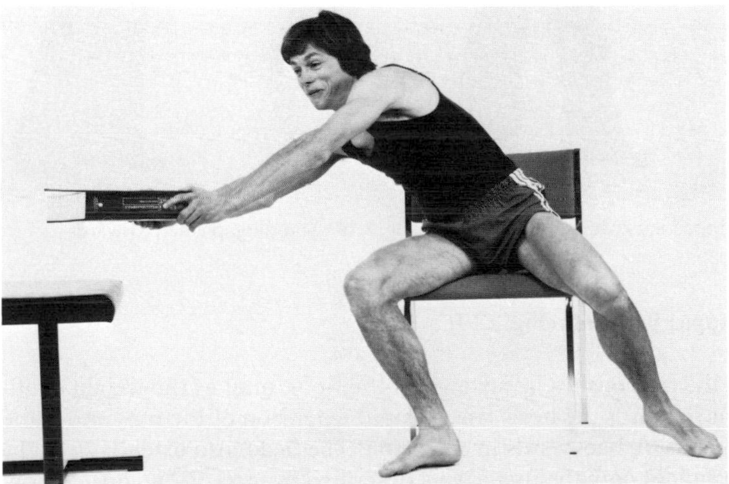

Fig. 2.17. Balance reactions modified to allow function

2.2.5 Sitting, Reaching out to Grasp an Object

The same reactions would take place but must be modified to perform a task such as reaching to lift a book (Fig. 2.17). The head-righting reaction is inhibited to allow the subject to turn and look at the book. The trunk side flexion and elongation are reversed, as is the trunk rotation. The arms cannot react in abduction and extension, as the hands must grasp the book.

2.2.6 Standing, Tipped Backwards (Fig. 2.18)

Small intrinsic muscles in the foot co-ordinate to adjust to the first slight change of posture. As the weight moves further back, the feet and toes spring into dorsal flexion, and the trunk is brought forward by the hips flexing slightly. The extended arms move forward from the shoulder as the spine flexes and the head comes forward.

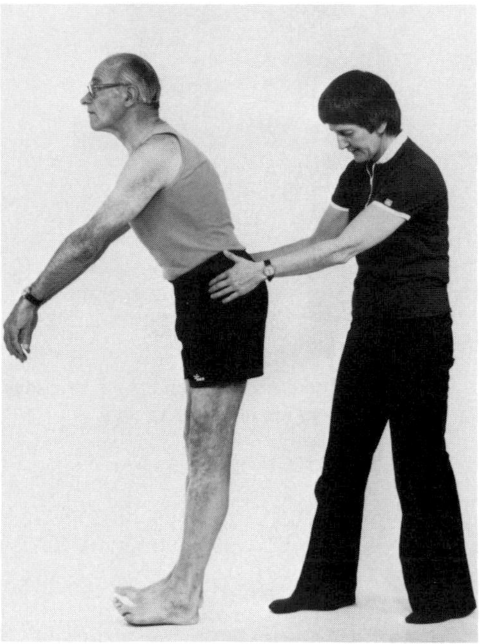

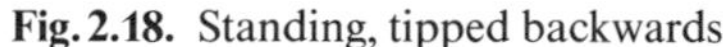

Fig. 2.18. Standing, tipped backwards

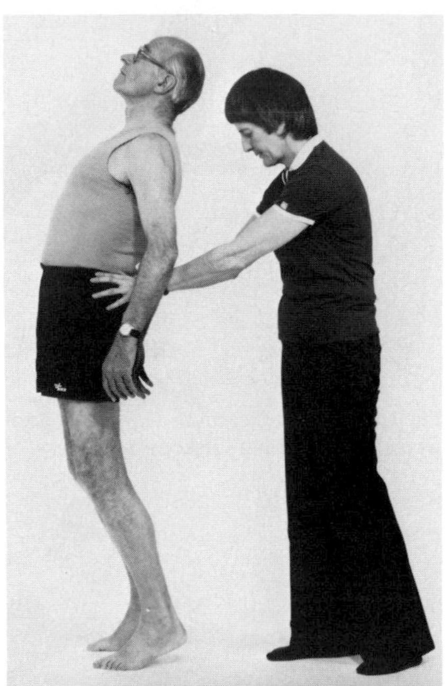

Fig. 2.19. Standing, pushed forwards

2.2.7 Standing, Tipped Forwards (Fig. 2.19)

The toes flex and the foot pushes firmly against the floor, until as the weight continues to be brought forwards the heels rise. A rapid extension of the hips and spine follow and the arms move backwards in extension. The head also extends strongly. In normal circumstances only the first events described in sects. 2.2.6 and 2.2.7 occur because it is then more economic for us to take a quick step to maintain our balance. The whole sequence would only occur if for some reason we were not able to take a quick step forward or back, e.g. when standing fully clothed on the edge of a swimming pool in winter, or when stopping abruptly at the pavement edge to avoid an oncoming car.

2.2.8 Standing, Tipped Sideways (Fig. 2.20)

The reactions which take place closely resemble those which occur in supine lying when the supporting surface is tilted. The whole side elongates over the weight-bearing leg, with the trochanter the most lateral point. As the weight is brought sideways the supporting foot rolls outward until only the lateral border is in contact with the ground. The toes flex strongly. The head rights to the vertical, maintaining its normal relationship to the shoulder girdle. The opposite side shortens, with the leg moving into abduction. Both extended arms move into abduction.

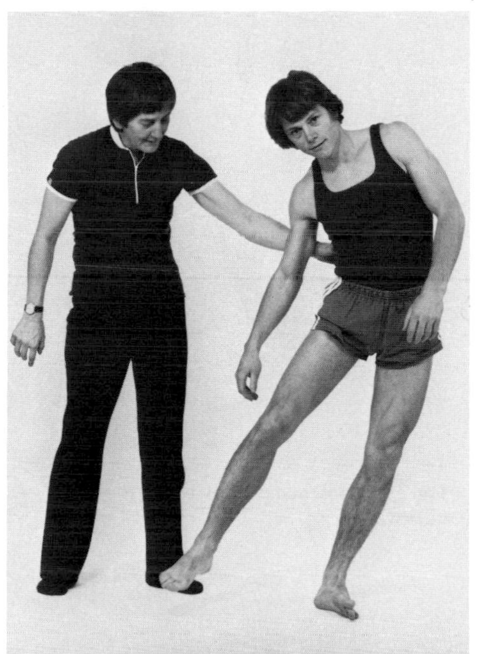

Fig. 2.20. Standing, tipped sideways until only the lateral border of the foot is on the ground. The head has righted beyond the vertical

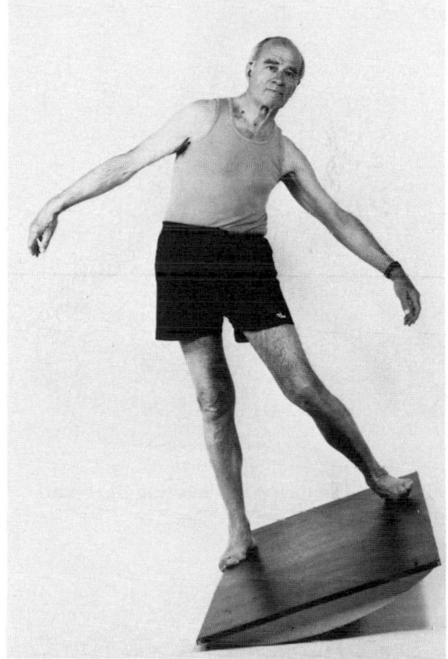

Fig. 2.21. Balancing while tilting the board sideways

2.2.9 Standing on a Tilting Surface, Such as a Tilt-Board

The reactions which occur when the subject is lying supine on a tilt-board are repeated when he is standing and tilting the board sideways (Fig. 2.21). The trochanter moves laterally to the side of the board which is lower and the trunk elongates on that side. The head rights to the vertical. The feet remain in contact with the board, with the knee on the uppermost side flexing somewhat. The extended arms abduct. When the board is tipped forwards, the pelvis comes well forward over the extended leg in front, and hips, trunk and head extend strongly. The arms move into extension (Fig. 2.22). As the surface is tipped backwards the hips flex and the trunk is brought forwards, with the extended arms also moving forwards from the shoulder (Fig. 2.23).

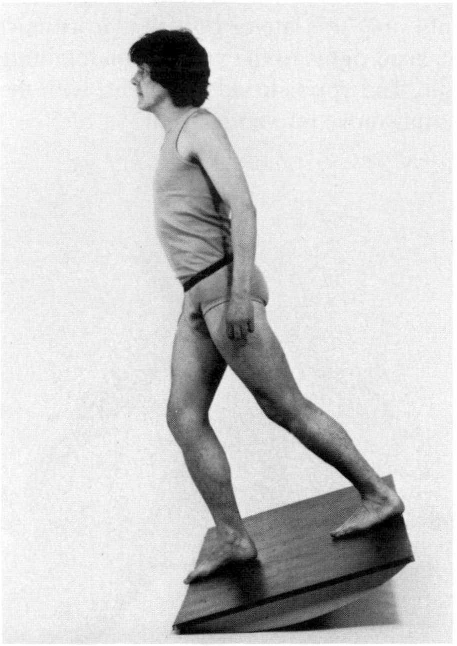

Fig. 2.22. Balancing while tilting the board forwards

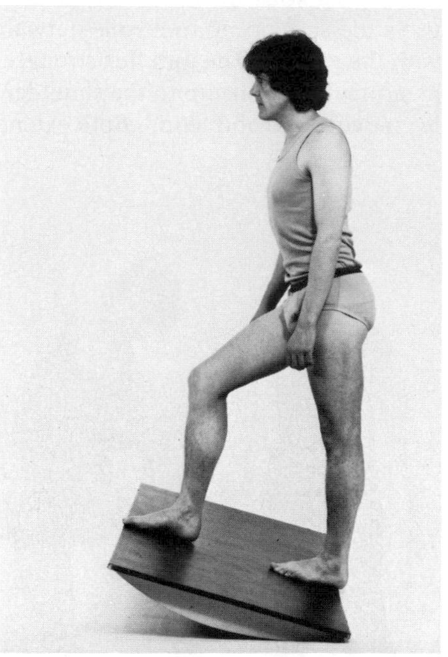

Fig. 2.23. Balancing while tilting the board backwards

2.2.10 Steps to Save

Normally, when reacting quickly and economically to maintain or regain our balance, we take a quick step in whichever direction is necessary: forwards, sideways or backwards. These steps are repeated, one foot following the other if we are still off balance. When stepping forwards the arms extend in front as if in preparation to save the face should we fall (Fig. 2.24). Stepping sideways one foot crosses in front or behind the other (Fig. 2.25). Taking quick steps backwards to regain balance, the trunk and head move forwards from the hips (Fig. 2.26).

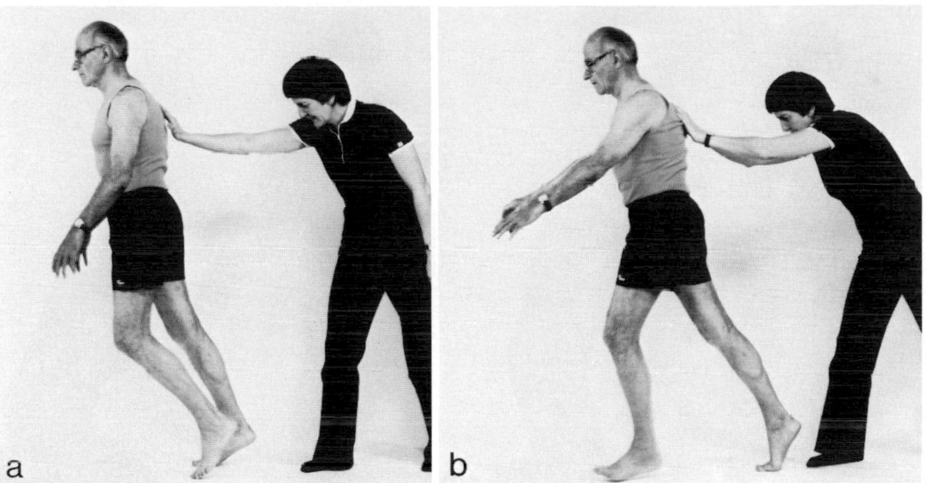

Fig. 2.24 a, b. Steps to regain balance. **a** About to fall forwards; **b** protective steps forwards

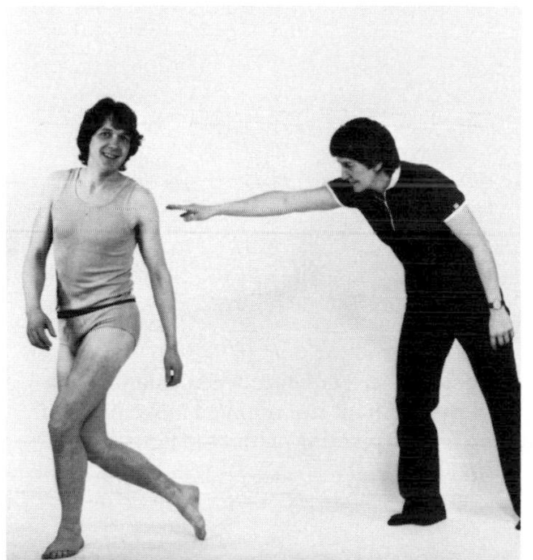

Fig. 2.25. Protective steps sideways

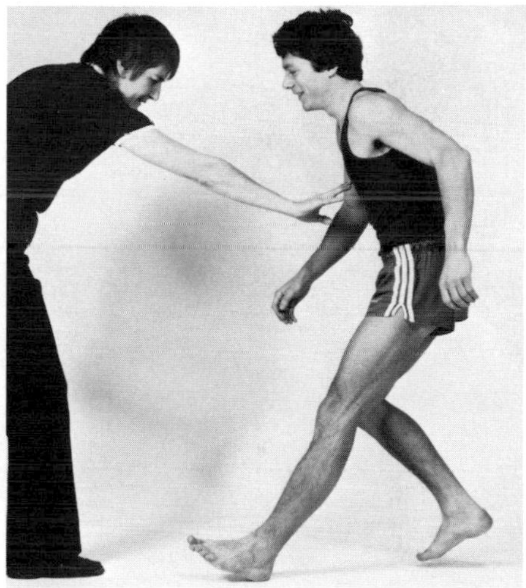

Fig. 2.26. Protective steps backwards

2.2.11 Balancing on One Leg

When we stand on one leg, the supporting foot moves pliantly and co-ordinatedly, adjusting to the changing shifts in the weight (Fig. 2.27 a). As the weight transfers further in one direction, we move by pivoting on the foot, a rapid movement alternating between weight being taken through the heel and then through the ball of the foot (Fig. 2.27 b). If the weight transfers further, and too rapidly to allow the pivot, we hop in the direction required to regain our balance (Fig. 2.27 c).

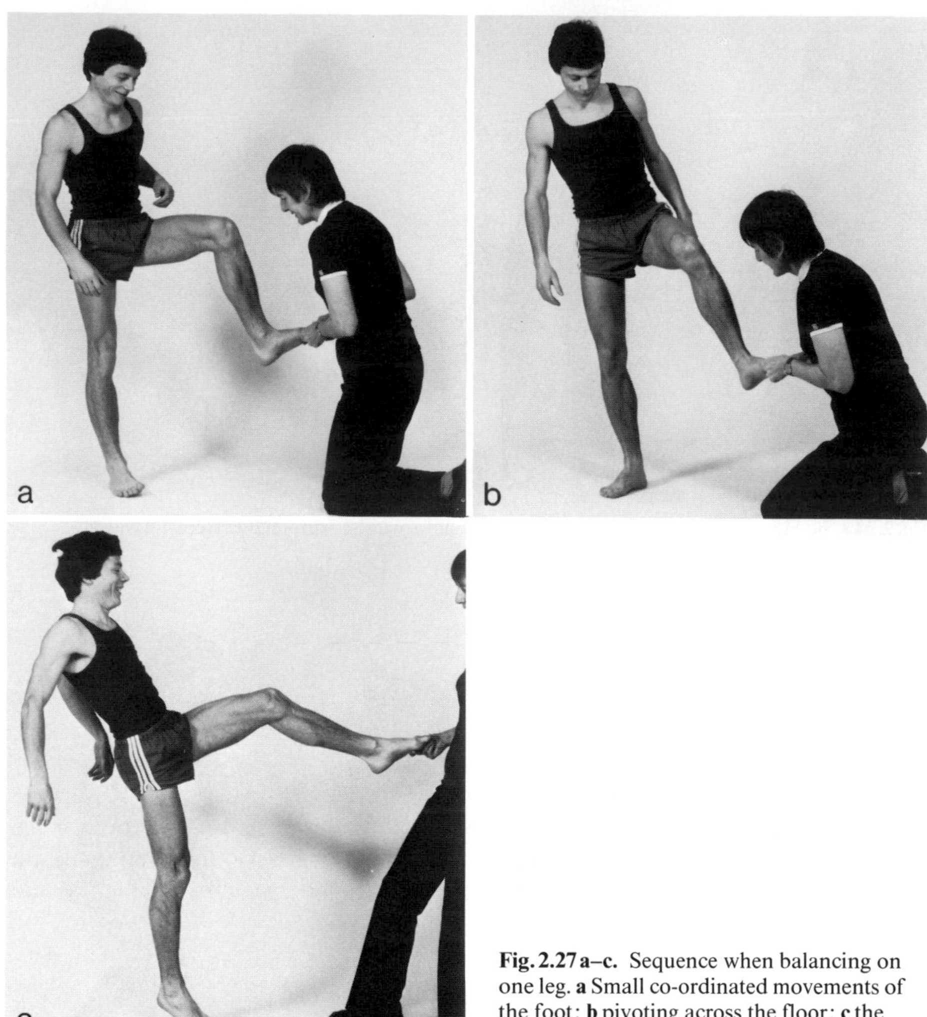

Fig. 2.27 a–c. Sequence when balancing on one leg. **a** Small co-ordinated movements of the foot; **b** pivoting across the floor; **c** the final hop

2.2.12 Protective Extension of the Arms

If all the reactions have failed to maintain balance and we fall, the outstretched hands spring to our protection, i.e. to save our head or face from hitting the ground or a fixed object in front of us (Fig. 2.28 a). This protective reaction occurs in whatever direction we fall and accounts for the numerous Colles' fractures, particularly among elderly people. We see the same protective reaction when a moving object approaches rapidly, e.g. something is thrown at us or falls towards us, or a door slams as we approach it (Fig. 2.28 b).

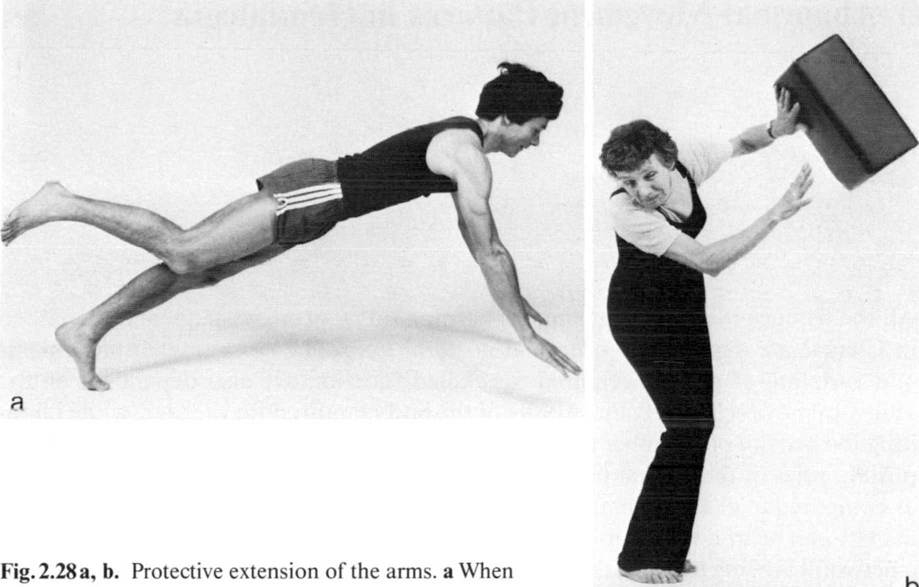

Fig. 2.28 a, b. Protective extension of the arms. **a** When falling; **b** when endangered by an approaching object

2.3 Considerations

Intact balance and saving reactions enable us to go about our daily life without the constant fear of falling. Free righting reactions of the head are a key factor in maintaining balance. Wyke (1983) emphasises the important role of the receptors in the apophyseal joints of the cervical spine in maintaining balance in adults. He reports an increased risk of falling in patients who wear a collar as part of the treatment of their cervical spine problems. Every activity in our daily lives is dependent on adequate balance and equilibrium reactions. Even lifting one arm requires an adaptation in other parts of the body. Although balance reactions are automatic they can be modified to allow functional activity. Each and all of the reactions can be voluntarily inhibited or controlled, so that they are reactions rather than reflexes in adults.

3 Abnormal Movement Patterns in Hemiplegia

All the balance reactions and smooth harmonious movement sequences described in Chap. 2 are dependent on normal postural tone. The co-ordinated movements and variation of posture required for skilled function are also dependent on the ability to move selectively those parts of the body required for the task, while inhibiting the activity of the other parts. Inhibition of over-activity is one of the most important roles of the central nervous system, hence the ratio of inhibitory pathways as compared to exitatory pathways in the brain-stem and spinal cord. Every skilled activity can be said to be surrounded by a "wall of inhibition" (Kottke 1978). When a new skill is being learned, the inhibition of over-activity increases as the performer becomes more skilled.

Learning to drive a motor car demonstrates clearly this process of increasing inhibition of excess activity as the learner becomes more adept. At first the steering-wheel is held in an almost vice-like grasp, and changing gear requires great effort and concentration. The movements of the feet on the accelerator, clutch and brake pedals are abrupt and forceful, so that the car moves somewhat erratically, in fits and starts. Later, the driver manipulates the controls with such appropriate strength, through inhibition, that the changes of gear and speed are smooth and barely perceptible, and he holds the steering-wheel lightly.

3.1 Persistence of Primitive Mass Synergies

Selectivity of normal muscular action is a function of cortical motor control guided by proprioceptive feedback (Perry 1969). Children are born with a high level of anarchy or over-activity in their motor control. As they mature, the over-activity disappears, and is absent in adults (Basmajian 1981). Reflex patterns are the bases for motion. The repetition of these reflex patterns in infancy teaches the child how to move. However, movement does not become effective unless and until the child learns how to inhibit the undesired components of movements in these reflex patterns at the same time that the desired components are excited (Kottke 1980).

"At birth, the body is under the unopposed control of the lower centres of the central nervous system, which basically generate involuntary reflex movements and postures." "The primitive, postural reflexes primarily involve changes in tone and distribution, which affect posture and movement. These the body responds to automatically and mechanically." "With maturation and integration of the lower centres contributing to the development of the higher centres, with more inhibitory control from the higher centres, the mass movements are integrated and goal-directed movements, which depend on the higher control within the central nervous system, are developed" (Fiorentino 1981).

The primitive but postural reflexes can still be observed in the intact human being, although they have become modified and changed by the activities of the higher centres (B. Bobath 1971). They reappear in an exaggerated form after a lesion to the central nervous system. "Damage to the highest or intermediate centres causes abnormalities in performance by releasing the activity of the undamaged next lower centre from control, rather than by generating a new form of activity originating from the damaged center itself" (Kottke 1980).

When a patient with hemiplegia can move his limbs at all, he does so in a stereotyped way, in total primitive mass synergies which Perry (1969) describes as the primitive pattern responses. These movement synergies should not be confused with the reflex patterns of spasticity. The very young baby moves in primitive mass synergies but is in no way spastic. Some hemiplegic patients may have no overt hypertonus, and are nevertheless unable to perform a certain selective or isolated movement. The therapist, moving the limb passively in the same direction, may encounter no resistance.

Perry differentiates between the two by describing a reflex as "an involuntary response to a sensory stimulus". The primitive pattern response, however, she describes as "a voluntary act, initiated when the hemiplegic patient wishes to perform a task. These synergies are stereotyped because the muscles that participate in patterned motion and the strength of their responses are the same for every effort, regardless of the demand." Naturally, the two overlap to a considerable extent and one or the other does not appear as an isolated symptom. So that it could be said that every patient who moves using primitive mass synergies will also have abnormal tone, and every patient who has abnormal tone due to a lesion of the central nervous system will move without full selection.

3.2 The Synergies as They Appear in Association with Hemiplegia

3.2.1 In the Upper Limb

3.2.1.1 Flexor Synergy (Figs. 3.1 and 3.2)

The Flexor synergy is seen when the patient attempts to lift up his arm, hold it in the air after it has been lifted, reach for an object or bring his hand to his mouth.)

Scapula	Elevates and retracts
Shoulder	Abducts and externally rotates (internally rotates)
Elbow	Flexes
Forearm	Supinates (pronates)
Wrist	Flexes
Fingers	Flex and adduct
Thumb	Flexes and adducts

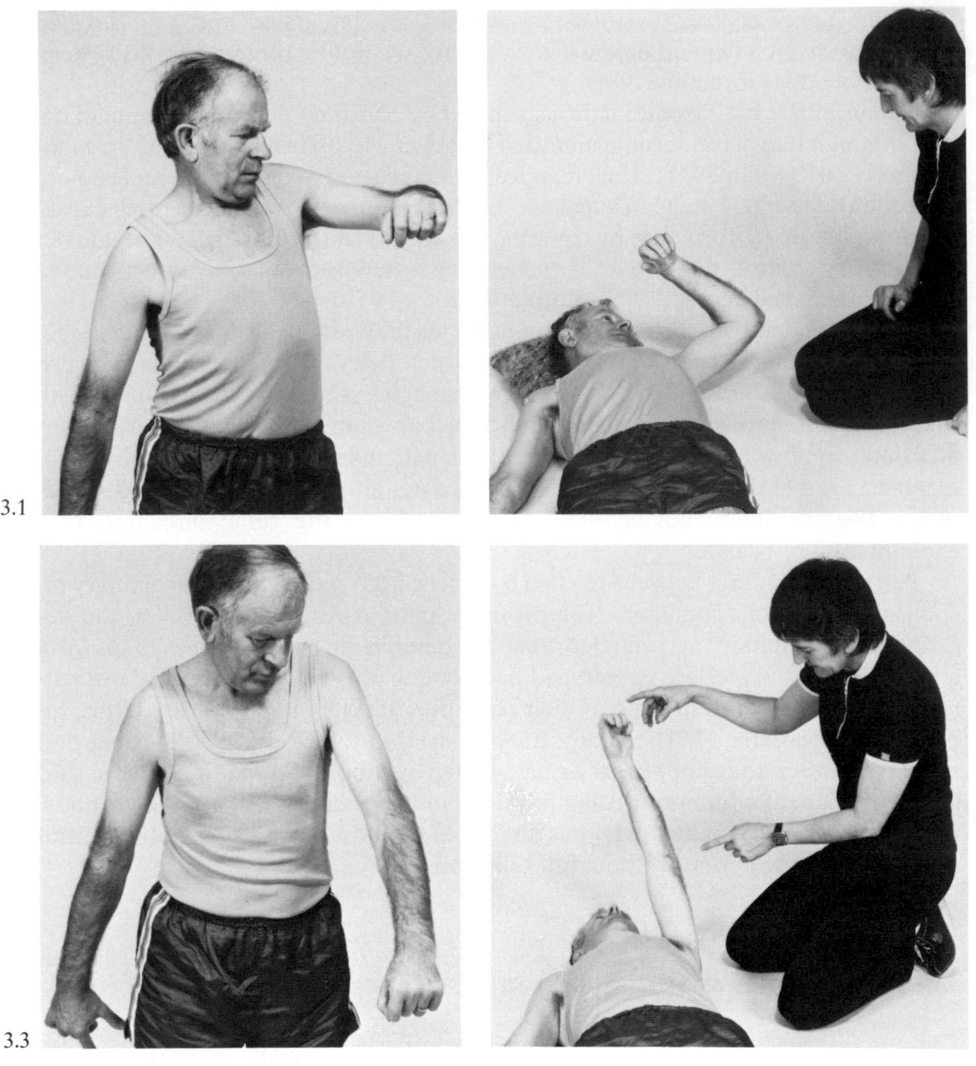

Fig. 3.1. Flexor synergy in the upper limb. The patient is trying to lift his extended arm. Because the shoulder is abducting (flexor component) the elbow flexes as well, instead of extending. In this case pronation rather than supination occurs with mass flexion (left hemiplegia)

Fig. 3.2. While lying, the patient tries to touch his head. The action of flexing the elbow causes the whole flexor synergy with retraction of the scapula and abduction of the arm. In this instance the shoulder rotates externally

Fig. 3.3. Extensor synergy is the upper limb – the patient is trying to straighten his elbow (left hemiplegia)

Fig. 3.4. While lying, the patient is trying to extend his elbow. The shoulder rotates internally and the forearm pronates strongly (left hemiplegia)

Because of hypertonus the flexion synergy will usually appear with internal rotation of the shoulder and pronation of the forearm.

3.2.1.2 Extensor Synergy (Figs. 3.3 and 3.4)

Scapula	Protracts and pushes downwards
Shoulder	Internally rotates and adducts
Elbow	Extends with pronation
Wrist	Extends somewhat
Fingers	Flex with adduction
Thumb	Adducts in flexion

Because of spasticity the wrist is often seen to be flexed.

3.2.2 In the Lower Limb

3.2.2.1 Flexor Synergy

Pelvis	Elevates and retracts
Hip	Abducts and externally rotates
Knee	Flexes
Ankle	Dorsiflexes in supination
Toes	Extend

Because of hypertonicity the toes usually flex. The great toe may be extended.

3.2.2.2 Extensor Synergy

Hip	Extends and internally rotates; adducts
Knee	Extends
Ankle	Plantar flexes with inversion
Toes	Plantar flex and adduct

Once again the great toe may extend.

"The great variety and manifold combinations of movement patterns necessary for skilled activities depend on the ability of any muscle or muscle group to function as part of a great number of patterns and not only as part of one or two total patterns" (B. Bobath 1978). "In damage to the central nervous system, as in stroke, the higher centers containing the complex patterns and the facility for the inhibition of massive gross patterns lose control and the uncontrolled, or partially controlled, stereotyped patterns of the middle and lower centers emerge" (Cailliet 1980).

3.3 Abnormal Muscle Tone

Tone can be described as the resistance felt when a part of the body is moved passively, i.e. lengthening or stretching those muscles which run in the opposite direction to that of the movement.

Normal tone is felt as an appropriate amount of resistance, allowing the movement to proceed smoothly and without interruption. The opposing or antagonistic muscles adapt instantly to the new amount of stretch, and "play out" accordingly. The amount of resistance felt varies slightly from one normal subject to another, and the therapist needs to experience and become familiar with the possible variations by moving the limbs of many different people.

Hypotonus is felt as too little or no resistance to the movement, and the limb feels limp and floppy. When released, the part being moved will fall in the direction of the pull of gravity.

Hypertonus is felt as an increased resistance to passive movement, ranging from a slight delay in giving way to considerable effort being required before the part can be moved at all. The limb feels heavy and when released is pulled in the direction of the spastic muscle groups. Hypertonus or spasticity is a release of tonic reflex activity and manifests itself in typical stereotyped patterns, either of flexion or extension.

Spasticity is never isolated to one muscle group. It is always part of a total flexion or total extension synergy (Atkinson 1979). So stereotyped are the patterns that they allow a patient to be identified instantly as hemiplegic. Although the patient may have hypertonicity with exaggerated reflex activity in all muscle groups following stroke, the recognised patterns result from the pull of the strongest muscle groups, and the influence of the tonic reflexes.

K. Bobath has often described the strongest muscles as being the philogenetically antigravity muscles – those in the upper limb which would be involved in pulling the body weight up into a tree, and those in the lower limb which support the body weight in standing.

3.3.1 The Typical Patterns of Spasticity

When considering spasticity, care must be taken to differentiate between the position in which the joints may find themselves and the resistance encountered when the limb is moved passively. For example, although the hip joint may be seen to be in some degree of flexion when the patient is standing, there will nevertheless be a resistance when passive flexion of the hip and knee is attempted in the presence of extensor spasticity.

Head	The head is flexed toward the hemiplegic side and rotated so that the face is toward the sound side.
Upper limb (flexion pattern)	The scapula is retracted and the shoulder girdle depressed. The shoulder is adducted and internally rotated. The elbow is flexed with pronation of the forearm (in some cases supination dominates). The wrist is flexed with some ulnar deviation. The fingers are flexed and adducted. The thumb is flexed and adducted.
Trunk	The trunk is rotated back on the hemiplegic side with side flexion of the hemiplegic side.

Lower limb (extension pattern)	The pelvis is rotated backwards on the hemiplegic side and pulled upwards. The hip is extended, adducted and internally rotated.

"Due to the rotation backwards (of the pelvis) the leg usually shows a pattern of external rotation in spite of extensor spasticity which, in cases with bilateral spasticity, is combined with internal rotation. A change of this pattern of external rotation can be observed if one moves the pelvis forward on the affected side, when internal rotation occurs" (B. Bobath 1978).

The knee is extended.
The foot is plantar flexed and inverted.

(The term "supination" is often used to describe the turning inward of the foot. Supination, however, is the movement which occurs when the foot is dorsiflexed and the unopposed pull of the Tibialis anterior is clearly seen. In the extension pattern the foot is plantar flexed and the tibialis anterior is not active. The term "inversion" can be used to differentiate between the two positions. Inversion is caused by the uninhibited activity of the tibialis posterior.)

The toes are flexed and adducted. (Occasionally the great toe extends in the presence of a marked positive Babinski sign.)

Although extensor spasticity usually predominates in the lower limb, in certain situations flexor spasticity may be more apparent. For example, patients who remain in the wheelchair for many months in a position of flexion will tend to have flexor spasticity in the lower limb. Any painful stimulus to the foot or leg will result in a flexor withdrawal response, with flexor spasticity being manifested. Any flexion contracture of the lower limb will tend to elicit a flexion pattern, due to the stretch reflex in the flexor muscle groups being stimulated earlier, each time the leg moves towards extension. The flexor pattern of spasticity is the same as the pattern of the mass movement synergy which has already been described. The difficulties caused by both the mass synergies and hypertonus can be easily observed when placing of the head, trunk or limbs is attempted.

3.4 Placing

The normal limb responds instantly to being moved by another person, without a verbal command being required. For example, if someone's hand is lifted into the air, it feels light because the subject immediately takes the weight of his own arm actively. The arm remains for a short time in the position which it is placed before returning to a relaxed position.

The arm can be placed in an enormous variety of positions and combinations of positions. The automatic response is dependent on normal tone and reciprocal innervation, and forms the basis of our ability to use the limb functionally and automatically. The reaction can be tested during assessment and also used as a treatment procedure. By comparing normal subjects with hemiplegic patients, the problems of abnormal tone and loss of selective movement (reciprocal innervation) can be observed. Placing is difficult if not impossible for the patients.

3.5
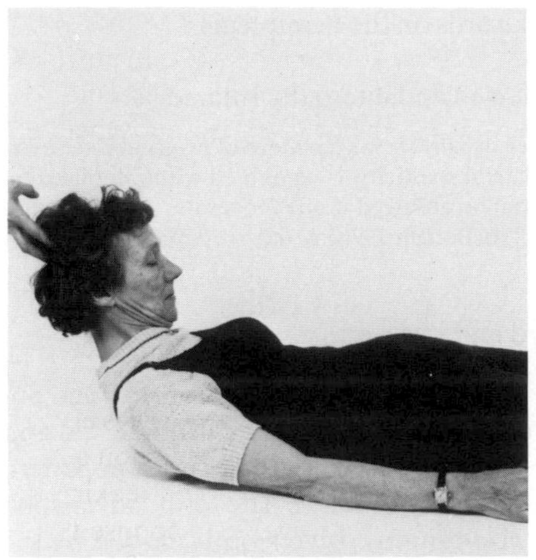

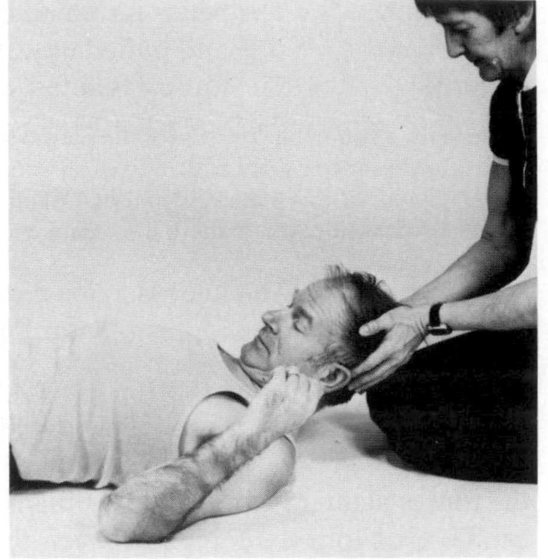
3.6

3.7
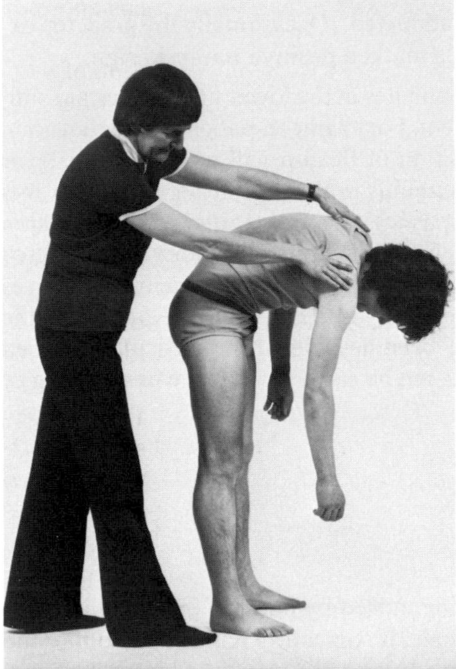

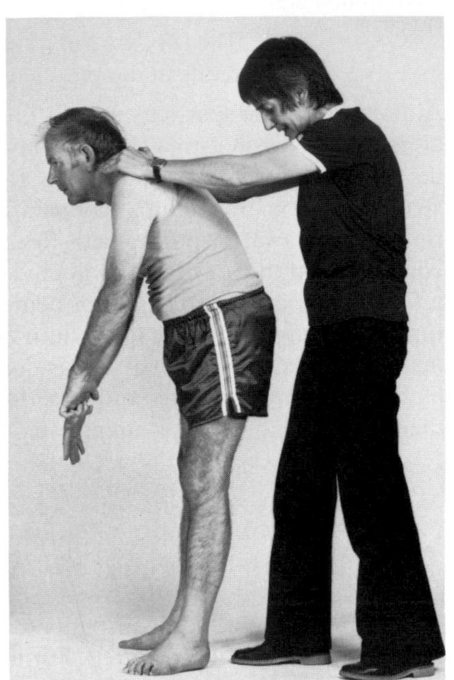
3.8

Fig. 3.5. Placing the head, normal subject. The arms remain relaxed at her side

Fig. 3.6. Placing the head, patient with left hemiplegia. As the head is lifted, the arm pulls strongly into flexion

Fig. 3.7. Placing the trunk in a standing position, normal subject

Fig. 3.8. Attempting to place the trunk, patient with left hemiplegia. A resistance is encountered by the therapist and she is not able to move the trunk into the various positions

When lying supine, the normal subject's head feels light and reacts at once to the therapist's touch. The model lifts her head without effort and it remains in any position indicated by the therapist (Fig. 3.5). The patient's head pushes back and feels heavy. It requires effort for the patient to maintain the position, and the therapist needs to assist the lifting movement before he can take over the activity. As the neck flexes the arm pulls up into flexion (Fig. 3.6).

While standing, the normal model's trunk moves forward without any resistance, and rotates easily in response to the slight pressure of the therapist's hand on one shoulder (Fig. 3.7). The model is able to hold any position which the therapist's hands indicate. The patient attempts to react to the therapist's hand, but there is a resistance to trunk and hip flexion. Because activity in the extensor muscle groups is required to support the patient against gravity, the whole extensor synergy is elicited with no selection. The foot pushes down against the floor in plantar flexion and so the patient's hip is also shifted backwards. The hip extensors overact, making the movement forwards impossible. No trunk rotation takes place in response to the therapist's hand on the left shoulder; instead, the scapula pushes back, and the arm flexes. The patient extends his neck strongly, which increases the extension in the lower limb (Fig. 3.8).

When lying, the normal model's leg can be placed in any combination of positions. In the example shown, the therapist has placed his leg in a position where the hip is flexed; the knee must hold with active extensor activity while the foot remains dorsiflexed (Fig. 3.9). The patient's leg, when placed in the same position, pulls into total flexion, as he cannot extend the knee actively while holding the hip in flexion (Fig. 3.10a). If he attempts to straighten his knee the total extension pattern is evoked, and the hip moves more into extension, the knee extends and the foot pushes into plantar flexion (Fig. 3.10b).

With the model seated, his arm is placed forward and remains in position when the therapist removes her hands. Without any effort he keeps his shoulder in active flexion, holds the elbow in position with active extension and is able to keep the wrist and fingers in active extension (Fig. 3.11). When the patient's arm is placed in a similar position he attempts to hold it there, but requires tremendous effort to do so. He elevates the shoulder girdle, has difficulty in stabilising the scapula and because he is maintaining flexion of the shoulder is unable to extend his elbow. Despite the activity in the elbow extensors the elbow pulls into further flexion. The fingers flex and the thumb flexes and adducts (Fig. 3.12).

The difficulties that the patient has when the limb cannot be placed in selected combinations are seen clearly whenever he moves actively. The degree of difficulty varies considerably, but the effect of the mass synergies can still be seen even when the patient has regained a significant amount of voluntary function in the hemiplegic limbs. The patient will not be able to extend his arm in front of him with the palm turned upwards. The activity requires a combination of movement patterns: holding the arm in the air is a flexor activity and the scapula therefore elevates and retracts. Straightening the elbow is an extensor activity and the forearm pronates as a result, with the wrist flexing and the fingers adducting with flexion (Fig. 3.13a).

The same difficulty can be observed when the patient tries to clap his hands together above his head. The activity requires flexion of the shoulder and extension of the elbow, but with supination of the forearm and extension of the wrist and fingers.

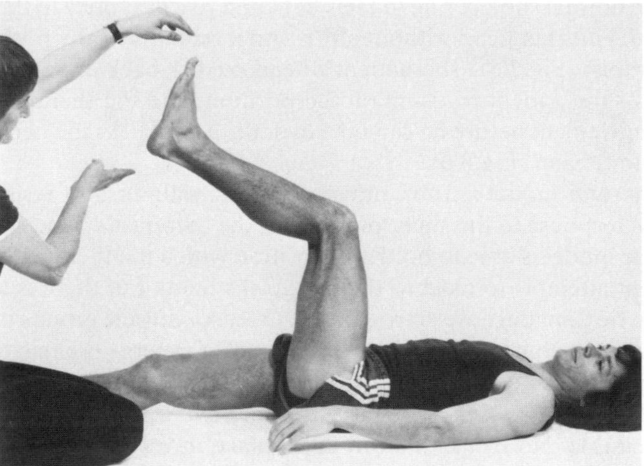

Fig. 3.9. Placing the leg, normal subject. The position requires selective hip flexion, knee extension and dorsiflexion of the foot

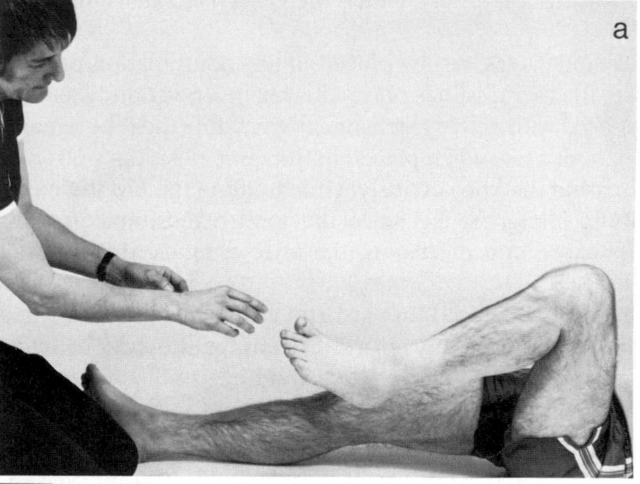

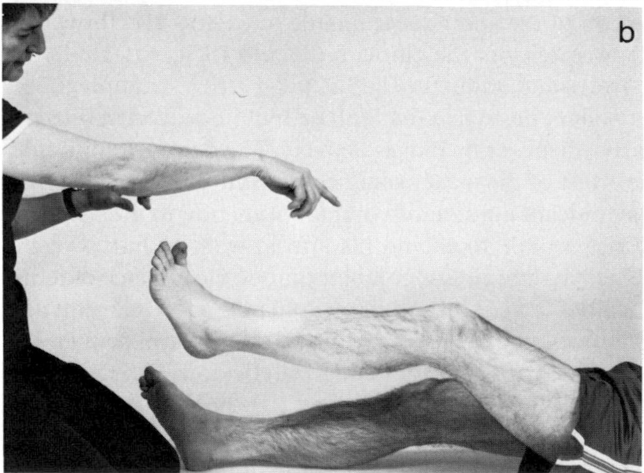

3.10

Fig. 3.10 a, b. Placing the leg, patient with left hemiplegia. **a** The leg pulls into the total flexion pattern without the knee extension component being possible while the hip is flexed. **b** The patient tries to extend his knee as required, and the whole limb extends in the total pattern. He is unable to keep the hip flexed as a result, and the knee extends further than it should

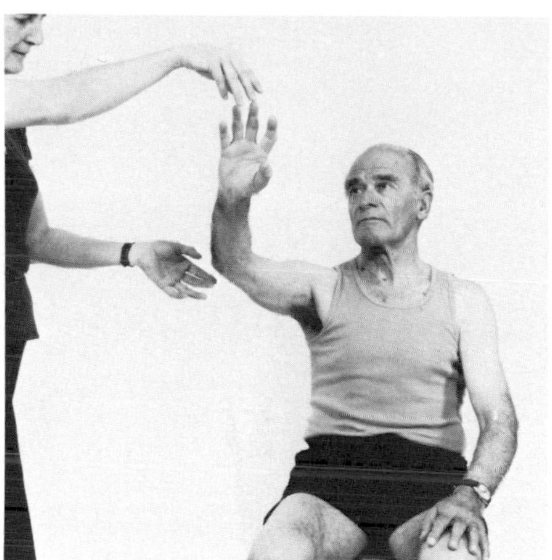

Fig. 3.11. Placing the arm, normal subject

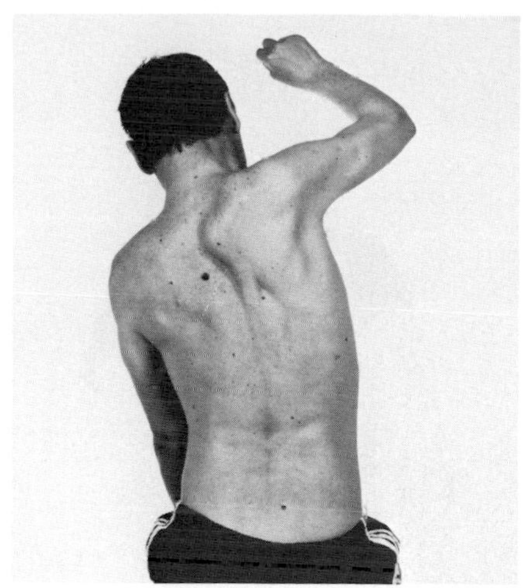

Fig. 3.12. Placing the arm, patient with right hemiplegia. Because the arm is being lifted flexor hypertonus increases and the total pattern of flexion makes the desired movement unattainable. The patient is unable to extend his fingers at all

(Fig. 3.13 b). Holding the extended arm horizontally abducted and outwardly rotated also requires full selective movement. The elbow is difficult to extend because holding the abducted arm in the air requires flexor activity. As the patient tries to extend the elbow, the shoulder rotates inwardly and the forearm pronates as part of the extensor synergy (Fig. 3.13 c).

The inability to move the leg selectively can be observed, for example, during the swing phase of gait. The patient brings the hemiplegic leg forward, but is unable to extend the knee for the last part of the swing phase. Because he is flexing his hip, the knee is also flexed and the foot is in supination (Fig. 3.14). The patient who extends his knee before placing the foot on the floor in front of him has difficulty in dorsiflexing his foot for heel-strike because the ankle is plantar flexing in the extensor synergy (Fig. 3.15).

These abnormal movement patterns arising in association with hemiplegia result from the combination of abnormal tone, the re-emergence of primitive mass synergies, a disturbed feedback system and other factors which are as yet unknown. Some variations may occur due to the patient using his abnormal movement patterns repeatedly for functional activities. "This will lead in time to the development of secondary or compensatory abnormal patterns of a greater variety" (K. Bobath 1971). Carr and Shepherd (1982) even go so far as to suggest that: "Practice of inappropriate muscle activity will result in the wrong movements being trained, and in a sense so-called "spasticity" is made up of habitual incorrect and unnecessary motor responses."

Many reflex mechanisms unleashed from the necessary inhibition are certainly responsible for causing increases in postural tone and for the reappearance of primitive movement synergies. "In essence, there are no pathological reflexes but

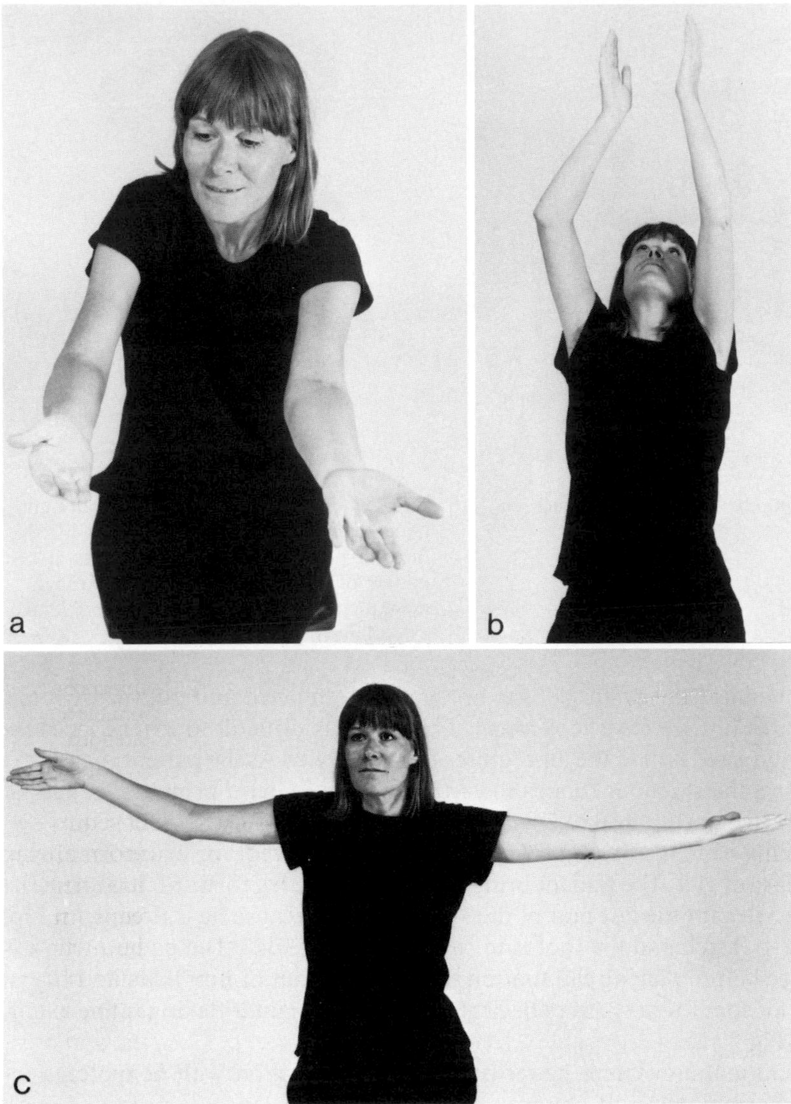

Fig. 3.13 a–c. Patient with right hemiplegia and active movement possible in the arm. **a** When she attempts to stretch both arms out in front of her with the palms facing upwards, the component of the flexor synergy can be seen. **b** When clapping her hands above her head the patient has difficulty in extending her elbow with the forearm supinated and the shoulder externally rotated. **c** When holding the arms in abduction, the patient cannot extend her elbow or turn the palm to face upwards

merely normal stereotyped lower spinal and middle supraspinal reflexes that are no longer activated, modified or inhibited" (Cailliet 1980).

The reflexes described in Sect. 3.5 would appear to be particularly relevant to the movement problems commonly encountered in hemiplegic patients. Understanding their influence will help the therapist in her treatment, which aims at in-

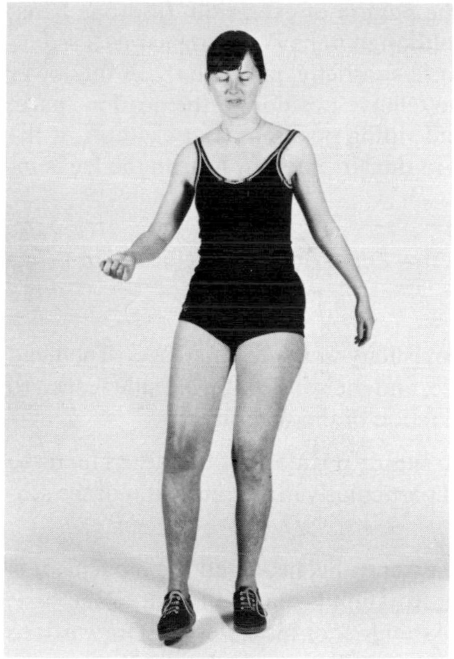

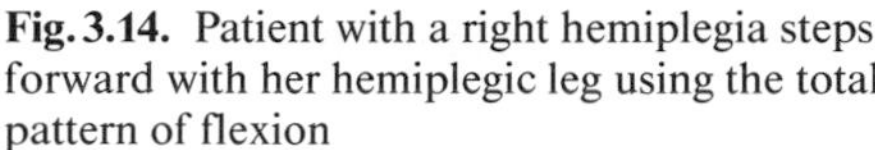

Fig. 3.14. Patient with a right hemiplegia steps forward with her hemiplegic leg using the total pattern of flexion

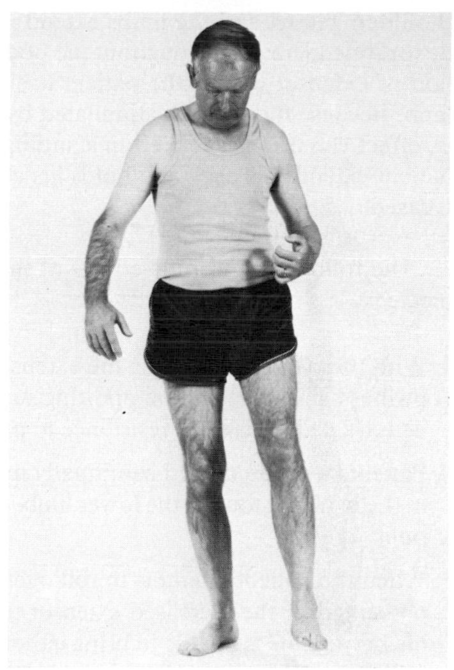

Fig. 3.15. Patient with a left hemiplegia brings his extended leg forwards and is unable to dorsiflex the foot with the knee extended

hibiting abnormal tonic reflex activity and facilitating normal movement sequences, including the higher integrated righting and equilibrium reactions. Abnormal postural reflexes can only be observed in patients with lesions of the central nervous system, where their release has led to their appearance in an exaggerated form. But even then it is difficult to isolate the various postural reactions, as the picture is usually complicated by the simultaneous action of a number of reflexes and by the patient's volitional efforts (B. Bobath 1971). Fiorentino (1981) describes the role of the postural reflexes in the normal development of movement in babies, and illustrates most clearly the results of their persistence in cerebral palsy as a typical neurological disability.

3.5 Relevant Tonic Reflexes

3.5.1 Tonic Labyrinthine Reflex

The tonic labyrinthine reflex is evoked by changes in the position of the head in space. It originates in the otolithic organs of the labyrinths, and is believed to be integrated at brain-stem levels (K. Bobath 1974; Fiorentino 1981). In supine, extensor tone increases throughout the body. The head pushes back as the spine extends, the shoulders retract and the limbs extend in the pattern of extension. In prone lying, flexor tone increases throughout the body, although it may only appear as a reduction of extensor tone if the patient has severe spasticity, particularly in the lower limb. Because the reflex is stimulated by the relative position of the head in space, its effect can also be noticed in standing and sitting positions. For example, if the patient extends his neck and holds his chin in the air, extensor tone in the leg is increased.

The following are some effects of the reflex appearing pathologically in hemiplegia:

1. With the patient in supine, the extensor spasticity in the leg increases. The head pushes back against the supporting surface, and the whole affected side is seen to be retracted. There is a resistance to protraction of the scapula.
2. Patients who are nursed continually in the supine position show marked increase in the extensor tone in the lower limb, and particularly in the retraction of the scapula.
3. When the patient attempts to roll over he extends his head and the movement is prevented by the increased extensor tone. Rotation is made difficult or impossible because he is unable to bring either his shoulder or his lower limb forwards to initiate turning over. If he flexes his head when rolling, the increased flexion prevents him from turning into the prone position. The lower limb and the arm remain flexed and block the movement, as does the trunk flexion.
4. When the patient sits for long periods in his wheelchair, the trunk is flexed and the neck must of necessity be extended to enable him to see. Extensor tone increases in the lower limb and the resulting hip extension causes his seat to slide forwards in the chair. The knee extends and the foot is pushed forwards off the foot-plate, so that eventually he may slip right out of the chair, or be left in a half-lying asymmetrical position in the chair.
5. When the patient attempts to stand up without sufficient preparation or adequate tone, he struggles to do so by extending his neck. The total extension pattern occurring in his leg as a result pushes him backwards, as does the retraction of the shoulder. The extending knee is unable to move forwards over his foot, and the necessary dorsal flexion of the ankle is prevented by the thrust of the plantar flexors.

   The same difficulty is experienced if he sits down with the head held in extension. Should he flex his head as he sits down, he collapses suddenly on to the chair as the total pattern of flexion is activated. The patient who can only maintain sufficient extension in standing by lifting his head will have difficulty in taking a step forwards with the affected leg when he walks. The increased extensor tone prevents the relaxation into flexion which is a prerequisite for the swing phase.
6. When the patient attempts to extend his elbow while lifting his arm, he reinforces the extension by pushing his head back. The movement is effortful and compromises functional use.

3.5.2 Symmetrical Tonic Neck Reflex

The symmetrical tonic neck reflex is a proprioceptive reflex, elicited by the stretching of the muscles and joints of the neck. Interacting with the labyrinthine reflexes, the symmetrical tonic reflex enables the baby to achieve the crawling position in normal development. In adults the reflexes interact to provide balance and equilibrium and orientate the head. When the neck extends, extensor tone in the arms and flexor tone in the legs increase. With the neck flexed, the extensor tone in the lower limbs increases, with more flexor tone in the arms.

The influence of the reflex seen in hemiplegia is as follows:

1. The patient who is nursed in bed in the half-lying position, with the head and trunk flexed by the supporting pillows, shows increased tone in the extensors of the affected leg and the flexors of the arm. Sitting with his head down while in the wheelchair produces the same pattern of spasticity.
2. The patient has difficulty when moving from lying to sitting because he must lift his head to initiate the movement, and the resulting increase in extensor tone at the hip resists the movement. Often, the whole leg will show marked extensor spasticity as he struggles to sit up, particularly if he attempts to do so symmetrically.
3. The patient who holds his neck flexed when walking and fixes his eyes on the ground has increased extensor tone in the leg. The knee hyperextends, the foot plantar flexes against the floor and the hip is pushed backwards during the stance phase. The patient has difficulty in relaxing the extensor activity to permit the necessary flexion of the hip and knee for the swing phase (Fig. 3.16).

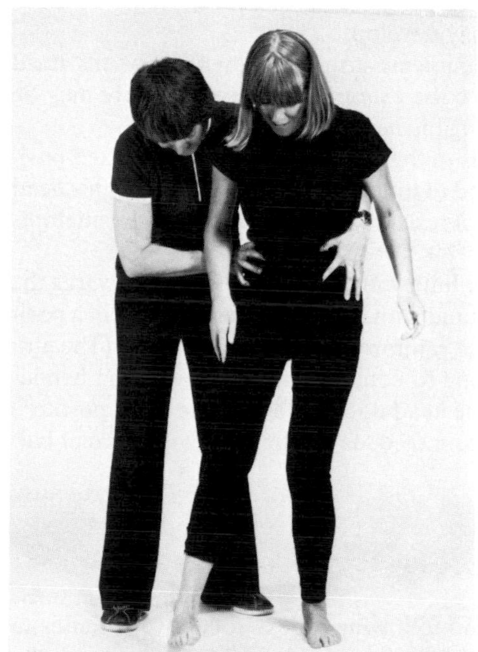

Fig. 3.16. Patient with a right hemiplegia flexes her neck to look at the ground when she walks. She is unable to release the hip and knee when taking a step and the position of the foot in the extensor pattern makes it difficult for her to place it correctly on the floor to initiate the stance phase

During walking the arm pulls strongly into flexion, the associated reaction reinforced by the position of the head.
4. When the patient attempts to transfer from his bed to the wheelchair he extends his head and his arms, and the affected leg may show increased flexor tone, either sliding under the bed, or lifting off the floor. He is unable to take weight on the leg.
5. When the patient attempts to kneel as he goes down on to the floor or stands up from the floor, he lifts his head and the affected leg collapses in total flexion.

3.5.3 Asymmetrical Tonic Neck Reflex

The asymmetrical tonic neck reflex is elicited as a proprioceptive response from the muscles and joints of the neck. When the head is turned, extensor tone increases in the limbs on the side towards which the face is turned. The limbs on the occiput side show an increase in flexor tone. In the normal baby, the reflex is fundamental to visual fixation, with the hand reaching out for objects. It also prepares the way for rolling over the prone with rotation at about 4–5 months in normal children.

Effects of the reflex seen pathologically in hemiplegia are as follows:

1. The patient's head is usually turned away from the affected side in lying and sitting and flexor tone increases in the hemiplegic arm as a result. Patients who remain in the wheelchair for many months, when standing and walking are delayed, often show increase in flexor tone in the hemiplegic leg as well. The leg shows flexor spasticity when the patient is helped to stand up. Even when the patient is lying supine, a resistance may be felt when passive extension of the leg is attempted. A flexion contracture of the knee may develop.
2. When attempting to straighten his hemiplegic arm the patient turns his head strongly to the affected side to reinforce the extension at the elbow. He may be unable to extend the arm without turning his head.
3. Although flexor spasticity predominates in the arm and it assumes a flexed position, the patient is unable to flex his hand to touch his head or face when his head is turned towards it. The therapist feels a resistance to flexion when she attempts to assist the correct movement.
4. The patient with hypotonus in the lower limb will often turn his head towards the affected side when he is attempting to stand with help. He fixes his head in a position of rotation to the hemiplegic side, to reinforce extension in the leg. (The attitude is often misinterpreted as being one to compensate for an existing hemianopsia, but when the patient is sitting the head does not adopt the same posture.) The fixed head position should be discouraged, as it interferes with normal balance reactions.

3.5.4 Positive Supporting Reflex

The positive supporting reflex is a reaction following an exteroceptive stimulus to the skin of the toe pads and the ball of the foot, often elicited as these touch the ground. A proprioceptive stimulus follows, due to the stretching of the interosseous muscles of the foot caused by the pressure on the ball of the foot. Extensor tone throughout the limb is increased, together with a simultaneous contraction of the opposing muscles to stabilise the joints for weight-bearing. In normal development the reflex is a precursor to standing and walking.

The effects of the reflex seen pathologically in hemiplegia are as follows:

1. Because the ball of the hemiplegic foot usually first makes contact with the ground, the exaggerated reflex causes an immediate increase in extensor tone throughout the limb in a total pattern. The leg becomes a rigid pillar, with the knee hyperextended, and the patient has difficulty in keeping his heel on the floor during weight-bearing, or releasing the hip and knee for the swing phase during walking. He also has difficulty in transferring weight over the hemiplegic leg at the start of the stance phase, as the plantar flexors push against the direction of the movement.
2. Attempts at maintaining dorsal flexion at the ankle by traditional passive movements fail because the therapist's hands on the ball of the foot increase the hypertonus in the plantar flexors, and the full range of movement is impossible.

3.5.5 Crossed Extensor Reflex

The crossed extensor reflex is believed to be a spinal reflex, causing an increase in extensor tone in one leg when the other leg is flexed. In normal developement it is a precursor to amphibian-type movement in preparation for crawling and walking (Fiorentino 1981).

B. Bobath (1971) discusses the animal experiments of Magnus and Sherrington, who describe the reflex as appearing when a painful stimulus is applied to one limb, causing a flexor withdrawal reaction. Extensor tone increases in the other leg(s) in order to support the additional body weight.

The effects of the reflex seen pathologically in hemiplegia are as follows:

1. When lying supine, the patient is able to lift his buttocks off the bed, the weight being supported by both his legs. If he lifts the sound leg off the bed in flexion, the affected leg is pushed into total extension pattern, and the "bridge" collapses.
2. When the patient stands from sitting with the weight only on the sound leg, the hemiplegic leg will often flex as the other leg extends actively. The patient has difficulty in transferring his weight over the affected leg in order to initiate walking.
3. A patient may be able to stand on his hemiplegic leg alone in the exercise situation. The leg remains mobile and he can even flex and extend the hemiplegic knee during weight-bearing without the toes flexing. However, during walking, when the sound leg is flexing forward to take a step, the hemiplegic leg pushes into total extension pattern, making balance difficult and the subsequent step forward with the affected leg stiff and effortful.

3.5.6 Grasp Reflex

The grasp reflex is elicited by tactile and proprioceptive stimuli in the palm of the hand and palmar aspect of the fingers, causing a grasp response with the fingers flexing and adducting. The reflex is present at birth in normal babies and disappears gradually as voluntary grasp develops. The reflex consists of an initial catching phase, elicited by a distally moving object in the palm of the hand in contact with the skin. The subsequent holding phase of the reflex results from a pull on the already contracting flexor muscles. "The stimulus for the proprioceptive phase is undoubtedly stretch, an increment of passive tension, acting on a centre already facilitated by deep cutaneous pressure" (Seyffarth and Denny-Brown 1948). The authors differentiate between the grasp reflex and the instinctive grasp reaction which is a "deliberate progressive closure of the whole hand made in a series of small movements, upon a stationary contact within the palm. This movement terminates in a final complete grip."

The effects of the reflex seen pathologically in hemiplegia are as follows:

1. Any object placed in the patient's hand will tend to increase flexor tone in the flexors of the wrist and fingers and cause flexion of the elbow, which is affected by the proximal insertion of the muscles involved. Patients with flexor spasticity in the hand are frequently treated by placing a firm roll in the hand to prevent flexion, or by applying a firm resting splint which includes the fingers. Both these procedures will tend to increase the spasticity by eliciting the grasp reflex and reaction.
2. The patient who shows some return of activity in the hand should not be encouraged to squeeze a rubber ball, as flexor tone will be stimulated and release of the grasp become increasingly difficult.
3. The patient may have difficulty in clasping his hands together in order to carry out his self-assisted arm exercises. As he attempts to interlace his fingers, the grasp reflex is stimulated by the fingers of the sound hand moving distally on the palmar aspect of his other hand. The fingers flex and adduct and resist the attempt.
4. The patient who has active extension of the fingers may also have an active grasp reflex which prevents him from releasing objects during functional activities. The inability to release or prevent the grasp is not necessarily related to weakness of finger extension.
5. Some patients have difficulty in preventing involuntary inappropriate grasping. The affected hand, even when not involved in an activity, may hold tightly to an object, e.g. the leg of the trousers, when walking.

3.6 Associated Reactions and Associated Movements

Associated reactions in hemiplegia are abnormal reflex movements of the affected side, and duplicate the stereotyped spastic patterns of the arm and leg (Fig. 3.17). Walshe (1923) described associated reactions as "released postural reactions de-

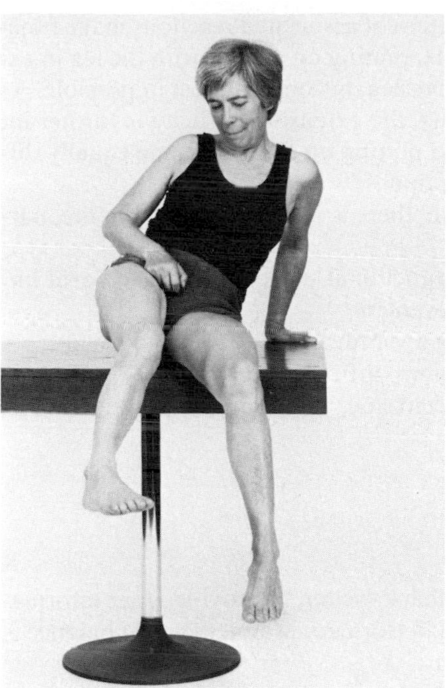

Fig. 3.17. Patient with a right hemiplegia shows typical associated reactions in the arm and leg when moving incorrectly and pulling herself back with her sound arm to sit on a table

prived of voluntary control". Riddoch and Buzzard (1921) defined associated reactions as "automatic activities which fix or alter the posture of a part or parts when some other part of the body is brought into action by either voluntary effort or reflex stimulation" (Brunnstrom 1970). The reactions are seen when the patient moves with effort, is trying to maintain his balance, or is afraid of falling. Mulley (1982) reports associated reactions in the hemiplegic arm in 80% of a group of patients, occurring in conjunction with yawning, coughing and sneezing. During functional activities, such as putting on shoes using the sound hand, associated reactions are prevalent in both the arm and the leg if attention is not given to inhibitory positions.

Associated movements are normal automatic postural adjustments which accompany voluntary movements. They occur in normal subjects, to reinforce precise movements of other parts of the body, or when an activity requires a great deal of strength. Associated movements can be observed in the unaffected limbs of the hemiplegic patient when he is trying to move his affected limbs. They should not be confused with associated reactions, which are pathological, and can be differentiated by the ability of the patient to alter or relax them. Associated reactions are stereotyped and occur even when no active movement is present in the limb. The patient is unable to relax them at will. The limb returns to its previous position only after the stimulus has ceased, and then often only gradually.

The detrimental effects of associated reactions in hemiplegia are as follows:

1. The abnormal flexed position of the hemiplegic arm is cosmetically unacceptable for the patient. It draws immediate attention to his disability.

2. The affected limbs in the fixed spastic position of associated reactions make functional activities more difficult. For example, putting on a shoe, with the leg in extension with the foot plantar flexed and inverted, becomes almost impossible. As the patient struggles to perform the activity, the extensor spasticity is further increased. Washing the hemiplegic hand and putting on a coat become equally difficult if the arm is pulling strongly into flexion.
3. If the arm is constantly pulled up in flexion, there is a danger of contracture, particularly of the elbow and the fingers.
4. The continuously flexed position makes functional use of the affected arm impossible, and return of activity may be prevented.
5. Balance reactions in both the arm and leg are prevented by the associated reactions, making the maintenance of equilibrium difficult.
6. Spasticity is increased throughout the affected side, hampering all movements.

3.7 Disturbed Sensation

All skilled movements require a refined feedback system to provide exact information as to the correctness of the activity being performed. Maintenance of balance is dependent on sensations throughout the body.

It is difficult if not impossible to know exactly what the hemiplegic patient feels, and what information he receives when he moves. Conventional testing of sensation can only provide a guide-line; the result, however, can be recorded, and changes noted at a later date. What is recorded states only that the patient at a specific time, in a given situation, gave the examiner information about what he was feeling. Even if all the answers he gave were correct as to the position of his limbs, the direction of their movements and the pressure or light touch he could percieve, he might be observed an hour later sitting with his hand trapped in the wheel of his wheelchair while attempting to move forwards.

Patterns of spasticity and mass movement synergies are closely related to sensation, either as cause or effect. The patient can only move in an abnormal way, so the feedback is of an abnormal movement. He moves in abnormal patterns because the sensation is inaccurate and inadequate.

3.8 Considerations

Movement is learnt through repetition and becomes more skilled as inhibition of unwanted activity increases. If the patient only moves in stereotyped mass movement synergies, he will learn only these, to the exclusion of more defined and selective movements. Abnormal movements reinforce the spasticity, which increases as a result. The treatment should aim at helping the patient to move in the most normal and economic way possible right from the beginning, so avoiding his learning abnormal movement patterns through constant repetition.

4 Practical Assessment – A Continuing Process

To assess the patient's abilities and difficulties fully and accurately, the therapist requires exact observation, ready hands, clear thinking and the time to listen to what the patient says. She needs to understand fully how people normally move and react in different situations or perform certain tasks, so that she can notice at once if the patient acts or reacts differently.

No scientific system of measurement is as yet available for the therapist when assessing a patient with a hemiplegia. A purely functional chart which can be ticked off briskly only provides quantitative information, stating what the patient can or cannot do. The recording of the patient's functional abilities alone is not sufficient for adequate treatment planning. For example, the statement "Patient cannot transfer from wheelchair to bed" does not answer the question "Why?". It only states that he is unable to perform the activity. In order to treat his particular difficulty, it is necessary to know whether his legs were too weak or his balance too poor, whether he was too spastic, or even whether he was too obese to lift his body from the seat of the chair.

Similarly, a patient might be described as having an adequate functional gait, of normal speed and with good balance, and able to use public transport. However, because of extensor spasticity, he may be unable to flex his knee while the hip is extended. In order to bring his foot forwards, he therefore circumducts his leg as he takes a step, and this is the information needed for treatment in order to overcome the difficulty.

A qualitative rather than a quantitative evaluation is necessary for appropriate treatment.

4.1 The Aims of Assessment

The assessment aims at:

Eliciting what is preventing the patient from moving in the normal way, in order to plan the treatment.
Making frequent reviews possible so that the treatment can be altered if necessary.
Enabling another therapist to continue the treatment effectively.
Recording the patient's condition accurately for future therapeutic or statistical purposes.

Assessment is always carried out in conjunction with treatment. The therapist is trying to discover where the patient's main problem lies and if she can change some factor. If she inhibits the spasticity, can he then move in a more normal pattern? What can he do if she helps him a little or supports him in a certain way? Assessment is therefore an integral part of the treatment itself. The therapist is constantly assessing and reassessing during treatment to see if she has reduced hypertonus, stimulated activity or enabled the patient to move in a more normal way during a certain activity.

Assessment involves far more than merely asking the patient to move his limbs while lying on a bed or plinth. The therapist should watch the patient as he arrives for his first treatment, and from this valuable moment onwards assessment is a continuous process, involving important variables which will come to light over a period. A full evaluation cannot be made on one particular day. Even a sleepless night or constipation can adversely affect the patient's performance.

The therapist notes how the patient enters, whether he is escorted, held or supported. If he is in a wheelchair, she notes how he pushes it or assists, how he is sitting, whether he looks alert or uninterested. The same would apply whether he is seen in bed, on the ward or in his home. She should take the trouble to put the patient at ease and speak in such a way that he understands what is required of him. Many assessments may be inaccurate simply because the patient is confused as to what activity the therapist wishes him to perform.

4.2 Immediate Observation

The therapist observes the patient carefully as he approaches and while he is talking to her, whether he is lying, sitting or standing. Figure 4.1–4.3 show patients as they might appear when arriving for their assessment and treatment. The following points can be observed, which could prove valuable later for treatment purposes.

In Fig. 4.1 the absence of facial expression is inappropriate to the situation, where the patient is greeting the therapist. The mask-like face and very wide-open eyes suggest a hypertonus of the facial muscles, as does the withdrawn upper lip on the left side. Her eyes are turned towards the therapist but her head remains turned to the right and side flexed to the left, and the hyperactivity apparent in the left sternomastoid muscle could account for the position.

She appears to have difficulty in lifting her head against the pull of the flexor spasticity in neck and trunk. She will certainly have problems with balance if her head is not free to move. The open mouth indicates that she will have problems with eating and drinking. Is it because of weakness in the jaw-closing muscles or is she unable to close her mouth due to hypertonus in the antagonistic muscle group?

The upper trunk is markedly flexed, particularly on the left side, and her weight is over the right side. The left side is probably more affected than the right. Her arms are in the pattern of flexor spasticity. Is it just spasticity or are there contractures or painful limitation of range? Can she use her arms at all? The patient's right arm is pressing heavily on the arm of the wheelchair. Is she unable to maintain the upright position without the help of her arm? Her legs are in adduction. Is this due to her position in the chair or is there a resistance to abducting them, caused by spasticity?

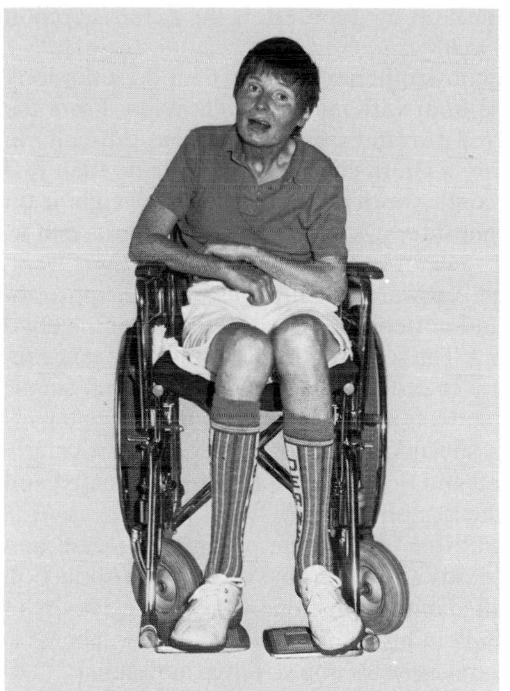
4.1

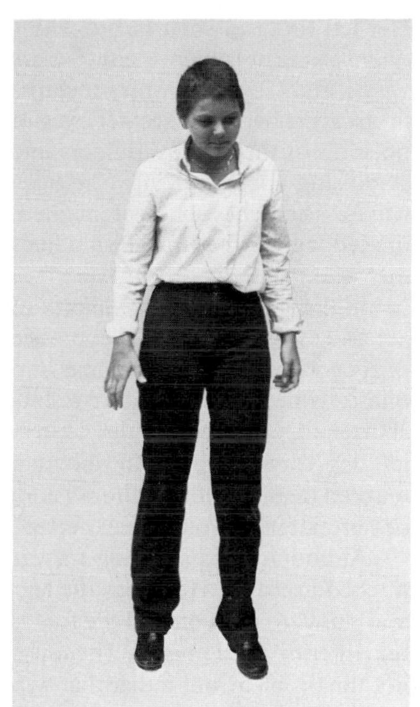
4.2

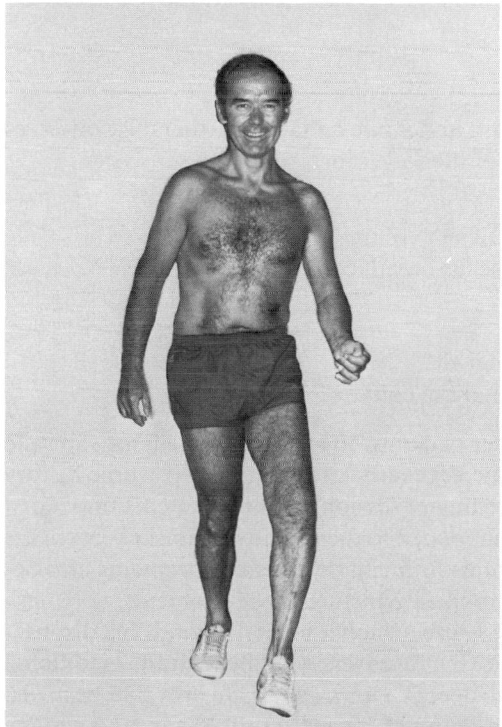
4.3

Fig. 4.1. Patient with bilateral hemiplegia following a thrombosis in both internal carotid arteries

Fig. 4.2. Patient with ataxia

Fig. 4.3. Patient with a left hemiplegia

Her left foot is plantar flexed with the heel off the foot-rest. Is the Achilles tendon only spastic or is there a contracture as well?

In Fig. 4.2, as she walks towards the physiotherapist, the patient does not look up to greet her but fixes her eyes on the floor with much concentration. From the position of the head, shoulders and arms it would seem that she has difficulty in stabilising and balancing. She takes only a short step, more to the side than forwards. The right foot has remained in contact with the floor until her weight is on the left leg. She has transferred her weight sideways rather than forwards as in normal walking.

In Fig. 4.3 the patient walks confidently towards the therapist with an appropriate and symmetrical facial expression and normal eye contact. His balance is obviously good, as he shows no fear of falling. The sensation in his left leg appears adequate, as he does not require to look at it in order to step forwards. His left side is shortened, with the shoulder depressed and retracted. With the effort of bringing his left leg forward, his arm shows an associated reaction in flexion, particularly marked distally with his thumb adducted and flexed. The forearm is supinated and not pronated as would be expected in the flexion pattern.

Although he is stepping forward with his left leg, the pelvis is retracted and hitched upwards. He brings the leg forwards in the flexion synergy with abduction and outward rotation and the foot is pulled into supination by the strong activity of the anterior tibial muscle. The muscle bulk in his whole leg shows that weakness is not the problem, but rather that hypertonus is restricting selective movement.

4.3 Subjective History

A short history is taken from the patient, and while he talks the therapist observes him carefully and gains an impression of the following:

1. Voice
   a) Does he speak clearly and with sufficient volume?
   b) Are his sentences very short because his breath control is inadequate?
   c) Is his voice hoarse or monotonous?
2. Facial expression
   a) Is it appropriate and does it change it all?
   b) Does he look at her and make normal eye contact?

If he is unable to speak at all, some other person who knows him well, for example his wife, should be present to provide the necessary information. The whole history should not be taken at the start of the treatment session, as many patients find it distressing to sit and talk about what has happened to them. The therapist observes the patient's abilities first, then uses her hands to facilitate certain movements and between activities gradually builds up a composite picture of the problems.

While listening to him, the therapist learns whether he understands his disorder and has a clear picture of the prognosis. She discovers what his attitude is to home and work, and whether he is prepared to accept a new way of life now that he is disabled. She hears from the patient what he thinks his main problem is, and why he has sought help. His subjective opinion of what he considers to be his main problem and what he hopes to achieve through the treatment is an important clue to how realistically he sees his disability.

It is also important for the therapist to compare her goals with those of the patient, because they must somehow be brought together to form a realistic aim. Failure to have a common goal will lead to disappointment and frustration for the patient or the therapist, or both. For example, where the therapist's aim is that the patient should learn to walk again, while his is to have a new wheelchair, success is only possible if they come to a mutual agreement. Similarly, if the therapist is concentrating on enabling the patient to walk without a walking-stick and his main wish is to be able to use his hemiplegic hand again, the treatment sessions will be disappointing.

4.4 Appropriate Clothing for Assessment and Treatment

The patient should always undress sufficiently and wear appropriate clothing for the assessment and all subsequent treatment sessions. Many significant problems may otherwise be overlooked. During treatment, adequate stimulation and observation is not possible if the patient remains fully dressed. A bathing costume or shorts and a vest are most suitable for assessment and treatment. How the patient undresses and dresses himself again and the amount of support or assistance he requires when doing so is an important observation in the assessment, e.g. with even a comparatively slight hemiplegia the patient may reveal balance problems in his inability to step out of his trousers. Through observation, the therapist can be building up a composite picture long before she handles the limbs or tests functions specifically.

4.5 Muscle Tone

While the patient is moving either to sit on the plinth or to stand up from his chair, the therapist can be gaining an impression of his muscle tone on a more automatic level, before he is conscious of being tested. She is looking and feeling all the time as he moves or is being assisted to move.

Muscle tone can be described as the amount of resistance to passive movement of the part; in other words, to stretch. Observation alone can be very deceptive, so the therapist must feel the resistances.

The muscle with normal tone responds to being moved by taking the weight of the part it affects and allowing the limb, head or trunk to be guided without resistance into a position which is spontaneously maintained with ease. In the presence of normal tone the part moved can be described as having a feeling of lightness. If placed in a certain position, the part will stay for a time before returning slowly to a resting posture.

Where hypertonicity is present, the limb or trunk feels heavy and resists movement to a greater or lesser degree. If released, the part will be pulled in the direction of the increased tone. Hypotonicity allows the movements with less than normal resistance, but the weight of the limb is not taken and it will fall in the direction of the pull of gravity (see also Sects. 3.3, 3.4).

4.6 Joint Range

Although there is variability in the measurement of joint range, it is an important record of the patient's state at the time and will influence the planning of the treatment. Care must be taken, however, to differentiate between spasticity and structural limitation of range, and also between soft tissue shortening and bony changes, as the information will be necessary for planning the treatment approach. When testing, it is effort saving to examine all parts of the body first in one position and then in another, but when the facts are recorded it is helpful to have them all grouped under the heading pertaining to the particular part of the body.

4.7 Muscle Charts

A specific muscle-testing chart is not included in the assessment. In the presence of spasticity, which is a varying force, it is not possible to estimate accurately the strength of a muscle acting against it. For example, a patient with possible grade 5 dorsiflexors may be unable to dorsiflex his foot against the hypertonus of the calf muscles, particularly when the leg is extended. Muscle strength may be adequate in certain positions, but if the patient can only move in synergistic, non-selective patterns he cannot use the limb or part functionally. The hemiplegic patient is often able to extend his elbow when lying supine with his arm above his head and the flexor spasticity inhibited. In this position the therapist may be unable to overcome the extensor activity, which could then be classified as a grade 5 in triceps (Fig. 4.4a). When the patient is standing or sitting, however, he is unable to extend his elbow, even though gravity is assisting the movement (Fig. 4.4b).

Both joint range measurement and muscle activity should be recorded under the heading pertaining to that part of the body. For example, it is far easier to refer to the section on upper limbs to see whether the elbow was contracted at the time of the last assessment than to have to search for a chart kept on a separate page.

A photograph or diagrammatic sketch of the movement possibility is often clearer than a recorded number of degrees. Actual measurement of a contracture can be noted by measuring the distance between two definite points, e.g. for a flexion contracture of the elbow the patient lies supine and his shoulder is held flat on the supporting surface. The distance between the dorsal aspect of his wrist and the plinth is measured and recorded.

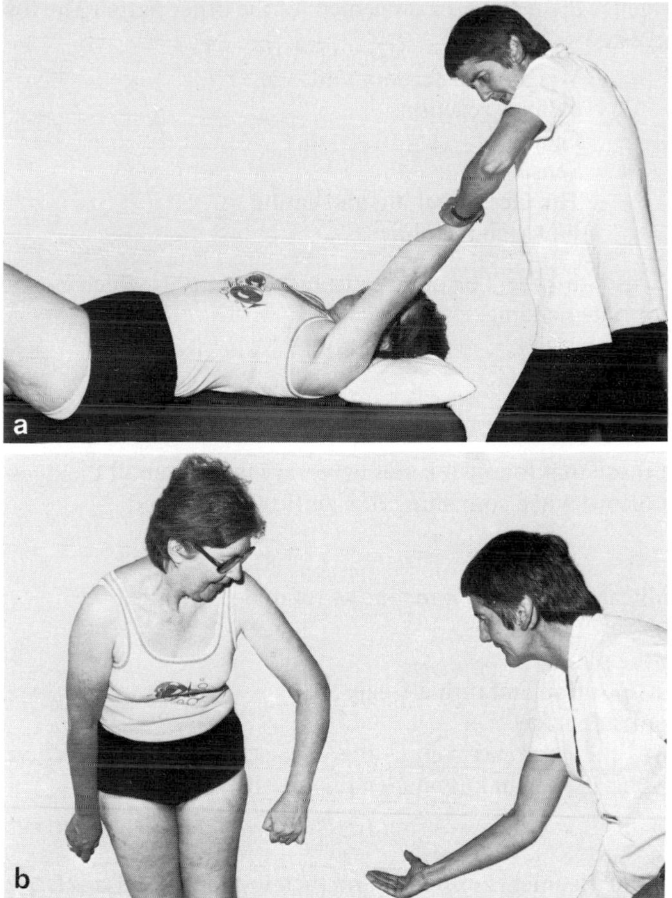

Fig. 4.4 a, b. Muscle strength cannot be tested by the traditional grading system. The patients' position and the variable tone in the antagonists give results which are not applicable to function. **a** A patient lying supine is able to hold her elbow extended against gravity despite considerable resistance from the therapist. **b** With gravity assisting the movement, in a standing position the patient is unable to extend her elbow to touch the therapist's hand

4.8 Recording the Assessment

There is no short cut to recording the assessment, no chart that would suit all patients and all therapists. The information should be clearly headed and neatly written or printed so that important facts are not overlooked. Recently, a carefully prepared assessment form for hemiplegic patients made no mention of tone or spasticity, so omitting one of the most relevant factors.

To make recording easier it is possible to have printed sheets giving headings and space, to ensure that each aspect is examined. (Any difficulty observed in one part of the body will influence the posture or movement of the other parts.) The following headings are suggested:

The head	Weight transference and
Thc trunk	balance reactions
The upper limbs	Gait
The lower limbs	Sensation
Sitting	The face, speaking and eating
Standing	Functional abilities.

Obviously, in individual cases there will be other outstanding features which can be recorded under an appropriate heading.

4.8.1 The Head

Under this heading and those that follow it is not necessary to answer all the questions separately, only to record when something of significance is noted.

In Supine

Does the head lie centrally at rest or does it incline or rotate to one side?
Does it remain flexed?
Does it push back on to the plinth?
Can the patient correct its position and turn it freely?
Can he raise it as if to look at his feet?
When the therapist moves the head passively is there resistance in any direction, and does the patient support its weight automatically himself?

In Sitting

The position which the head assumes is observed and then tested to see if it is freely movable. Is there resistance to passive movement, and can the patient move it actively?

In Standing

The same tests should be made with the patient in a standing position.

4.8.2 The Trunk

In Supine

Does the body lie symmetrically or is it shortened on one side?
Is the pelvis rotated?
Has the lumbar spine a fixed lordosis, and if so, can it be corrected passively by flexing the hips and tilting the pelvis?
Can the patient sit up from lying without using his arms?
Can he roll over to both sides?
Can he roll from supine to prone and back again over either side? How does he do so?

4.8.3 The Upper Limbs

In Supine

What position do the arms assume at rest?
Can the patient move them voluntarily in a normal manner? If not, state the pattern of movement.
When moved passively, is there resistance to movement in any direction?
Do the arms move involuntarily on effort or when the patient yawns or coughs? If so, in what pattern of movement?
Does the tone in the arms change according to which way the head is turned?
Is contracture present at any joint even after release of spasticity?

In Prone Lying

Can the patient bring his arms forwards, or is there too much flexion in this position?
Is full elevation of the shoulders and extension of the elbows possible in this position?
Can he support his weight on his elbows?
Can he support his weight on extended arms?

In Sitting and Standing

The tests carried out in supine and prone lying should also be done with the patient sitting and standing. Many patients have comparatively good movement when lying fully supported, and the problems may only be obvious when he has to hold himself upright against gravity and maintain his balance at the same time.

It is even more important to know how the patient actually uses his hands. Testing the different movements in a free exercise situation will not provide the information as to what happens when he performs a task. For example, the patient is asked to carry out an everyday activity which normally requires the use of both hands, such as opening a bottle, pouring himself a drink and then drinking it. He could also be asked to cut a slice of bread, spread it with butter and then eat it. The therapist observes if he performs the activity in any way differently from other people. Even how hard he has to concentrate to perform the relatively simple task will indicate whether he has problems when using his hands.

4.8.4 The Lower Limbs

In Supine

Active and passive movements are tested in a similar way to the upper limbs. In addition the following are observed with the patient lying prone.

In Prone Lying

Can the patient flex his knees actively without flexing his hips as well?
Is there resistance to flexing the knees passively, and do the hips flex if this is done?
Do the knees remain flexed easily if left in this position?
Can the patient perform isolated ankle movements with the knee flexed?

In Sitting

The patient moves his leg actively in different directions, e.g. crossing the leg over the other one. The therapist also moves the leg passively to note any resistance.

In Standing

The patient lifts his leg in different directions and can be observed while he takes a step or kicks a football with the hemiplegic foot. The therapist should also feel the resistance as she moves the leg passively.

4.8.5 Sitting

Can the patient come to a sitting position from lying unaided, and how does he do so?
Does he sit with the trunk flexed or does he push or fall backwards?
Does he lean more to one side than to the other?
Does he bear weight equally through each buttock?
Is the trunk rotated, for example is one shoulder or one side of the pelvis drawn backwards?
Is one shoulder lower than the other?
Do the legs hang in a normally flexed position over the side of the bed or couch, or do the knees extend, showing hypertonus?
How is his balance in this position? Does he have normal balance reactions when he is moved to either side?
Can he move his head, arms and legs, or have them moved passively, without falling over?
Can he save himself from falling?

4.8.6 Standing

How does the patient stand up from sitting? Does he push backwards in his effort to assume the upright position? Does he come up more over one side than the other?
Once upright, does he bear weight equally on both legs?
Does his posture deteriorate as he comes upright against gravity? For example, what posture does he assume?
Does the pelvis tilt in an anterior or posterior direction or shift laterally?
Does he show associated reactions in the rest of the body due to his efforts to maintain the upright position?
Does he require a caliper for standing, and if so, how does he manage without it?

4.8.7 Weight Transference and Balance Reactions

While lying prone with elbow support, can the patient transfer weight to either side, freeing the opposite limb for movement?

While sitting, can he shift weight to either side without the support of his arms and lift or free the opposite leg for movement? When his weight moves over to the side does the head right freely and adequately to the vertical position? Does the trunk lengthen and shorten adequately when the weight is transferred to either side?

While standing, can he move his weight over one leg and is the supporting leg hyperextended or flexed to permit this? Can he stand on one leg and move the other leg? In step position, can he transfer weight easily from the front leg to the one behind? Can he take steps to regain his balance – sideways, forwards and backwards? When the therapist steers the patient in different directions, with her hands placed lightly on his shoulders as he walks, does he follow quickly and automatically?

4.8.8 Walking

It is difficult to give an accurate description of walking, but it is probably best done by describing variations from the normal. The walking pattern is recorded as vividly as possible, describing also the ease with which the patient walks, the speed, rhythm and length of stride. The arm swing gives a good indication as to how freely he walks and if rotation takes place. Do the arms assume a fixed position during walking, either due to associated reactions or in the patient's attempt to maintain his balance?

The description of the walking pattern is far clearer when the weight-bearing phase and then the step forward are described separately.

Can the patient move his head freely while walking, and is he able to talk and walk at the same time?

Can he walk freely out of doors, even on uneven surfaces?

Is he able to walk in the street when there is traffic, and can he negotiate the pavement without hesitation?

Approximately how far does he walk without being unduly tired? (It is useful to record how long it takes the patient to walk a certain distance for comparison at a later date.)

Does the patient require support when he walks, manual support from another person, a stick or a crutch and does he wear a caliper? (It is also important to describe what happens when he walks without these aids if it is possible for him to do so, and when he walks barefooted.)

4.8.9 Negotiating Stairs

Can the patient go up and down stairs? Does he do so in a normal manner, i.e. with one foot on each step? Is he able to manage without holding on to the bannister?

4.8.10 Getting up from the Floor

Can the patient get down on to the floor unaided? How does he do so? Is he able to come from lying through kneeling to standing again?

4.8.11 Comprehension

Does the patient understand verbal instruction, or is he merely imitating or anticipating what is required rather than actually understanding thc words? IIis ability to understand simple verbal commands can be tested by showing him two objects, for example a cup and a spoon. Without the therapist giving him any non-verbal cues she can ask him to look at either the cup or the spoon. If he follows correctly she can give him a two-part instruction by asking him to do something with the spoon, e.g. "Take the spoon and tap it against the side of the cup before replacing it." His response will give an idea of his ability to follow a command. Often, as the therapist reaches out a hand expectantly, while saying, "Give me your hand", the patient responds correctly, and she may think he has full comprehension when he is, in fact, responding to non-verbal cues in a known situation.

4.8.12 The Face, Speaking and Eating

While listening to the patient giving his subjective history, the therapist will already have formed an opinion as to the patient's ability to speak and to vary his facial expression appropriately. In addition:

Does the patient sound different when the therapist assists breathing, indicating that poor breathing is handicapping his speech?
Does his position influence voice production because spasm is limiting speech, making it sound effortful and/or monotonous? Is neuromuscular dysfunction slurring his speech and rendering him incapable of producing certain sounds? For example, are labials impossible for him due to the facial paresis? He can be asked to whistle or blow out his cheeks and move the air from one cheek to the other.
Can he move his tongue from side to side equally?
Can he move his tongue up or down outside his mouth? If he cannot, the chances are he cannot do it inside his mouth. Is he able to put his tongue in his cheek and to put its tip behind his upper front teeth?
Can he eat and drink without difficulty? If not, it may be that he cannot move the food around in his mouth preparing it for swallowing, rather than be actually unable to swallow.
Are his teeth and mouth clean or are pieces of food left stuck anywhere?
Can he pronounce easily and rapidly the consonants "t", "g" and "k"? The first requires that he be able to place the tip of his tongue up behind his front teeth and the two latter that he raise its posterior portion. These movements are necessary for transporting the prepared food back for swallowing.

Many patients with hemiplegia have inadequate or inappropriate facial expression, which can be a most distressing handicap. They may be misinterpreted as a result and thought to be depressed, unmotivated, or unfriendly. The patient and his relatives are very sensitive to facial abnormalities, particularly should dribbling occur or pieces of food remain unnoticed on his lips or chin. The movement, tone and sensation of the face and mouth should be included for treatment should difficulties exist (see Chap. 13).

4.8.13 Sensation

Testing of sensation is often totally omitted by the therapist, although it may well hold the key to the problem being treated. All tests for sensation must be done without the patient being able to see at all. A towel should be held in front of him, as he may otherwise obtain clues by seeing movement if the eye closure is not complete. Without going into too much detail, the therapist should test the following:

1. Light touch, deep pressure, and differentiation between hot and cold. It is not sufficient for her merely to touch various parts of the patient's body with her hand, saying, "Can you feel me touching you here?" She should ask the patient to acknowledge each time she touches him, and to inform her where she is touching or pressing.
2. Position sense. The patient should be able to describe the direction in which the joint is being moved or the position in which it is placed. The therapist moves the hemiplegic limb into certain positions and the patient then places his sound limb in exactly the same positions. The test is performed in two ways:

   The patient moves his sound limb simultaneously as the therapist places his affected limb in a position.

   The therapist selects a position and then asks the patient to copy it with his other arm or leg.
3. Stereognosis. Can he identify a familiar object placed in his hand, for example a key? If he has speech problems, he can indicate a duplicate object near at hand. Where there is inability to manipulate the object the therapist can move the patient's hand for him to simulate his own grasp.

For the hemiplegic patient, the testing of sensation may be a complex performance, and he may fail due to other reasons than his poor sensation. Testing first with visual control will ensure that he understands what is required, and that he is able to perform the task. Then his vision can be excluded and the actual test for sensation carried out.

4.8.14 Functional Abilities

The therapist must record the patient's ability to carry out the routine activities of daily living. It is one of the few objective measurements of his progress and capability that she has. She should assess thoroughly the activities concerned with personal hygiene, dressing and eating, and note how long each activity takes him. The patient should be observed while he performs these tasks, to avoid any discrepancies. Careful discussion with those people nearest to him at home may bring other difficulties to light, which is particularly important if the therapist is unable to assess the patient in his own environment. Recording the patient's profession, age and hobbies gives the therapist an idea of his life before the hemiplegia. The information will also be a guide to his life-style and his expectations from the rehabilitation.

4.8.15 Considerations

The assessment which has been described is a very full one and is not necessarily carried out during the first treatment session. If the patient is seen during the acute phase of his illness many of the tests will not be applicable. In the same way a patient who has not had adequate treatment and has a painful shoulder or is afraid of moving will not be tested in the prone position, or asked to kneel down on the floor. The therapist estimates which of the tests are feasible at the time.

When a patient comes for treatment at a later stage in his progress, the whole assessment may be necessary to discover exactly where his difficulties lie. It should also be noted how much treatment he has already had, and of what type. Although the assessment may seem long, time is actually saved by accurate assessment, and without it full rehabilitation is impossible. Even if the information is not fully recorded, the therapist nevertheless needs to observe all the points that have been mentioned.

A "scribe" writing down the observations during the assessment can be a great help. Alternatively, a small tape-recorder could be of assistance and the actual writing be done afterwards. Perhaps one of the greatest aids to recording movement is the ciné or video film. A short film of a patient performing an activity will describe the action far more vividly than words, and can be used for comparison later. Even a photograph, as shown earlier, can be a clear record of some aspects of the patient's disability.

Compensatory or "trick" movements can allow a degree of independence, but once they become established they may inhibit the return of normal activity. Care should be taken to assess whether the trick movement is really necessary, or if it has become a habit which could possibly be changed and so allow a more normal and economic movement sequence.

A detailed neurological assessment separate from a functional assessment is recommended because it is the only way in which the therapist can treat the condition itself, rather than merely pushing for rapid independence, possibly at the expense of the patient's chances of regaining more normal function and complete recovery of the affected parts.

When the results of the assessment show a marked discrepancy from the patient's ability to perform independently the activities of daily life, the problem could be a perceptual one (see Chap. 1). For example, where the therapist has recorded that the patient can move his arms and legs and balance in a sitting position, he may be unjustly labelled "unmotivated" when he fails to put on his shoes and socks unaided. It is important to understand the complex requirements for carrying out such tasks and understand why the patient is unable to manage them alone. For the patient there is a huge step between the recognition level, for example putting on the shoe handed to him by the therapist, and producing the whole sequence on his own when he dresses in the morning. The same applies when any person is learning something new. He recognises what is required or is correct long before he can reproduce what has been taught without any cues being provided.

5 The Acute Phase – Positioning and Moving in Bed and in the Chair

Successful rehabilitation depends not only on the various therapy sessions but also very much on what happens to the patient during the remaining hours of the day and night. Even the position in which he sleeps can make a remarkable difference to the end result. No matter how good the therapy, if during the rest of the time the patient moves with effort in abnormal patterns of movement, spasticity will increase and most of what he achieves during therapy will be lost and not carried over into his daily life. Rehabilitation should therefore be regarded as a 24-hour management or way of life.

It is more satisfactory and easier for all concerned if such a concept is adopted from the very beginning, immediately following the stroke. However, even if a patient comes for treatment at a later stage, some months after the stroke, the same principles apply, and he too must be helped to achieve what he has missed. It will merely require more time because he will have established other habits, some of which may be difficult for him to change. The following positions and ways of moving him, or helping him to move, are recommended whether the patient is being nursed in an intensive care unit, in a general ward, in a rehabilitation centre or at home.

5.1 The Arrangement of the Patient's Room

How the patient's bed and chair are placed in relation to his surroundings can play an important role, particularly in the early stages of the illness when his ability to move about on his own is restricted. It is well worth going to considerable trouble to change the arrangement of the room if it is not ideal. Because of the lesion, the hemiplegic patient's head turns away from the affected side and he tends to neglect not only that half of his body but also the space on that side. Often the sensory modalities of feeling, hearing and seeing are reduced on the hemiplegic side. Intensive stimulation is necessary to counteract the resultant sensory deprivation. The room must be so arranged that the hemiplegic side automatically receives as much stimulation as possible during the day.

If the bed is so placed that the patient's affected side is against a wall or where little activity will take place, the sensory deprivation will be reinforced. All nursing duties will be carried out from the unaffected side, and doctors and visitors will approach from that side too. When he starts sitting out of bed, he will transfer towards the sound side, look to that side and neglect the hemiplegic side still further. Merely by altering the position of the bed so that all activity and interesting events take place on the patient's hemiplegic side, the situation can be changed remarkably. The nurse will approach from his affected side, to wash him to help him with brushing his teeth, or when she brings him his food and assists him with eating, to mention but a few instances. The doctor, likewise, will sound his chest, take his blood pressure and carry out other regular examinations and observations from the hemiplegic side. If the patient has difficulty in turning his head at first, all who work with him can assist him to do so by placing a hand flat on the side of his face, and then holding the head in the corrected position until they feel the resistance subside.

Because the room is arranged in this way the patient is constantly encouraged to turn his head toward his hemiplegic side to look at the people attending to him. The hemiplegic side will be required to react and will have input throughout the day. The bed-side table should be placed on his affected side so that he will need to turn his head to look at objects on the table and must move his arm across the mid-line to reach for anything he requires. Transferring to the chair next to his bed will also be a movement towards the affected side.

Many patients enjoy watching television, as they may be unable to read at first. The television set should also be placed so that the patient turns his head to the affected side when watching it. Relatives and friends can be of great assistance if carefully instructed. They should sit next to the patient on his hemiplegic side, or in front of him but more to that side. The patient will then turn his head in their direction when they are talking to him and the visitors can encourage him to move his eyes and look directly at them during the conversation. Normal eye contact with other people and fixation of objects may otherwise remain difficult, as the eyes are pulled towards the sound side. Close relatives or friends can also hold his hemiplegic hand while talking with him, providing further stimulation (Fig. 5.1).

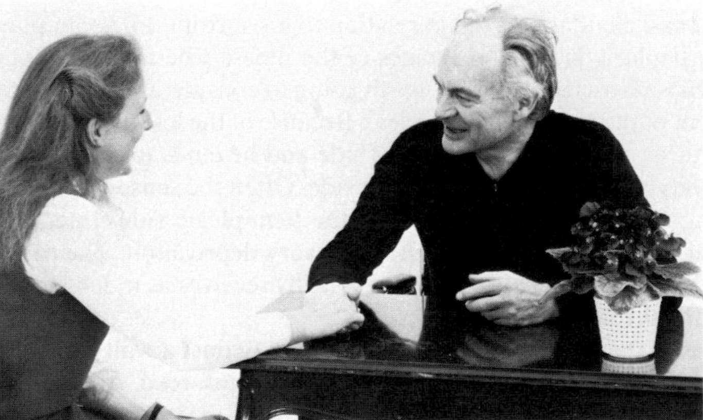

Fig. 5.1. A friendly visitor encourages the patient to turn his head toward the hemiplegic side (right hemiplegia)

5.2 Positioning the Patient in Bed

In the early stages, the patient will spend most of his time in bed, and how he lies will therefore be of great importance. As soon as possible, he should sit out of bed, and in fact there are very few circumstances which would necessitate his staying in bed for more than a few days. Many serious complications can arise as a result of prolonged immobilisation in bed, particularly for older patients: thrombosis, pressure sores and hypostatic pneumonia, to name but a few. Even patients who are out of bed during the day will still be spending 8 hours or more in bed at night.

If an infusion is necessary, it is not a contra-indication to turning the patient regularly and positioning him correctly in bed or in a chair.

5.2.1 Lying on the Hemiplegic Side (Fig. 5.2)

Lying on the affected side is the most important position of all and should be introduced right from the beginning. In fact, most patients seem to prefer it in the end. Spasticity is reduced by the elongation of the whole side, and the awareness of the side is increased because the patient is lying on it. Another obvious advantage is that the more skilled hand is free to carry out tasks such as pulling up the bedcovers or arranging the pillow.

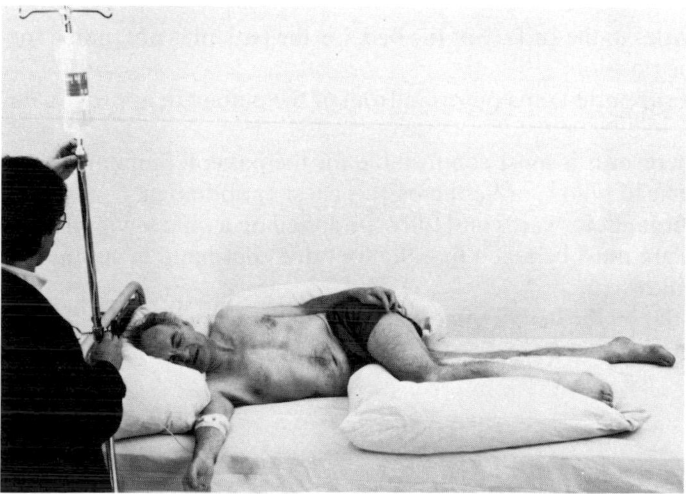

Fig. 5.2. Lying on the hemiplegic side in the correct position. The intravenous drip does not prevent the patient from lying on his side (right hemiplegia)

The head is well supported. If the head lies comfortably, the patient is far more likely to remain in the correct position and sleep. The head should be flexed in the upper cervical region and not pushed back into extension.
The trunk is rotated somewhat backwards and supported from behind by a firmly placed pillow.

The hemiplegic arm is drawn forwards until it lies at an angle of not less than 90° to the body. The forearm is supinated and the wrist lies in passive dorsiflexion. The assistant, working from the front, places one hand under the patient's shoulder and scapula and brings the latter forwards into protraction. The patient's body weight maintains the protraction, and when the shoulder-blade is protracted flexor spasticity in the entire arm and hand is reduced, enabling the correct position to be maintained. To check that the scapula is indeed protracted, the assistant should always feel across the back of the thorax. When the patient is correctly positioned the medial border of the scapula lies flat against the chest wall. Without sufficient protraction, the patient will often complain of shoulder pain or discomfort, as he is lying on the point of his shoulder.

The other arm rests on the patient's body or on the back pillow. If this arm lies in front of the patient, it brings the whole trunk forwards, which will cause retraction of the hemiplegic scapula.

The legs lie in a step position, the sound leg flexed at the hip and knee and supported on a pillow. The pillow also maintains the position of the hemiplegic leg, which is extended at the hip and lightly flexed at the knee.

5.2.2 Lying on the Unaffected Side (Fig. 5.3)

The head is again well supported on a pillow, to ensure that the patient is comfortable.

The trunk is at right angles to the surface of the bed, i.e. the patient is not pulled forward into a semi-prone position.

The hemiplegic arm is supported on a pillow in front of the patient in approximately 100° elevation.

The other arm lies wherever it is most comfortable for the patient. Sometimes it is flexed underneath the head pillow, or lies across his chest or abdomen.

The hemiplegic leg is brought forwards and fully supported on a pillow with flexion at the hip and knee. Care must be taken that the foot does not hang in supination over the edge of the pillow.

The other leg remains flat on the bed in some extension of the hip with slight flexion of the knee.

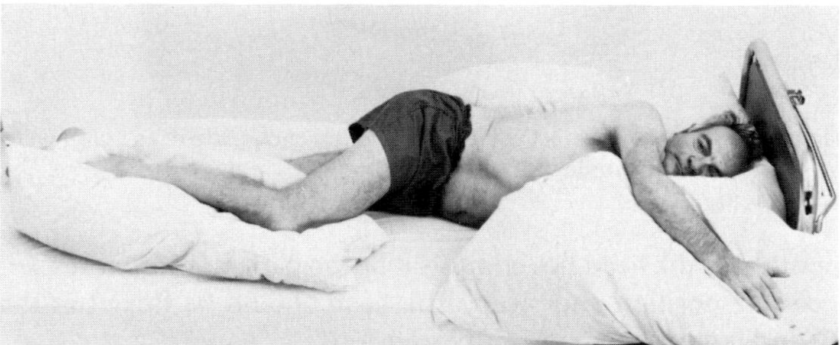

Fig. 5.3. Lying on the unaffected side. The hemiplegic arm is well supported by the pillow (right hemiplegia)

5.2.3 Lying Supine (Fig. 5.4)

The supine position should be used as little as possible, because in this position abnormal reflex activity is at its highest due to the influence of the tonic neck and labyrinthine reflexes. For hemiplegic patients it also involves the highest risk of pressure sores developing on the sacrum and, even more commonly, on the outside of the heel and on the lateral malleolus. The pelvis is rotated backwards on the hemiplegic side and pulls the hemiplegic leg with it into outward rotation, causing pressure on the two sites mentioned.

However, it may be necessary to use the position as an alternative, particularly

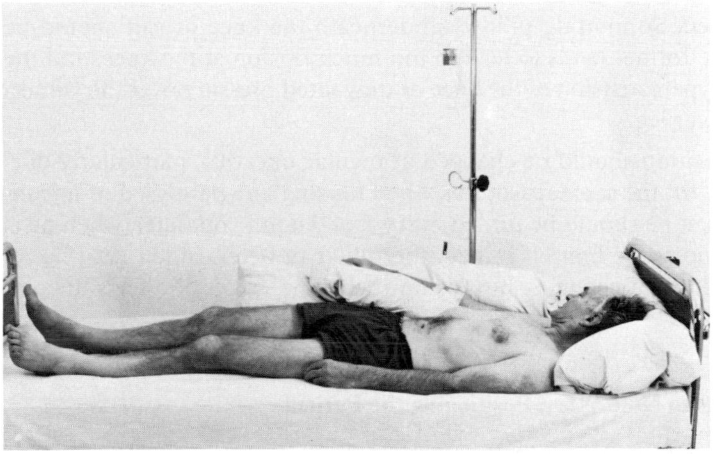

Fig. 5.4. Lying in a supine position. The pillows beneath the hemiplegic buttock and scapula keep the whole side forwards and correct the position of the limbs. The head is turned to the affected side (right hemiplegia)

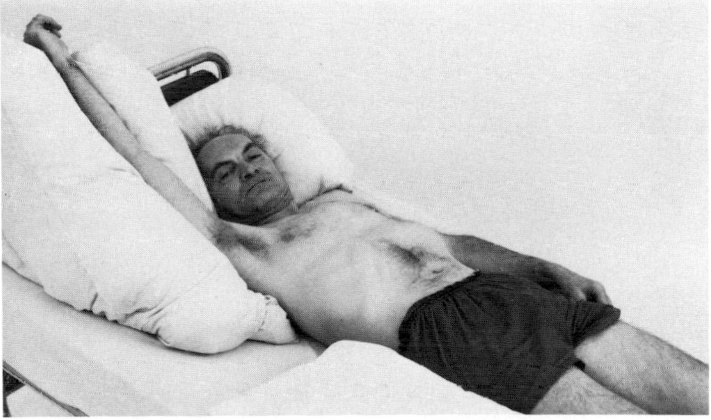

Fig. 5.5. An alternative position for the arm when the patient is lying supine. The position is used for short periods during the day (right hemiplegia)

for those patients who have been nursed for a long time only on their backs, and find it difficult to tolerate side-lying at first.

The head is well supported on pillows, care being taken that these do not flex the thoracic spine.
A pillow is placed beneath the hemiplegic buttock and thigh to bring the side of the pelvis forward and thus prevent the leg from pulling into outward rotation.
A pillow placed beneath the hemiplegic scapula maintains protraction and allows the arm to lie in a corrected, raised position, i.e. extended at the elbow and with the wrist in dorsiflexion and the fingers extended.
A useful alternative is to place the extended arm above the patient's head for certain periods during the day. Some patients use this position later when reading in bed (Fig. 5.5).
The legs lie extended. Supporting pillows underneath the knee or calf should be avoided because the former tends to lead to too much flexion at the knee, and the latter could cause hyperextension of the knee or unwanted pressure over the vulnerable veins of the lower leg.

The patient's position should be changed at regular intervals, particularly during the acute phase, for the same reasons as when nursing any paralysed or unconscious patient. At first he should be turned every 2 or 3 hours, but later, when he is able to turn over and move himself in bed, the time can be extended until he resumes a normal routine of changing his position when he wakes and feels uncomfortable.

5.2.4 General Points to Note When Positioning the Patient

1. The bed should be kept flat and the head-end should not be raised at all. The half-lying position should be avoided at all times as it reinforces unwanted flexion of the trunk with extension of the legs (Fig. 5.6). In the preferable side-lying positions the patient tends to slide down the bed if the head of the bed is raised.

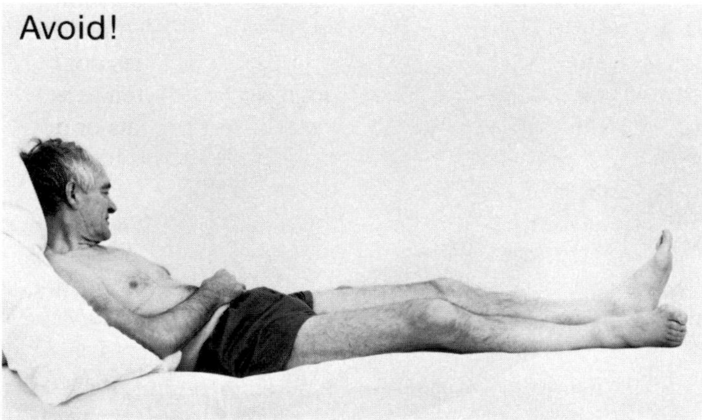

Fig. 5.6. The half-lying position should be avoided, at all times. It reinforces the patterns of spasticity (right hemiplegia)

2. Nothing should be placed in the hand in an attempt to counteract flexor spasticity. The effect will be just the opposite, as the influence of the grasp reflex causes the hand to close on an object placed in the palm. In a study comparing electromyographic (EMG) activity in the finger flexors of the hemiplegic hand when using a volar splint, a foam rubber finger-spreader and no device at all, Mathiowetz et al. (1983) write that "..." the effects of positioning devices over time generally show that no device evokes the least amount of EMG activity." The volar splint appeared in fact to increase EMG activity while it was being put on and during the period when the patients were grasping something with their sound hand. The correct positioning proximally will allow the hand to remain open, particularly as the patient is at rest, and not exerting himself against gravity.
3. Many patients have difficulty in aligning their body in relation to other objects. It is helpful to position the patient in bed so that he lies parallel to the sides of the bed, and not diagonally across it, as so often happens when he is left to his own devices.
4. Pillows vary considerably in size and consistency in different countries. Ideally, they should be large and well-filled with a soft material, e.g. down, which will mould to support and maintain the part of the body in the desired position. Most positions require about three to four continental pillows or five to six English/American pillows. It is confusing for staff and for patients and their relatives to have pillows of various sizes and shapes to support different parts of the body.
5. Nothing should be placed against the balls of the feet in an attempt to avoid a plantar flexion deformity. Firm pressure against the ball of the foot increases unwanted reflex activity in the extension pattern. The hemiplegic patient will shift himself away from the uncomfortable fixation, in any case. Heavy or tightly tucked-in bedclothes should be avoided, and a bed-cradle used to support their weight, if necessary.

5.2.5 Sitting in Bed

It is difficult to sit in bed with a good upright posture, and so the position should be avoided whenever possible. Flexion of the trunk is encouraged and the hips remain in some degree of extension. However, in the acute phase it is sometimes not feasible for the nursing staff to transfer the patient to an upright chair as often as would be necessary during the day. The patient needs to sit up every time he eats or drinks (Chap. 13), a minimum of five times a day. He has to sit when he brushes his teeth or needs to empty his bladder or bowels.

When sitting in bed is not avoidable, it should be made as optimal as possible. The hips should be flexed as near to a right angle as is feasible and the spine extended. Sufficient pillows, firmly stacked, help to achieve the erect position, and the head should be left unsupported so that the patient learns to hold it actively. An adjustable table placed across the bed, beneath the patient's arms, will help to counteract the pull into trunk flexion. If the pull is strong, a pillow should be placed beneath his elbows to avoid pressure.

Some modern hospital beds have an adjustable back-rest that can be brought almost to a vertical position. A pillow behind the patient's back will provide trunk ex-

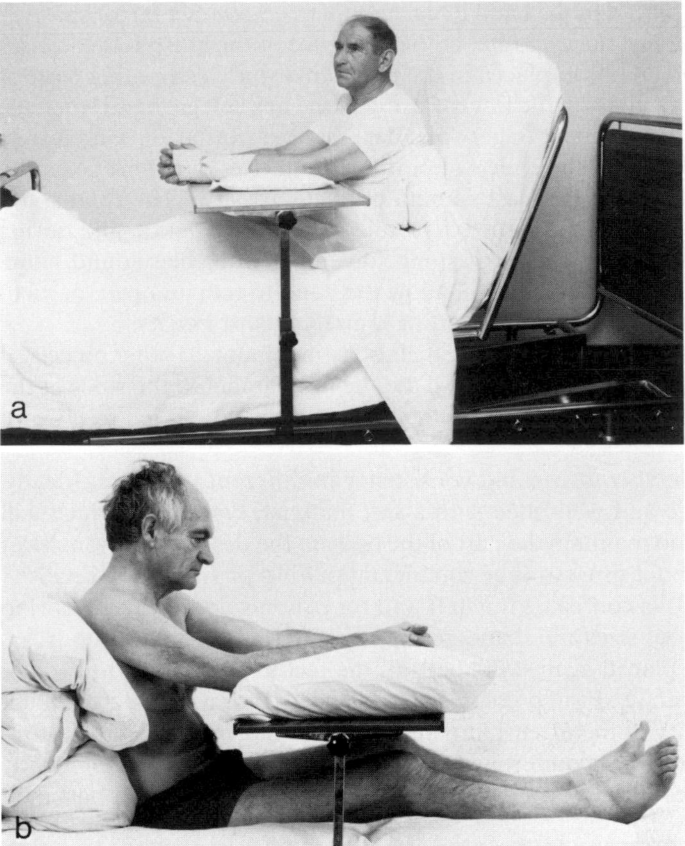

Fig. 5.7 a, b. Sitting upright in bed (right hemiplegia). **a** Easily achieved in a modern hospital bed with a fully adjustable back-rest. **b** If the head-end is not sufficiently adjustable the bed is left flat and the patient is moved up the bed and supported by pillows

tension and the recommended upright sitting posture is achieved (Fig. 5.7 a). If, however, the back-rest can only be adjusted to slope upwards, it should be left flat and the patient moved so that he is supported against the head of the bed and sufficient pillows (Fig. 5.7 b). In this way the detrimental half-reclining position is avoided. The patient should not be left for long in the sitting position because he will slide down the bed and assume very undesirable postures over prolonged periods.

5.3 Sitting in a Chair

In a suitable chair a far more upright posture can be achieved and maintained, and it is therefore advisable to transfer the patient from bed as soon as his general condition allows. If the patient is unable to stand and walk at all even with assistance, a

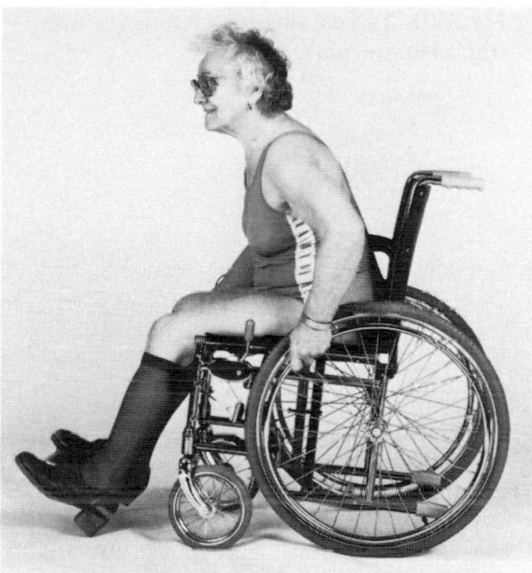

Fig. 5.8. Pushing the wheelchair with the sound hand and foot (right hemiplegia)

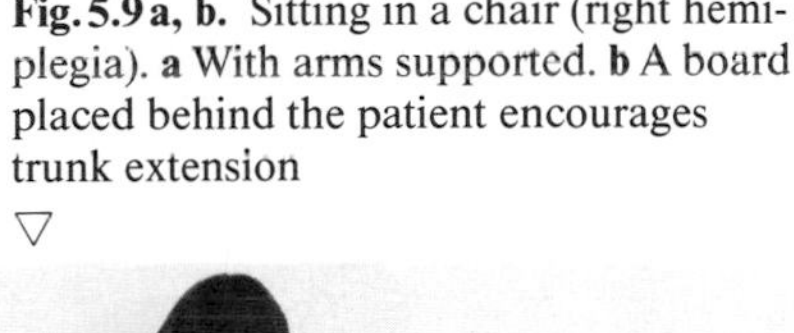

Fig. 5.9 a, b. Sitting in a chair (right hemiplegia). **a** With arms supported. **b** A board placed behind the patient encourages trunk extension

▽

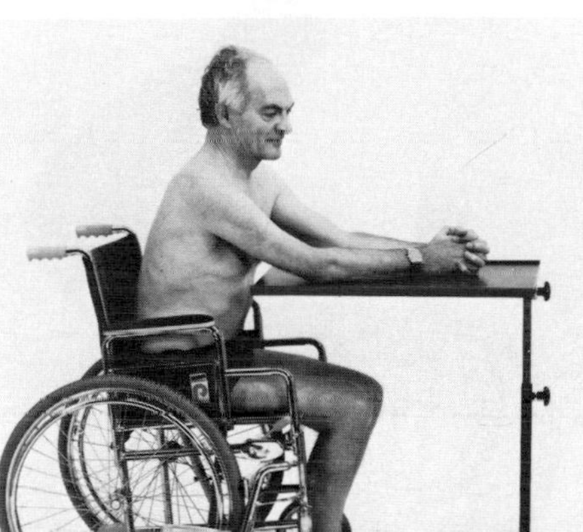

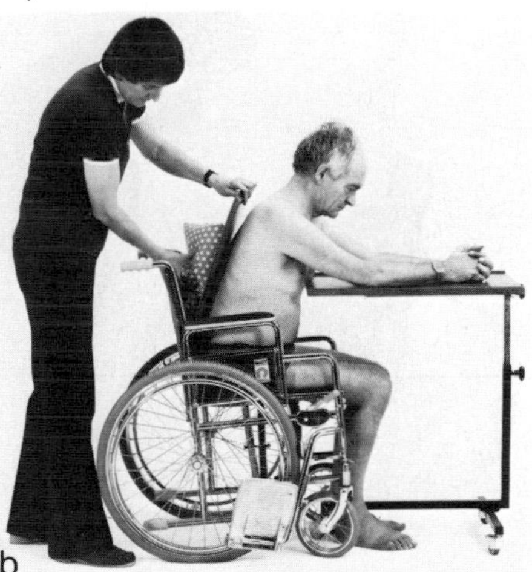

wheelchair is the best answer. He can then be easily transported to therapy sessions or to X-ray or other investigations, and can also enjoy the change of scene. He can learn to move about on his own, pushing the wheelchair with his sound leg and helping with his hand, if necessary (Fig. 5.8). Because the back-rest of the wheelchair encourages too much flexion of the trunk, a board should be placed in the chair to help the patient to maintain an upright position. The board should be adjustable so that it can be tilted forwards when the patient is sitting at a table. Whenever he is not moving from place to place he is positioned with his arms on a table in front of him, spine extended and hips flexed (Fig. 5.9). When positioned in this way, there is far less tendency for him to slide his seat forwards and half lie in his chair (Fig. 5.10). In the corrected position he can stay erect far longer, watching television, talking to visitors or other patients, or even reading and writing. However, it must be realised that in the early days following a stroke the patient will tire quickly, particu-

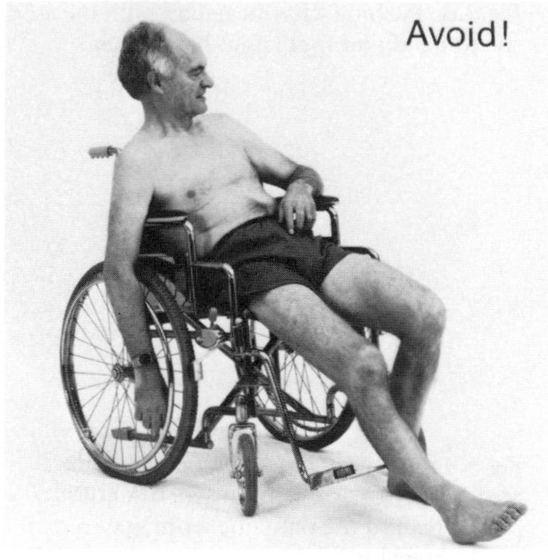

Fig. 5.10. Typical incorrect sitting posture (right hemiplegia)

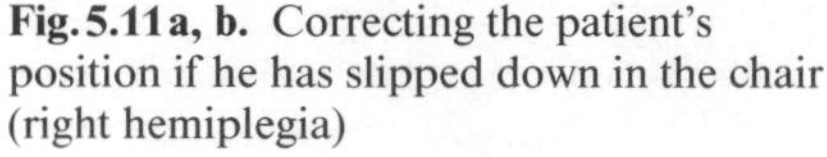

Fig. 5.11 a, b. Correcting the patient's position if he has slipped down in the chair (right hemiplegia)

▽

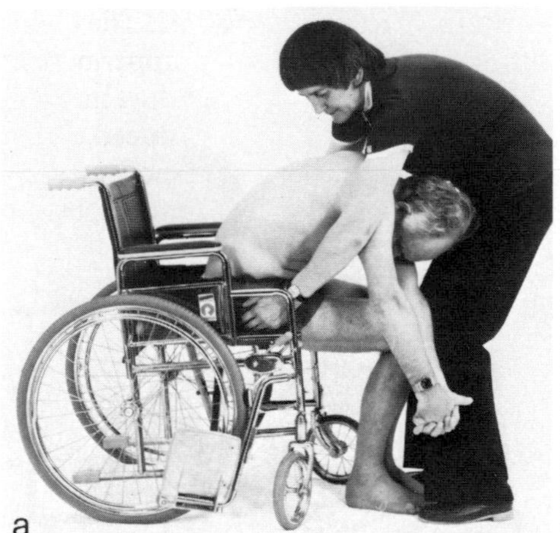

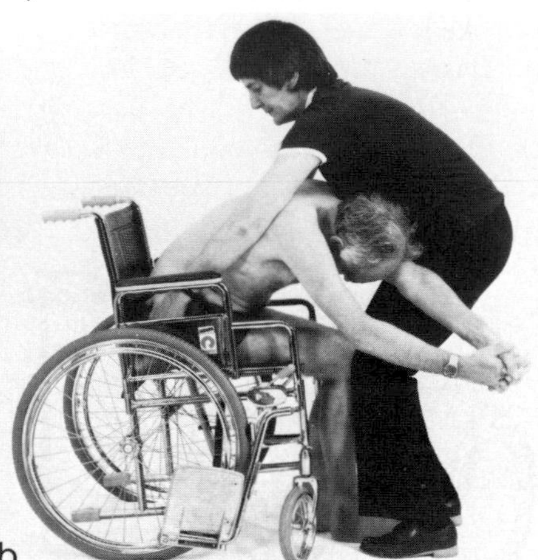

larly if left on his own, and it will be necessary to let him rest in bed frequently. It is better to sit him up again for short periods than to let him sleep uncomfortably in the chair in a position which emphasises abnormal tone and posture.

Gradually, the time which the patient spends out of bed can be increased, and the more stimulation he receives the longer he will be able to tolerate sitting up. He should not be left to his own devices but be kept occupied with appropriate activity in the company of others. Should he slip down in his chair he is helped to correct his posture again.

To correct the patient's position in the chair the therapist or nurse places both his feet flat on the floor with his knees flexed. She stands in front of him with her knees against his knees to prevent him from sliding still further forwards in the chair as she helps him to lean forwards with his hands clasped together. The patient is asked to lean forwards as far as he can and the therapist guides his hands to one side so that she can lean over far enough to grasp his hips on either side at about trochanter level (Fig. 5.11 a). She then leans back to lift his weight from the seat of the chair, and pushing her knees against his knees places his buttocks right back in the chair (Fig. 5.11 b). Because the therapist is using her body weight to lift the patient, her own back is protected. The patient can help more actively until he is able to adjust his own sitting position in the same way. The method is also a preparation for standing up from sitting, as it teaches him to lean well forwards and take weight over his feet while lifting his buttocks.

5.4 Self-Assisted Arm Activity with Clasped Hands

From a very early stage the patient is taught how to release the spasticity in his arm and around the scapula, and how to maintain full passive elevation of his shoulder (Fig. 5.12 a). Due to its special construction, allowing for functional mobility in daily life, the shoulder is a vulnerable joint and reacts badly to immobilisation. Following a stroke it is therefore necessary to keep it moving, passively if need be. The hands are clasped together, fingers interlaced with the hemiplegic thumb uppermost in some abduction (Fig. 5.12 b). Because the fingers of the sound hand abduct the fingers of the hemiplegic hand, the flexor spasticity in the whole arm is reduced.

Whether lying, sitting or standing, the patient is taught to start the movement by pushing his clasped hands well forward, assuring protraction of his scapula, before

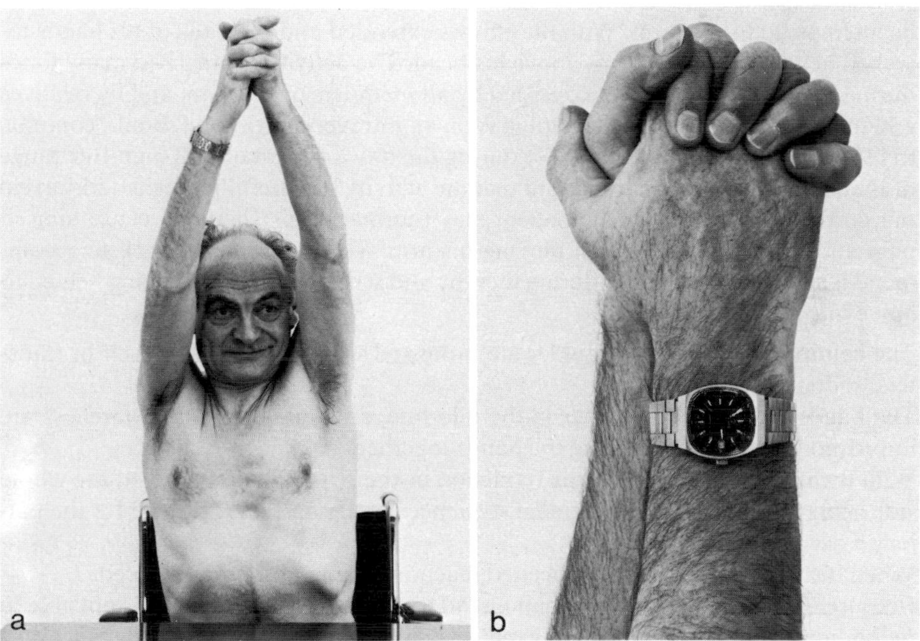

Fig. 5.12 a, b. Self-assisted arm activity with the hands clasped together maintains full pain-free range of shoulder movement and inhibits spasticity (right hemiplegia)

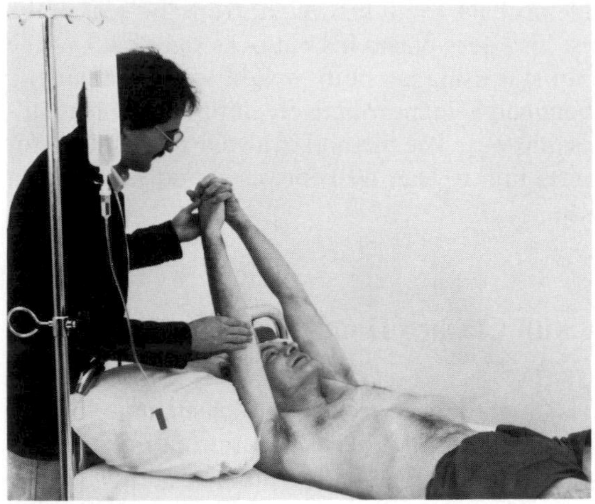

Fig. 5.13. Even the doctor can encourage the patient to move his arm after adjusting the infusion (right hemiplegia)

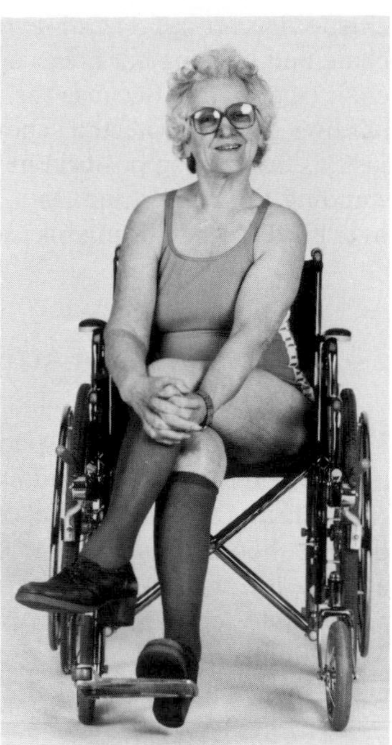

Fig. 5.14. Patient sitting with her clasped hands over one knee. The hemiplegic arm is prevented from pulling into flexion and the weight is over the affected side (right hemiplegia)

he attempts to lift the arm. With the elbows extended and the balls of his hands together, he then raises his arms above his head. The activity is practised many times during the day, and can be encouraged by all members of the team and by relatives and other patients. Even if the patient is on an intravenous drip he should continue to lift his hemiplegic hand carefully during the day to maintain full pain-free range of motion (Fig. 5.13). It is important that the activity be carefully taught and carried out correctly, as otherwise the patient may traumatise his shoulder, cause himself pain and be discouraged from moving his arm. The activity has much to recommend it and can also be used during therapy and when the patient is being helped to move into different positions.

The hemiplegic hand and shoulder are protected while he moves himself or transfers.

The hands are brought together in the mid-line, and sensation and awareness are improved by the act of clasping the hands together.

With the hands held forward, the retraction of the scapula and in fact of the whole side is prevented, making movement sequences easier and less effortful for the patient.

When the patient is moving, associated reactions in the arm are prevented.

Because the patient is using his sound hand to hold the other hand, he is not able to pull or push with it as he moves. He therefore uses other parts of the body more normally, and trunk activity is stimulated and symmetrical movement and weight-bearing are improved.

The stiff contracted hand is avoided by the simple manoeuvre, as it enables the patient to perform several exercises to inhibit and elongate the spastic muscles himself. The patient can sit with his legs crossed and his clasped hands over his knee to help him to maintain a correct posture during the day (Fig. 5.14).

5.5 Moving in Bed

If the patient is unconscious or still unable to help actively, he must be turned into the side position by an assistant. The turn is easier if both legs are flexed with the feet remaining on the bed, and the knees then turned to one side. The shoulders and trunk follow. He can also be moved passively into the upright sitting position by two people, using the Australian lift:

The assistants stand on either side of the patient, facing in the opposite direction to him.
The hands nearest to the patient are placed beneath his thighs and the assistants grasp each other's wrist.
Placing their shoulders under his shoulders and leaning towards each other the assistants straighten their knees to lift the patient off the bed (Fig. 5.15 a).
With their free hands the assistants can support themselves on the bed to avoid straining their backs, or can adjust the bedclothes or pillows (Fig. 5.15 b).

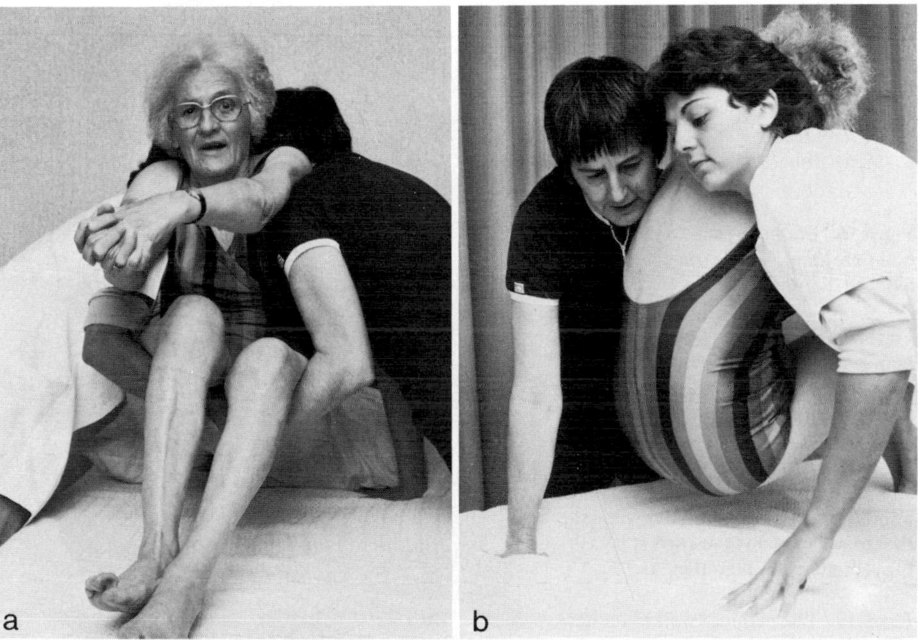

Fig. 5.15 a, b. Moving the patient passively in bed using the Australian lift (left hemiplegia)

This method of passive lifting is recommended because it is comfortable and safe for the patient and will not traumatise his shoulder. It can also be used to lift the patient back into bed if the height of the bed is not adjustable. Very soon, however, the patient is able to assist, and activity should be encouraged, but with sufficient facilitation to allow the movement to take place in a normal pattern, without his having to struggle. Because the aim is to re-establish normal movement patterns, a monkey-chain should never be used. If it is there the patient will naturally reach for it and try to pull himself into position with his sound hand. Immediately, an abnormal one-sided response follows, leading to increased tone on the hemiplegic side.

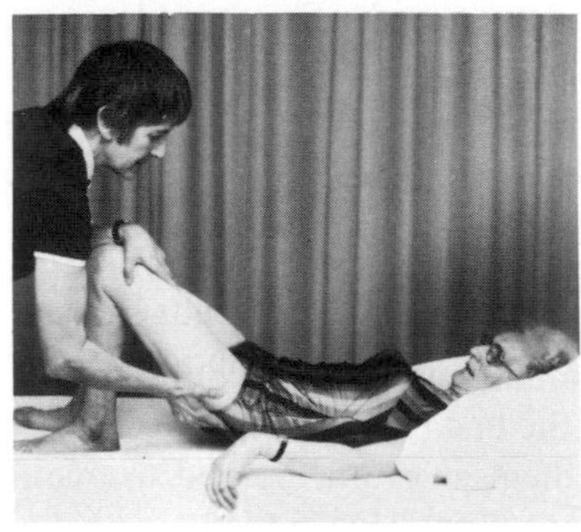

5.16

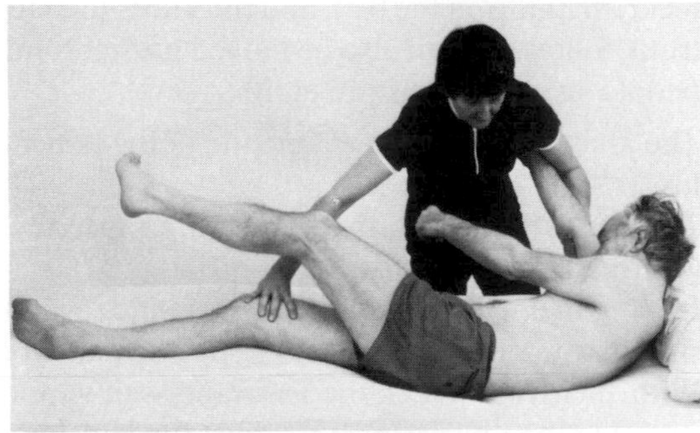

5.17

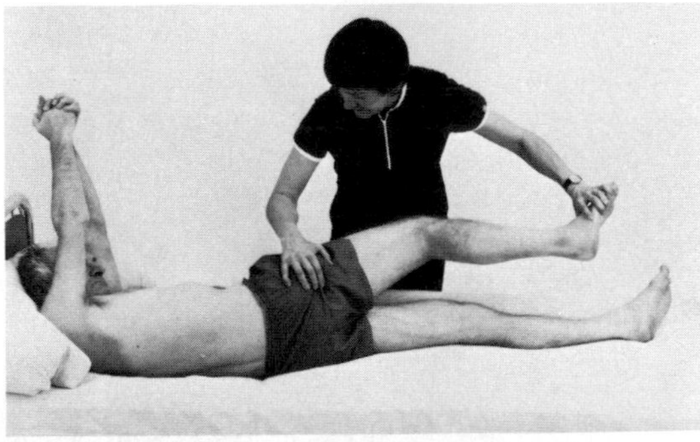

5.18

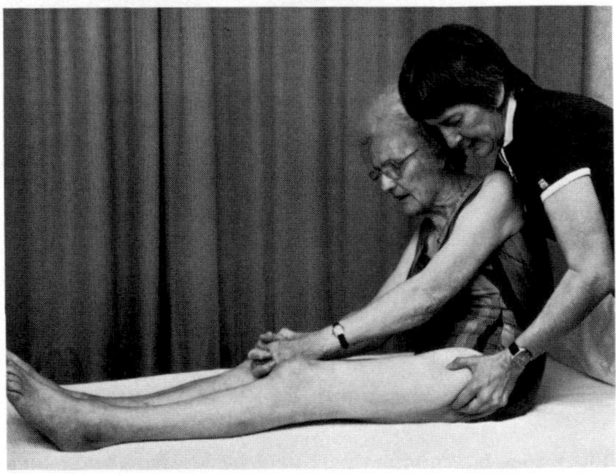

5.19

Fig. 5.16. Bridging used to move in bed (left hemiplegia); see also Fig. 6.5, 6.6

Fig. 5.17. Turning over on to the hemiplegic side. The therapist protects the hemiplegic shoulder from injury (right hemiplegia)

Fig. 5.18. Turning over on to the sound side. The patient clasps his hands to protect his shoulder while the therapist facilitates the correct leg movement (right hemiplegia)

Fig. 5.19. The patient "walks" on her buttocks to move up and down the bed (left hemiplegia)

5.5.1 Moving Sideways

With his legs flexed and his feet on the bed, the patient raises his buttocks off the bed and moves them to the side. The assistant facilitates the movement by pressing down on his hemiplegic knee, drawing the knee forwards over his foot as she does so (Fig. 5.16). The patient then moves his shoulders into line, help being given to prevent the scapula from retracting. The same assistance can be given when the patient needs to move up or down the bed.

5.5.2 Rolling over on to the Hemiplegic Side (Fig. 5.17)

Rolling is most therapeutic, as it stimulates reactions and activity throughout the body. How it can be used during therapy will be described in Chap. 11. When the patient is turning towards the affected side, it is important that the assistant support the hemiplegic shoulder while the patient rolls over. He lifts his sound leg off the bed and swings it forward, without pushing off from behind. His sound arm must also swing forward and he should be discouraged from grasping the edge of the mattress to pull himself over. The assistant facilitates the lateral rotation of the hemiplegic leg with her hand placed over his knee.

5.5.3 Rolling over on to the Unaffected Side (Fig. 5.18)

The patient clasps his hands together, so that the hemiplegic arm is supported. The assistant facilitates the correct movement of the hemiplegic leg, helping him to bring it forward over the sound leg, which plays no active part in the movement.

5.5.4 Moving Forwards and Backwards While Sitting in Bed

With help, the patient moves up the bed by transferring his weight first over one buttock and then the other. The opposite side, when relieved of weight, is moved backwards, as if the patient were walking on his buttocks. The assistant stands on his hemiplegic side, holds his trochanters, and using her body to help him to transfer his weight facilitates the walking action (Fig. 5.19).

The patient should use the same movement pattern when moving himself to the edge of the bed before transferring into a chair, or later, before standing up from the bed. In this case, help is given from the front. The assistant places one hand over the trochanter and the other over the opposite shoulder, to prevent him leaning backward. She helps him to transfer his weight and then brings the hip on the freed side forward, or backward when he is returning to his bed (Fig. 5.20 a). She then changes hands, to facilitate the step with the buttock on the other side.

The patient soon learns to move himself in this way unaided, and by so doing avoids the extensor spasticity in his hemiplegic leg which is strongly increased in an associated reaction if he pulls himself with his sound hand to move to the edge of the bed. The same sequence is used later when he moves to sit further back on the

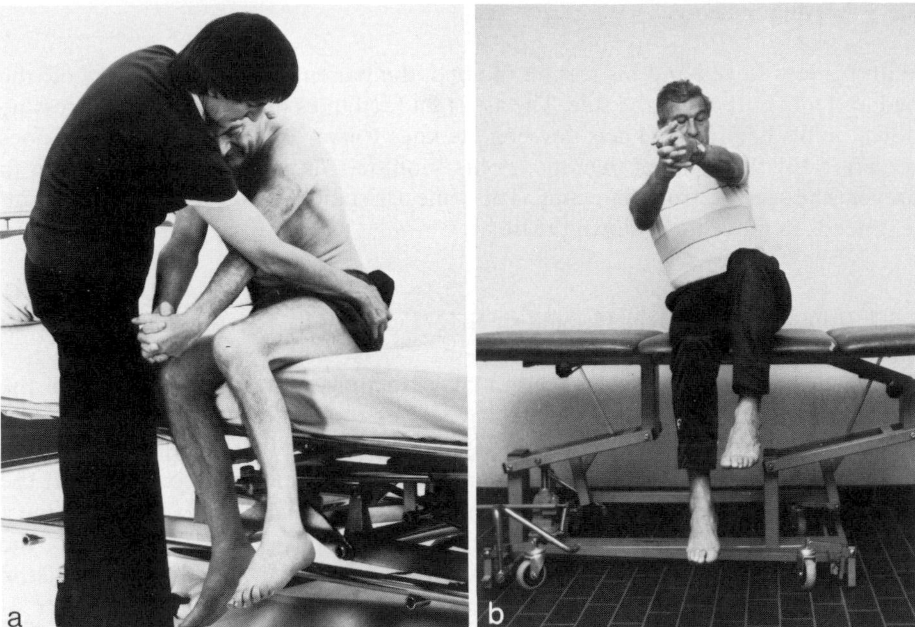

Fig. 5.20 a, b. Moving to the edge of the bed or back again (right hemiplegia). **a** The therapist facilitates "walking" on the buttocks. **b** Patient moving back on a plinth unaided

plinth in the physiotherapy department (Fig. 5.20b). The activity is not only functional but can also be used therapeutically, as it stimulates automatic weight transference and active trunk movement with rotation and balance reactions.

5.5.5 Sitting up over the Side of the Bed

Sitting up over the hemiplegic side is stressed because of the therapeutic effect. When we sit up over one side normally, that side is forward when we reach the upright position. For the patient this will mean that his hemiplegic side is forward instead of in its usual retracted position. The sequence starts with the patient lying on his back. He brings his hemiplegic leg over the side of the bed keeping the knee flexed, with the assistant facilitating the movement at first. He then brings the sound hand forward across his body to push on the bed on the hemiplegic side, rotating the trunk in order to do so. He pushes himself up to the sitting position, swinging his sound leg out simultaneously to aid the movement by its counterweight (Fig. 5.21). The head rights to the vertical and the hemiplegic side elongates during the movement, and the weight-bearing through the side is beneficial.

The assistant facilitates the movement by placing one hand on the sound shoulder, which she presses down, and the other hand on the iliac crest, doing the same. Should the patient require more help, she can encircle his head and hemiplegic shoulder with one arm, and lean her body weight sideways to bring him to the up-

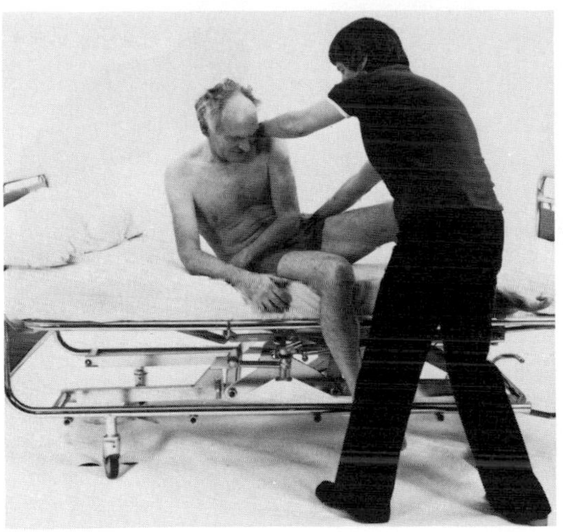

Fig. 5.21. Sitting up over the side of the bed. The same pattern is used when the patient lies down (right hemiplegia)

right position. To lie down in bed the patient uses the same movement sequence in reverse. The assistant facilitates the movement by drawing his hemiplegic shoulder forward as he lies down.

5.6 Transferring from Bed to Chair and Back Again

Transferring correctly and without undue effort will later enable the patient to stand up easily, and will assist in achieving weight-bearing through the hemiplegic leg without using the total pattern of extension. If transferring is easy for the patient and nursing staff alike, the problem of incontinence will be far easier to overcome.

Transferring is greatly assisted when the patient is nursed in a bed of adjustable height which can be lowered until it is approximately the same height as the chair. When at home, the bed is usually low enough, but in a hospital where the beds cannot be lowered both patient and staff are at risk of being injured. The therapist will need all her ingenuity to find a safe and easy method of transfer if the bed is too high.

5.6.1 The Passive Transfer

When the patient is unable to help actively, the following method can be used to transfer him into his chair. The assistant moves him to the edge of the bed until both his feet are flat on the floor. With her feet beside his feet, she supports his knees with her knees, from the front, and at the same time prevents his knees from falling into abduction. She rests his forearms on her shoulders and places her hands over his scapulae, gripping their medial borders to keep them forward. She splints the patient's arms with her extended arms. She then brings his weight forwards over his

5.22 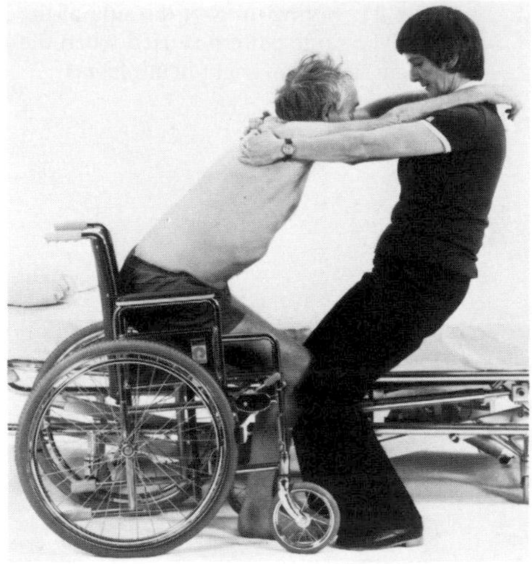

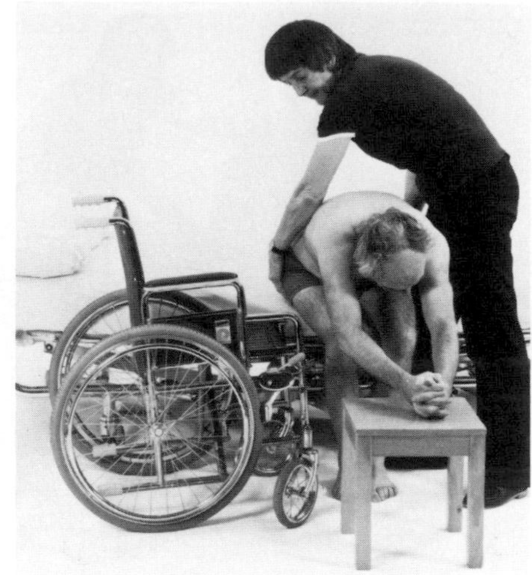 5.23

5.24 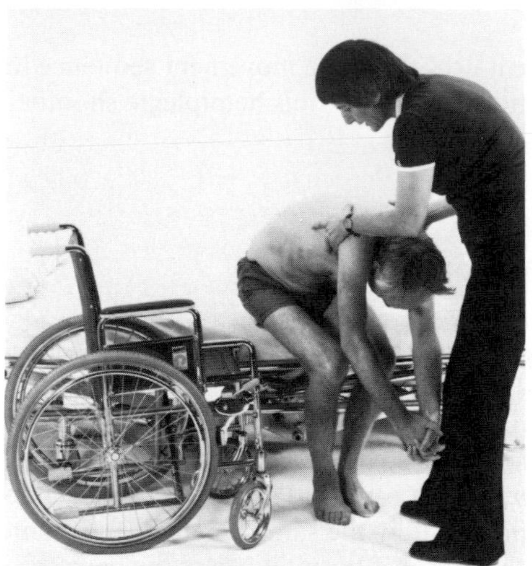

Fig. 5.22. The passive transfer (right hemiplegia)

Fig. 5.23. Transferring more actively with the patient's clasped hands supported on a stool in front of him (right hemiplegia)

Fig. 5.24. The active transfer (right hemiplegia)

feet and presses downward on his scapulae until his seat lifts off the bed. Weight-bearing through his legs is assisted if he lifts his head. The assistant pivots the patient round and lowers his seat far back into the chair (Fig. 5.22). The patient should not clasp his hands round the helper's neck because he would pull too hard and come to the upright position with total extension of his leg. The chair should be so placed that the patient transfers towards his hemiplegic side. Moving back into bed, the same procedure is followed.

5.6.2 The More Active Transfer

As soon as the patient is able to help at all, the transfer becomes more active. A stool or chair is placed in front of him on which he supports his clasped hands. The stool should be sufficiently far away so that when his hands rest on it, his head is over his feet. The assistant grasps his trochanters and two separate movements follow to facilitate the transfer. The patient first lifts his seat from the bed, and then turns to sit in the chair (Fig. 5.23). The assistant gives only as much help as the patient requires to carry out the movement easily and smoothly.

5.6.3 The Active Transfer

When the patient can transfer with the help of a stool in front of him, he can learn to do the same movement, only now with his clasped hands held actively in the air. The assistant facilitates by placing her hands lightly on his scapulae, helping him to remain forwards and to turn his seat to the chair (Fig. 5.24). Some patients may require help to keep the hemiplegic foot flat on the floor. The assistant then places her hand on his knee, presses down on it and draws the knee forwards over the foot as he transfers.

5.7 Incontinence

In the acute phase of the disease some patients may have difficulty in controlling both urine and faeces. Once the patient is more mobile and able to help himself the difficulties usually disappear, so that they are seldom a problem after the first 3 months. Persisting difficulties are associated with perceptual problems or pre-existing urological conditions.

The patient with severe perceptual difficulties is unable to plan sufficiently to be continent. The incontinence is not an isolated problem but will appear in conjunction with failure to perform tasks of a similar complexity (see Chap. 1). The patient will also be unable to dress himself or carry out other activities of daily living independently. The uncontrolled bladder can be likened to that of an infant who has not yet learned to inhibit its emptying appropriately, rather than being regarded as pathologically neurogenic.

Because many patients who suffer a hemiplegia are in the older age group they may already have been experiencing difficulties with micturition, e.g. due to prostatic enlargement or sphincter weakness. Under normal circumstances careful planning and anticipation assured continence, as did the ability to move easily and independently within a known environment. With loss of mobility following stroke, and in the unfamiliar hospital routine, the patient becomes incontinent or may have retention. Once the patient is able to walk and arrange his own clothing once more, he usually regains continence by re-establishing his former routine.

Whichever of the problems is causing the patient to be incontinent before he is sufficiently able to manage on his own, those who are looking after him should assist him at regular, timed intervals so that the humiliation of incontinence is avoided. When an indwelling catheter has been used in the acute phase, it should be removed as soon as possible, i.e. when the patient has progressed in his ability to move and care for himself. If necessary, specific problems such as urinary tract infection or persisting prostatic difficulties will need to be treated accordingly.

5.8 Constipation

Constipation is almost always a problem in the early stages of hemiplegia. The patient is immobile in bed, his diet is restricted due to eating difficulties, his fluid intake is reduced as he has difficulty swallowing liquids and psychologically he is inhibited by the presence of the person who is required to assist him. His usual timing is altered by the hospital routine, and he misses the dietary or medicinal aids he used at home.

Constipation is distressing for the patient and may affect him in other ways:

He has difficulty in concentrating on his rehabilitation and may become depressed.
He may have apparent diarrhoea, as he is unable to empty his bowels completely.
The pressure from the loaded bowel may interfere with urination or catheter drainage.
If severe, the constipation may lead to obstruction or to difficulties with breathing.

Continence of faeces is easily re-established if constipation is avoided right from the beginning by using appropriate doses of a laxative. The patient should be transferred on to the toilet or a commode next to his bed, as it is extremely difficult to "perform" in bed.

5.9 Considerations

If the patient is taught to move in normal movement patterns right from the beginning his whole rehabilitation will be easier and quicker. It is always difficult for adults to change an established habit. When assistance is given in the ways described in this chapter, the patient will not be afraid to move and his shoulder will have been protected from trauma. Each position and way of moving is a preparation for independent movement later. Although it is not possible to prevent spasticity altogether, the correct positioning and handling of the patient in the acute phase will reduce its development considerably.

The positions in which the patient lies in bed are those which he should use even when he is at home and independent. He will then no longer require all the supporting pillows, but the basic side-lying positions remain the same and serve to inhibit hypertonus. During his rehabilitation he is taught to turn himself in bed and achieve the correct position without the help of another person.

Time spent in the acute phase is time well spent because it will shorten the duration of the whole rehabilitation programme.

6 Normalising Postural Tone and Teaching the Patient to Move Selectively and Without Excessive Effort

Perhaps the most important and difficult task for the therapist is the normalisation of tone, which is necessary before the patient can be expected to move easily in a normal pattern. When the tone is too low, the patient will be unable to support himself or parts of his body against gravity. Where tone is too high and spasticity is a problem, the patient will only be able to move with great effort in stereotyped patterns against the resistance. One or other of these problems may be predominant, but very often there is a mixture of the two, or a state of muscle tone which fluctuates between the two. How the patient moves or is positioned throughout the day will influence the tone considerably (Chap. 5 and 10). From the beginning he should be assisted sufficiently so that spasticity is reduced to a minimum and abnormal patterns of movement do not become a habit. During treatment the principles of facilitation should be followed, after tone has been made as normal as possible. The treatment is not a series of isolated exercises but a sequence of activities to achieve a specific aim. When an activity has normalised tone, a selective movement is practised and then used in a functional way. Although one part of the body cannot be treated in isolation, as each part influences the others, this chapter deals more specifically with trunk and lower limb activity and Chap. 8 with the trunk and upper limbs.

The activities which follow are a preparation for walking and the selective movements are necessary for a correct stance phase and swing phase during walking. They will also help to improve an already established abnormal pattern of walking. While working for control of the leg it is important that the arm should not pull into flexion, and should remain instead at the patient's side (see Fig. 6.2). The therapist may have to inhibit the spasticity first, and then the patient is asked to leave the arm there consciously. He should perform the activities in such a way that associated reactions do not occur. In so doing he is learning to inhibit the associated reactions which can often be a problem during walking and other functional activities.

Such intrinsic inhibition of spasticity is preferable to having him clasp his hands together and maintain the arms in extension above his head or stretched out in front of him while practising lower limb activities. Using the sound hand to hold the hemiplegic arm in an extended position has several disadvantages:

Often considerable effort is required and the sound shoulder may suffer as a result of the prolonged holding. A supraspinatus tendinitis is not uncommon.

The effort increases the tone in the lower limb which the patient is concentrating on moving selectively and without over-exertion.

In standing, holding the hands clasped in front of him increases flexion of the trunk and hips while he is trying to extend them.
The position cannot be carried over into function, where he will need his sound hand for more skilled tasks.

6.1 Activities in Lying

6.1.1 Inhibiting Extensor Spasticity in the Leg

The patient lies with both legs flexed and encircles his knees with his clasped hands. Lifting his head from the pillow, he rocks gently into more flexion and then less (Fig. 6.1). The movement reduces the extensor spasticity in his leg and simultaneously brings the scapula into protraction and inhibits flexor spasticity in the arm. Lifting his clasped hands he tries to hold the legs in flexion, and then to flex them actively as he replaces his hands over his knees. The same activity can be performed holding the hemiplegic leg alone, while the other lies flat on the plinth.

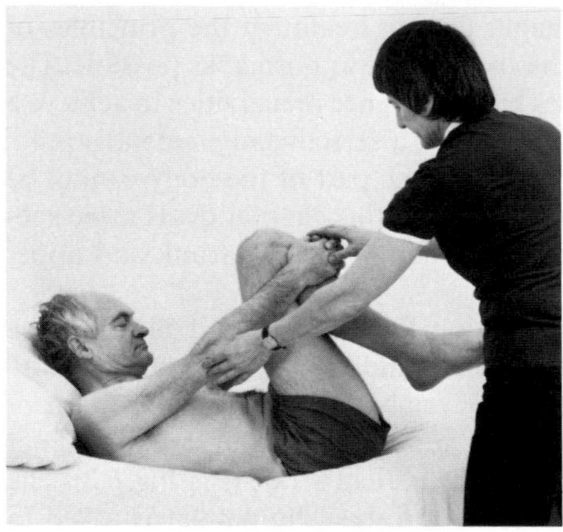

Fig. 6.1. Inhibiting extensor spasticity in the leg. The patient learns to carry out the activity on his own (right hemiplegia)

6.1.2 Control of the Leg Through Range

The therapist holds the patient's foot in dorsiflexion with pronation, with the leg flexed. She guides the leg toward extension, and the patient holds the weight of his leg actively, avoiding the influence of the mass movement synergies. He tries to maintain the position of the leg in flexion without abduction and external rotation at the hip, and as the leg is moved toward the plinth he tries to prevent it pushing into adduction with internal rotation as it extends (Fig. 6.2). If the therapist feels that the leg is pushing into extension she quickly asks him to lift it again a little before proceeding. The activity is practised until the patient can eventually control it all the way down to lie flat on the plinth.

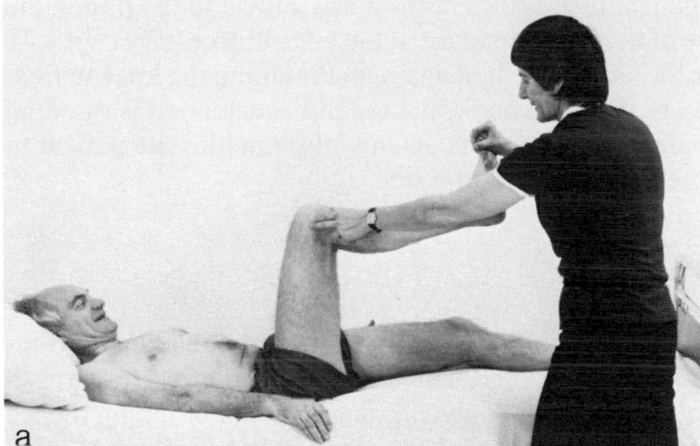

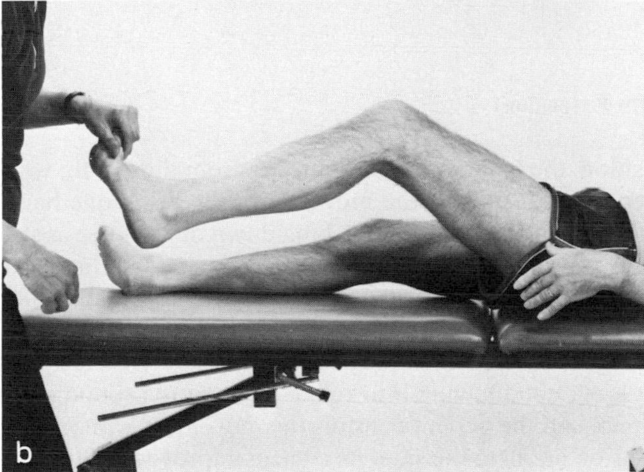

Fig. 6.2 a, b. Learning to control the leg actively. **a** At first it is easier for the patient to hold his leg in a flexed position (right hemiplegia). **b** Later he must learn to maintain control in increasing extension (left hemiplegia)

6.1.3 Placing the Leg in Different Positions

The therapist places the leg in various positions and the patient maintains the position. At first only full flexion of hip and knee may be possible, and positions where the foot is supported on the plinth. As control improves, the positions can be made more demanding. Flexion of the hip with internal rotation and adduction is important for function, and also hip flexion with various degrees of knee extension, i.e. selective knee extension.

6.1.4 Inhibition of Knee Extension with the Hip in Extension

The patient's hemiplegic leg is brought to lie over the side of the bed or plinth. The therapist inhibits plantar flexion fully by lifting the toes into full dorsiflexion with her fingers and giving counter-pressure with her thumbs over the tarsal area (Fig. 6.3). At the same time she eases the knee into flexion until all resistance to the movement disappears. The patient then brings his foot actively on to the plinth, the therapist having released one of her hands to assist at the knee if necessary (Fig. 6.4). He then lowers his foot over the side of the bed again, maintaining the knee in flexion as he does so. The ability to flex the knee while the hip is extended is essential for the start of the swing phase in walking. The activity also enables the patient to bring his leg out of bed before sitting up over the side.

6.1.5 Active Control at the Hip

Lying with his feet supported on the plinth and his knees flexed, the patient brings the hemiplegic knee away from the other knee, which is kept stationary. He learns to do so smoothly and to stop the movement at given points, instead of letting the leg fall into abduction. He can also practise keeping the affected knee still while moving the other knee.

6.1.6 Bridging (Selective Hip Extension)

From the same starting position, the patient lifts his buttocks from the plinth, with the pelvis held level. The therapist facilitates the movement by placing one hand over the patient's thigh on the hemiplegic side and pushing down on his knee as she draws the femoral condyles forwards towards his foot. With the extended fingers of her other hand she helps him to extend his affected hip by tapping to stimulate activity in the gluteal region (Fig. 6.5). The patient is then asked to lift his sound foot off the plinth, so that all weight is on the hemiplegic side (Fig. 6.6). He must still maintain the pelvis on one level, not allowing it to rotate back on the sound side. The therapist reduces her help, and the patient controls the movement without letting his knee push into extension or fall to the side. As control improves, the patient can raise and lower his buttocks with the weight only on the hemiplegic leg. When the patient can perform the activity easily, he will be able to prevent his knee locking when walking. During bridging activities, the further away the feet are placed the greater is the amount of selective activitiy required to maintain knee flexion as the patient extends his hips.

6.1.7 Isolated Knee Extension

Lying with his foot held in full dorsiflexion by the therapist's body, the patient extends his knee isometrically, with a static contraction of the extensor muscles. The therapist stimulates the activity and asks the patient not to push against her with his foot or toes as he tenses his thigh (Fig. 6.7). It usually helps the patient if he performs the activity first with his unaffected knee. It may also be helpful for the therapist to flex his knee slightly before the attempt at extension, but once he can do this the isometric contraction should be practised with no movement of the knee at all. Apart from enabling the patient to stand without the foot pushing into plantar flexion, the activity also inhibits spasticity in the calf muscles, and can be used before stimulating active dorsiflexion of the foot.

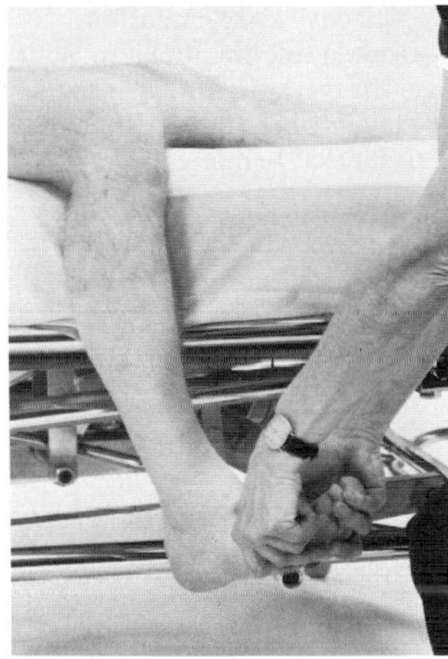

6.3

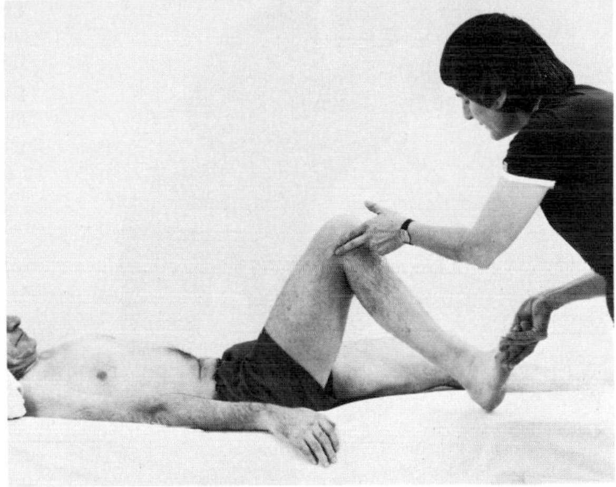

6.4

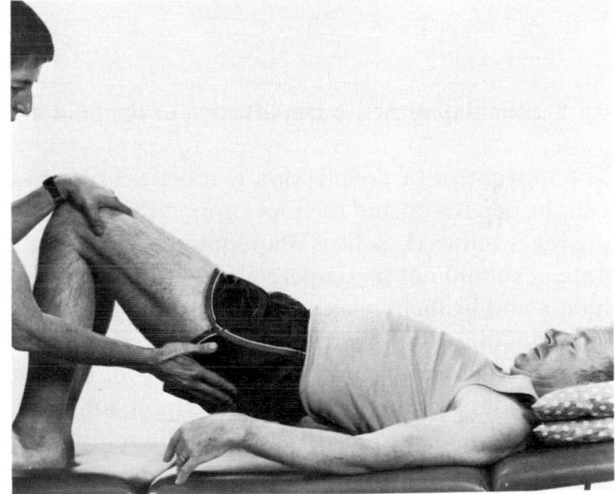

6.5

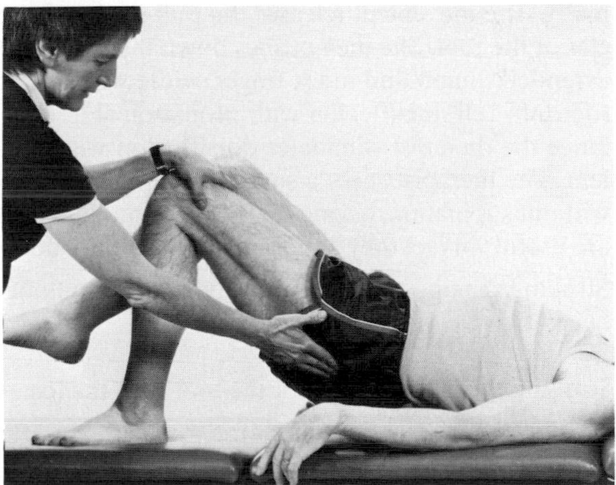

6.6

Fig. 6.3. Inhibition of knee extension with the hip extended. The therapist also inhibits plantar flexion of the ankle. She avoids touching the ball of the foot, as this would stimulate extensor spasticity (right hemiplegia)

Fig. 6.4. Selective movement of the leg over the side of the bed after inhibition. The arm remains at the patients side without pulling into flexion (right hemiplegia)

Fig. 6.5. Bridging with facilitation (left hemiplegia)

Fig. 6.6. Bridging, lifting the sound leg (left hemiplegia)

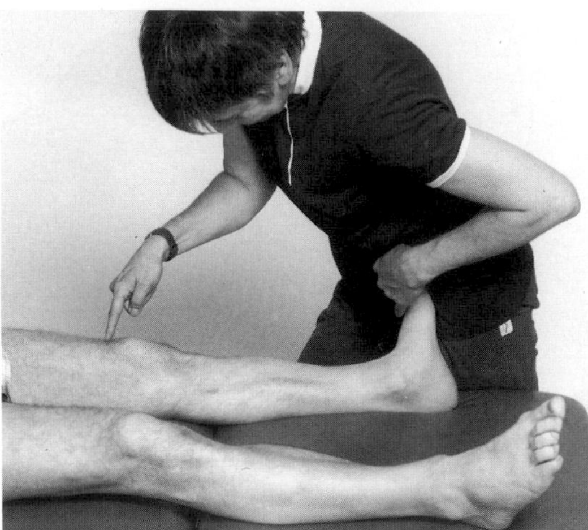

Fig. 6.7. Selective knee extension, with the foot in full dorsiflexion. With her finger the therapist indicates to the patient exactly where the activity should occur (left hemiplegia)

6.1.8 Stimulating Active Dorsiflexion of the Foot and Toes

The movement of dorsiflexion is most easily stimulated when the patient is lying with his leg flexed and the foot supported on the bed. In lying extensor spasticity in the leg is reduced, as he is not required to hold himself upright against gravity. The patient should not try desperately to pull his foot up, but should just lift the toes up lightly and let them relax again. If he struggles to perform the movement the tone in the antagonists will increase, making the desired movement impossible or causing the foot to pull into supination. Showing the patient exactly what is required on his sound foot helps him to move correctly. To inhibit the hypertonus in the antagonists before attempting the movement, the therapist holds the whole foot in front of the ankle firmly down on the plinth, and then moves the patient's leg over it from adduction into abduction, i.e. the foot is pronated by the movement of the leg proximally. The movement releases the pull into supination and relaxes the small muscles of the foot. She then pushes down through the ankle with the web between her extended thumb and index finger, while with her other hand she lifts the toes and foot into full dorsiflexion with pronation (Fig. 6.8). When the foot offers no resistance the therapist stimulates dorsiflexion with the active participation of the patient. The therapist seeks a stimulus that will elicit dorsiflexion in a normal pattern without supination, asking the patient simultaneously to lift his toes. The following are useful; in fact they almost always elicit the desired response:

Stroking the tips of the toes briskly with a chunk of ice, or even pushing the ice between the two most lateral toes (Fig. 6.9).

Stroking the lateral border of the foot with the ice.

Brushing the tips or dorsum of the toes with a bottle-brush.

Tapping the dorsum of the foot laterally with the bottle-brush.

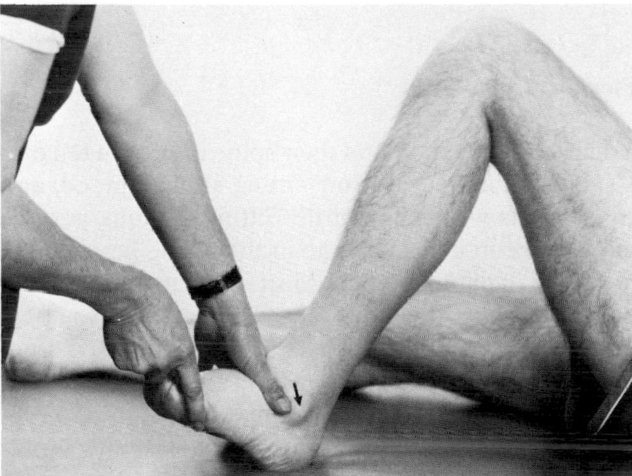

Fig. 6.8. Inhibiting plantar flexion of the foot. The toes are held in full dorsiflexion (left hemiplegia)

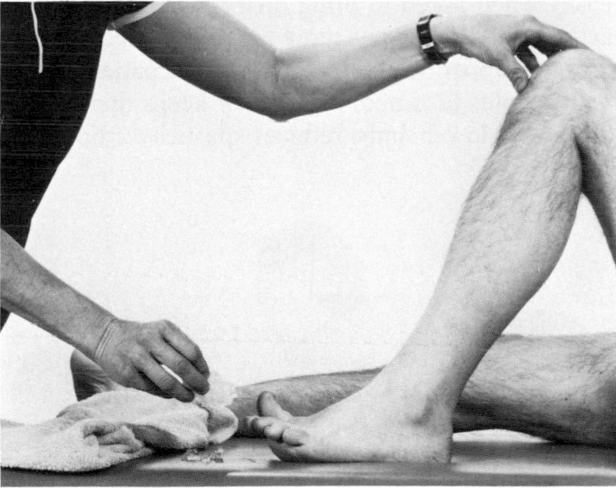

Fig. 6.9. Stimulating active dorsiflexion with ice after inhibition of the antagonists. The towel is not placed under the patient's foot as it tends to stimulate plantar flexion (left hemiplegia)

Sometimes the whole foot needs to be immersed in melting ice before the bottle-brush is effective. Some patients may need less stimulation and merely tickling the toes or flicking the lateral toes upwards will evoke a response. Whichever stimulus is effective, the patient must learn to reproduce the movement actively on his own. He feels the movement or gets feedback from the therapist informing him when the movement is correct. She then reduces the intensity of the stimulus and asks him to perform the movement again until eventually only her verbal stimulus is required. Once the movement is established she stimulates the activity in the same way with the patient in a sitting position, after inhibition, and ultimately when he is standing. The ability to dorsiflex the foot actively without supination means for the patient that he will not have to wear a calliper at all times, so is a very important aspect of the treatment.

6.2 Activities in Sitting

6.2.1 Isolated Extension and Flexion of the Pelvis

Patients nearly always sit with their hips extended and their spine in flexion to compensate. As a result, activities such as standing up from sitting are hampered, and the patient rounds his back to bring his weight forwards. Sitting for long periods with extended hips leads to an increase in extensor tone in the whole leg, making function more difficult. It is of no use to tell the patient to sit up straight, as he will pull his shoulders back and only hold the correction for a very short time. The posture needs to be corrected from its base, by helping the patient to adjust the position of his pelvis (Fig. 6.10). The therapist stands or kneels in front of the patient, and with one hand in his lumbar spine she assists him to extend it, with his trunk vertically over his pelvis (Fig. 6.11). With her other hand she helps him to keep his shoulders still, while he flexes his lumbar spine and then extends it again. Patients understand what is required more easily when asked to bring their navel forwards and then let it go backwards. The activity should become more and more selective until no additional movement occurs in the upper trunk. According to the patient's individual problem, the therapist either holds his knees together or keeps them apart. The movement of his trunk against the lower limbs reduces spasticity around the hips and knees.

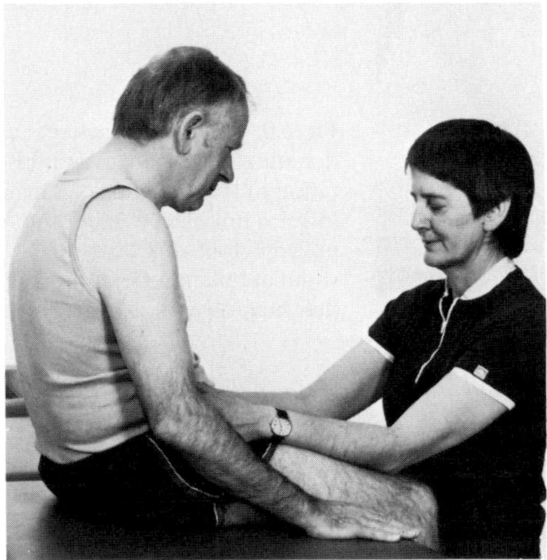

Fig. 6.10. The typical sitting posture with insufficient flexion of the hips, should be corrected from its base (left hemiplegia)

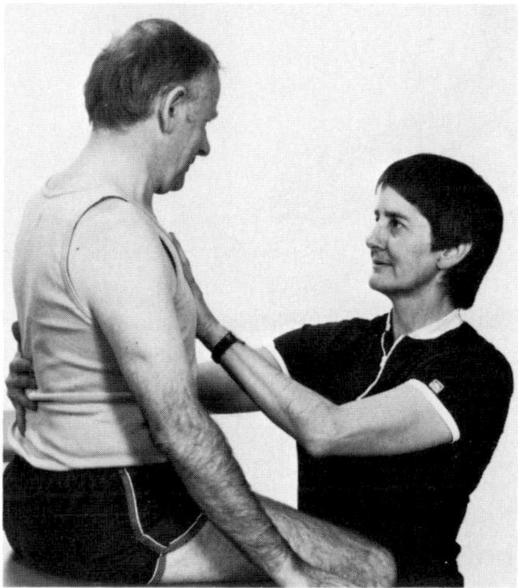

Fig. 6.11. Correcting the patient's sitting posture (left hemiplegia)

6.2.2 Placing the Hemiplegic Leg and Facilitating Crossing It over the Other Leg

The therapist holds the patient's toes in dorsiflexion with one hand and helps him to lift his leg without external rotation and abduction with her other hand. The pat-

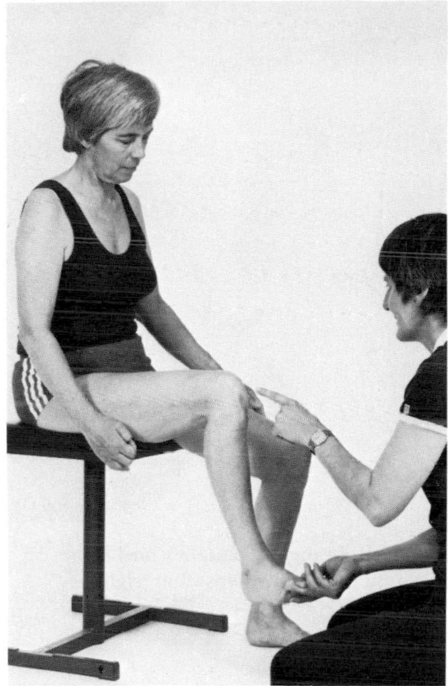

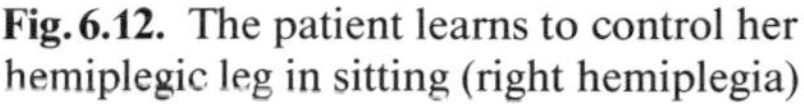

Fig. 6.12. The patient learns to control her hemiplegic leg in sitting (right hemiplegia)

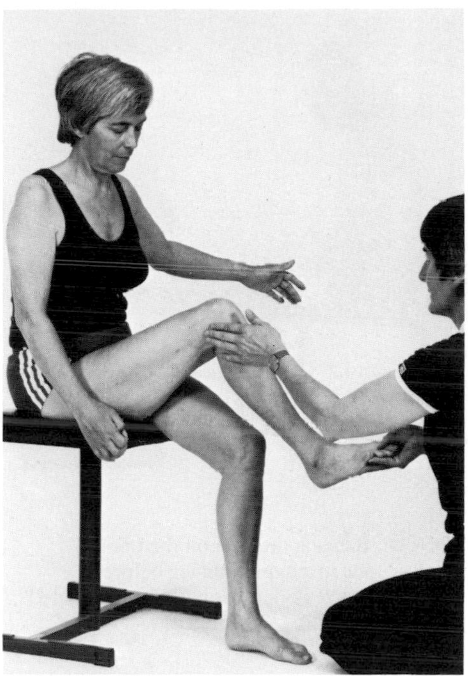

Fig. 6.13. Learning to cross the hemiplegic leg actively over the other one without pulling it with the sound hand (right hemiplegia)

ient takes the weight off his leg and tries to lower it slowly to the ground (Fig. 6.12). He maintains his upright sitting posture while doing so, and does not lean back or allow the hemiplegic side to retract. The therapist facilitates the action of crossing the leg over the sound leg (Fig. 6.13), a movement he will need in order to put on his trousers, shoes and socks (see Chap. 10). He must cross and uncross the leg without pulling it with his unaffected hand and without pushing the heel of the sound foot off the floor.

6.2.3 Stamping the Heel on the Floor

When the patient's heel is banged on the floor, tone in his knee extensors is built up and dorsiflexion of the foot stimulated. He also becomes aware of his heel on the ground and the activity is a very good preparation for standing up and bearing weight on the affected leg for patients whose leg is hypotonic and who have poor sensation. The therapist holds the patient's foot and toes in full dorsiflexion with one hand and her other hand is placed over his knee. She lifts his leg from the foot, and then pushes down on his knee to bang the heel on the floor. The ankle must remain firmly dorsiflexed so that the ball of the foot does not make contact with the ground (Fig. 6.14).

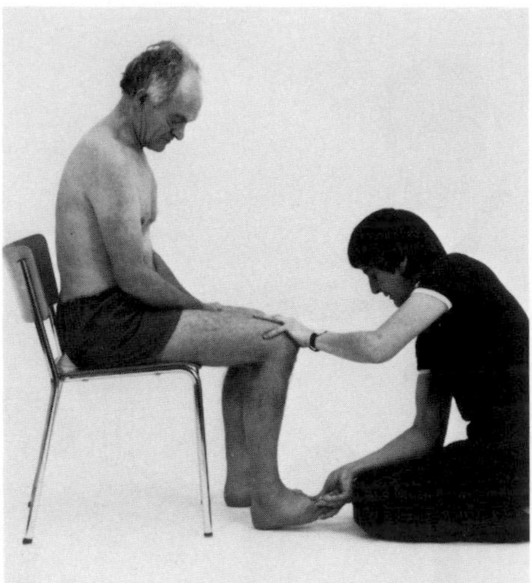

Fig. 6.14. Banging the heel on the floor to increase tone in a hypotonic leg before standing. Active dorsiflexion is also stimulated (right hemiplegia)

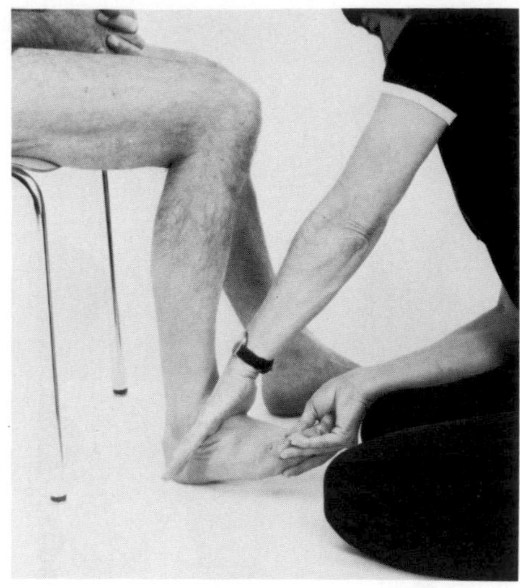

Fig. 6.15. Rubbing the patient's heel firmly on the ground to improve sensation (right hemiplegia)

The patient can also try to participate actively with the stamping movement, as it facilitates selective hip extension, with the knee and foot flexed. If the patient does not feel his heel on the ground, the therapist can rub it against the floor backwards towards him. She maintains full dorsiflexion of the foot with the web between her extended thumb and index finger pushing down through his ankle, and with the other hand holding his toes in extension (Fig. 6.15).

6.2.4 Weight-Bearing with Selective Extension

Once the patient's lower extremity has been carefully prepared for weight-bearing, he should practise coming up to the standing position using the normal pattern of movement. Most patients, if not trained correctly, push themselves up with the unaffected hand, most of their weight over the sound side, while the hemiplegic leg thrusts into the total extension pattern. The weight is therefore too far back, the activity is effortful and the resulting posture is asymmetrical and emphasises the spastic pattern.

Sitting with his feet flat on the floor, the patient places his clasped hands on a stool in front of him. The stool should be so positioned that when his hands rest on it with the elbows extended, his head is further forward than his feet to ensure the normal pattern of standing up. The therapist guides him as he lifts his hips off the chair or low plinth, drawing his knee forward over his foot with one hand, and helping him to lift his weight with her other hand over his opposite trochanter. With her shoulder against his scapula she prevents him from pushing back with his trunk

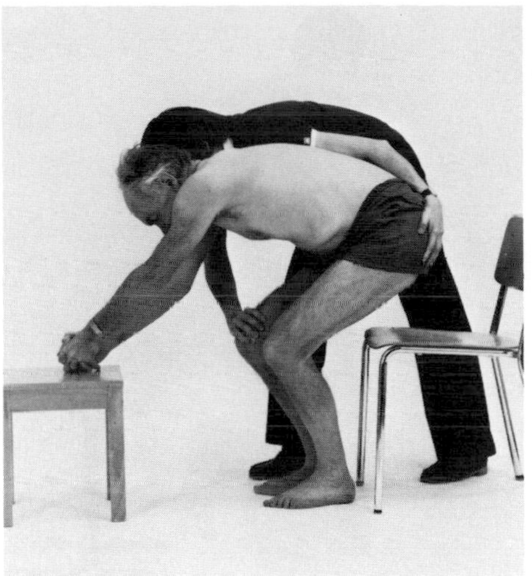
6.16

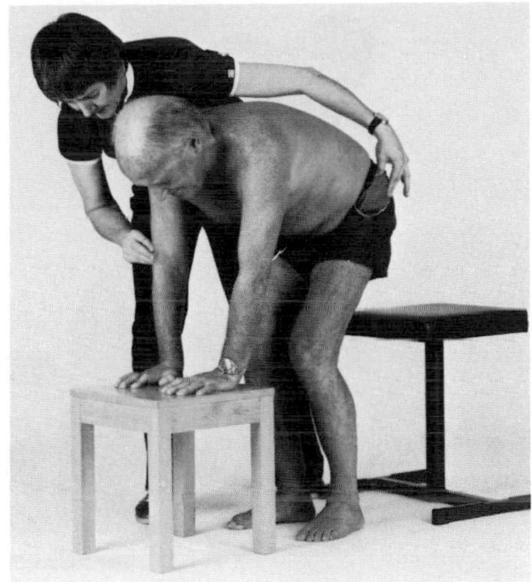
6.17

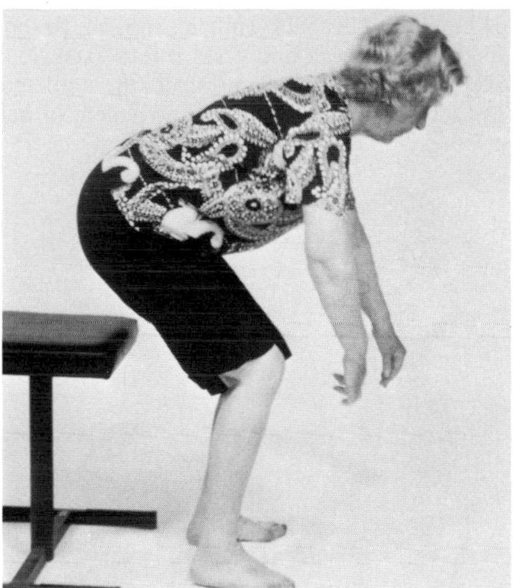
6.18

Fig. 6.16. Teaching the patient how to stand up from sitting using the normal pattern of movement. The stool is so placed that his head is in front of his feet. The therapist assists the forward movement of the hemiplegic knee (right hemiplegia)

Fig. 6.17. Preparation for coming to standing. The patient lifts his hips while his hands remain in place on the stool (right hemiplegia)

Fig. 6.18. Standing up with the arms swinging freely (right hemiplegia)

(Fig. 6.16). He learns to maintain this position as she withdraws her support, and practises moving his hips from side to side and then back on to the plinth.

When the patient can perform the activity easily, his hands can be placed separately flat on the stool, and he lifts his hips while the hemiplegic hand remains in place, without the arm pulling into flexion (Fig. 6.17). Finally, without the stool, the patient practises the movement either with his clasped hands extended in front of him or with both arms swinging lightly forward (Fig. 6.18). The patient often needs help to flex his hips sufficiently and to bring his trunk forward with the spine extended. The therapist achieves the extension for him first passively by pressing on his spine (Fig. 6.19 a), and then asks him to straighten his back actively (Fig. 6.19 b).

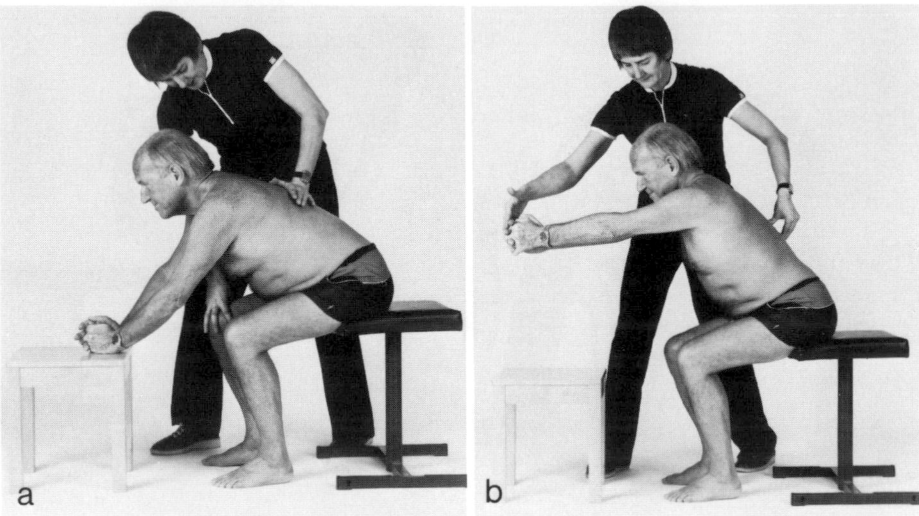

Fig. 6.19 a, b. In a sitting position the patient is helped to extend his back while his hips are flexed. **a** Passively: the therapist presses down on the patient's flexed spine and eases it into extension. **b** Actively: when passive extension has been achieved the patient lifts his hands from the stool and extends his back actively. The therapist indicates the activity with a squeezing movement of her thumb and fingers over his spine (right hemiplegia)

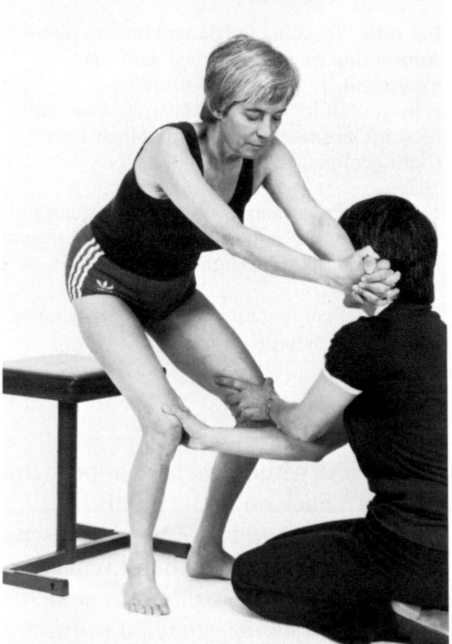

Fig. 6.20. Standing up without the hemiplegic leg adducting. The therapist facilitates the correct movement and the patient tries to keep her knees apart (right hemiplegia)

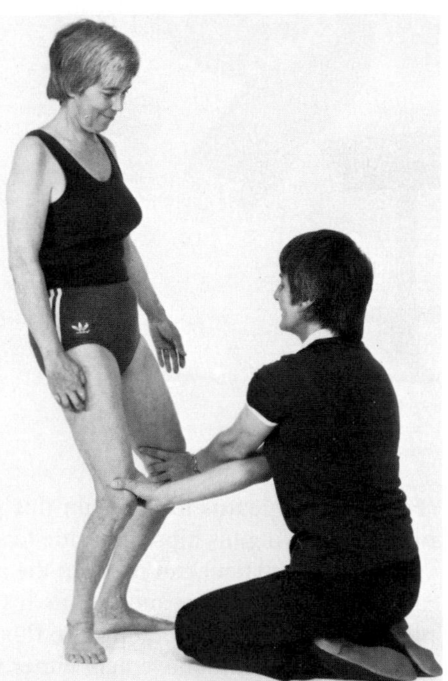

Fig. 6.21. Standing with the hips in extension, abduction and external rotation. The patient flexes her knees and practises tilting her pelvis selectively (right hemiplegia)

Patients whose tone is on the low side will use the total extension synergy in the leg when they stand from sitting. The affected leg adducts and inwardly rotates, and the heel may be raised up off the floor. The therapist facilitates the correct movement, kneeling in front of the patient and drawing his knees forwards and away from each other as he stands up. She does so by crossing her hands over and grasping his thighs at the femoral condyles (Fig. 6.20). She slowly withdraws her assistance, making the patient aware that he must not push against her hands.

When standing the patient maintains his hips in extension with abduction and external rotation, and bends his knees as far as he can without the heels coming off the floor (Fig. 6.21). With more advanced patients it is possible to go right down to the squatting position, or for them to sit down on a low step and rise to a standing position again with their knees apart.

6.3 Activities in Standing to Train Weight-Bearing on the Hemiplegic Leg

6.3.1 Improving Extension of the Hip with External Rotation

The patient stands on his hemiplegic leg and places the sound foot in front of it and at a right angle. He does not transfer his weight on to the foot, but places it accurate-

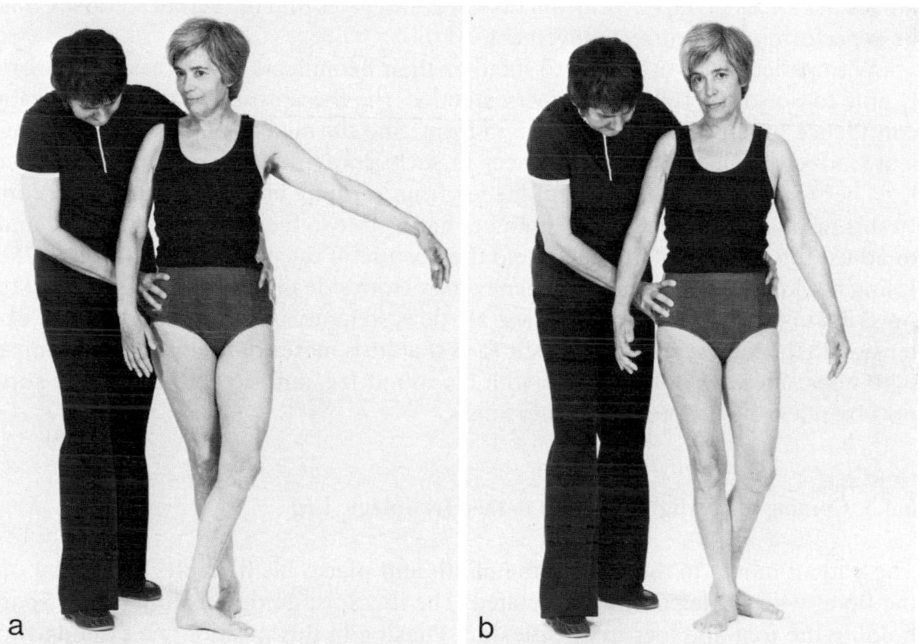

Fig. 6.22 a, b. Weight-bearing on the hemiplegic leg, with the hip extended and outwardly rotated (right hemiplegia). **a** The sound foot is placed across the front of the supporting foot, at a right angle. **b** The sound foot is placed at a right angle behind the other foot. The left side of the patient's pelvis remains forwards

ly while trying to keep his pelvis forwards on both sides (Fig. 6.22a). The foot is then placed at right angles behind the heel of the hemiplegic foot (Fig. 6.22b).

6.3.2 Standing with a Rolled Bandage Under the Toes to Maintain Dorsiflexion

With a bandage rolled to an appropriate size and placed under his toes (Fig. 6.23), the patient stands up and transfers all his weight on to the hemiplegic leg. With the other leg held in the air he bends and straightens his affected knee, extending it as far as he can without letting it snap back into extension, and then flexing it again. The therapist maintains the correct position of his pelvis, with her hands over his iliac crests. The activity is very useful to inhibit the clawing of the toes during weight-bearing, and in fact inhibits plantar flexion of the foot so effectively that often active dorsiflexion can be stimulated immediately afterwards. It is also a good way of preventing any shortening of the Achilles tendon.

Patients with disturbed sensation in the hemiplegic leg should feel correct weight-bearing and so learn to reproduce it alone. At first the therapist may have to facilitate the movement with total support. She stands on the patient's hemiplegic side and supports his knee on that side between both her knees. With her arms round him, she draws him towards her and asks him to lift his sound leg in the air (Fig. 6.24). She then moves his supported knee into flexion and extension by adducting and abducting her legs alternately. When she feels him move actively, she moves her knees slightly away from his knee, and gives him the verbal feedback that he is performing the correct movement.

With patients who are afraid to stand on their hemiplegic leg, or feel they are only able to do so with the knee hyper-extended, the therapist can help them to gain confidence by supporting them from in front. She sits on a stool and holds the patient's affected knee between her knees in such a way that, when she adducts her legs, her femoral condyles prevent his leg from pushing back into hyperextension. In this position the therapist has both her hands free to facilitate hip extension and to adjust the position of the pelvis and the posture of the patient's trunk (Fig. 6.25). Using her knees, she moves the patient gently from side to side, and asks him not to press against her leg with his good leg. He does so to use adduction to reinforce extension in the total synergy. When she feels that he is more confident she asks him to take steps sideways or backwards with his sound leg, and slowly reduces the support by releasing the pressure of her knees.

6.3.3 Coming off a High Plinth on to the Hemiplegic Leg

The patient moves to the edge of the plinth and places his hemiplegic foot flat on the floor, with the leg outwardly rotated. The therapist guides his foot to the floor, holding the foot and toes in dorsiflexion. Pausing in this position, he extends and flexes his knee selectively, moving it as far as he can into extension without it snapping back, and without his toes clawing. The therapist facilitates the knee movement with her other hand, and ensures that the patient remains vertically upright and does not lean over the plinth towards his sound side, or support himself with

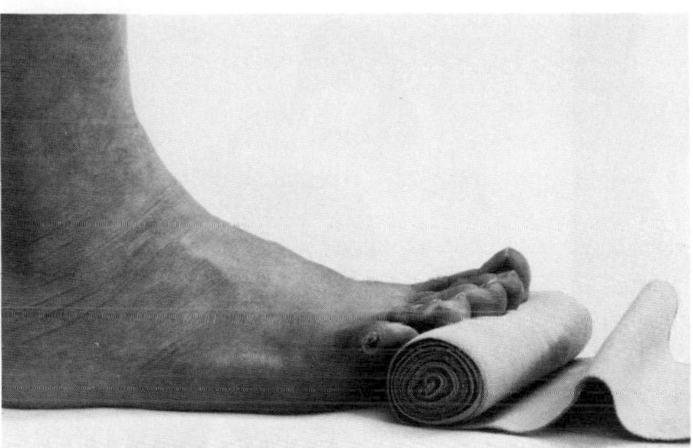

Fig. 6.23. Bandage placed under the patient's toes to inhibit flexion. The size of the rolled bandage is increased as spasticity releases (right hemiplegia)

6.24

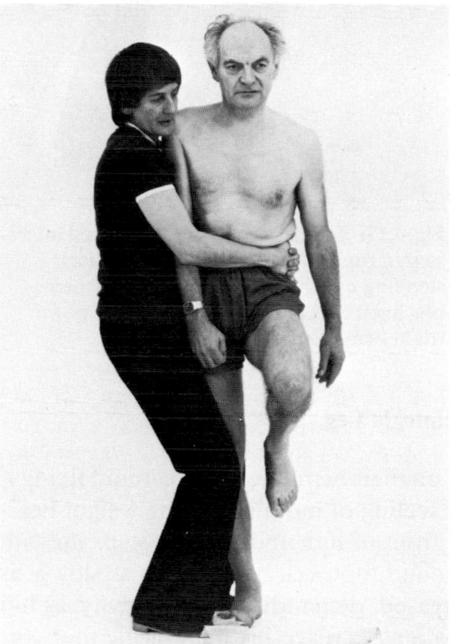

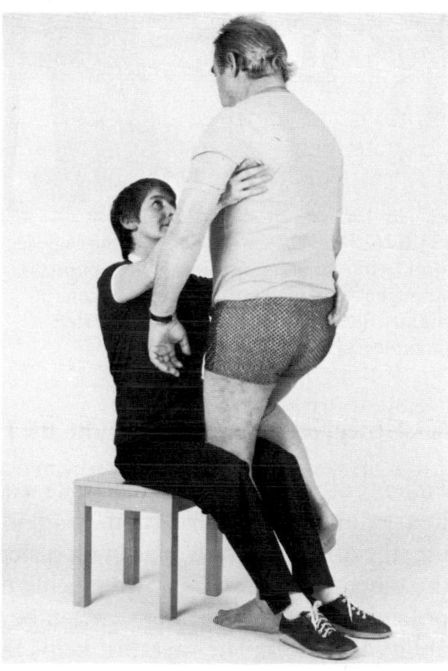

6.25

Fig. 6.24. Weight-bearing on the hemiplegic leg with full support. The therapist uses her legs to facilitate flexion and extension of the knee and the patient starts to join in actively. His weight must be transferred right over the hemiplegic leg (right hemiplegia)

Fig. 6.25. Patient supported so that he stands confidently on the hemiplegic leg without hyperextending the knee. The therapist lengthens the spastic side during weight-bearing (left hemiplegia)

his hand. The patient lifts his other leg from the plinth and comes to stand with his feet together, still with his affected knee in some degree of flexion. He then lifts the sound leg into the air and rotates his pelvis to sit back on the plinth again (Fig. 6.26). The activity is valuable because it requires extension of the affected hip independent of the rotation component.

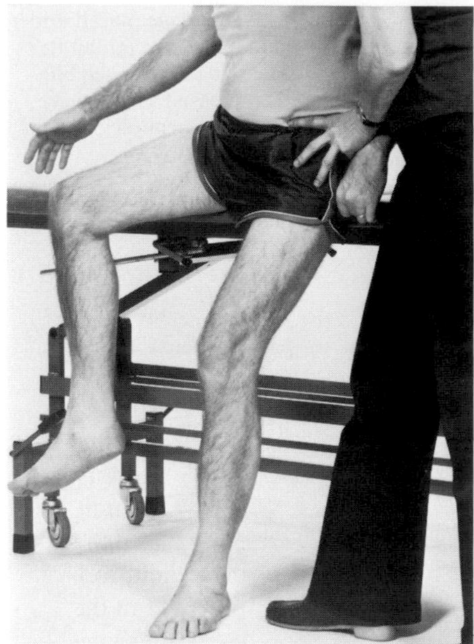

Fig. 6.26. Weight-bearing on the hemiplegic leg alone while standing up from a high plinth, or sitting back on it again. The knee remains slightly flexed throughout the activity (left hemiplegia)

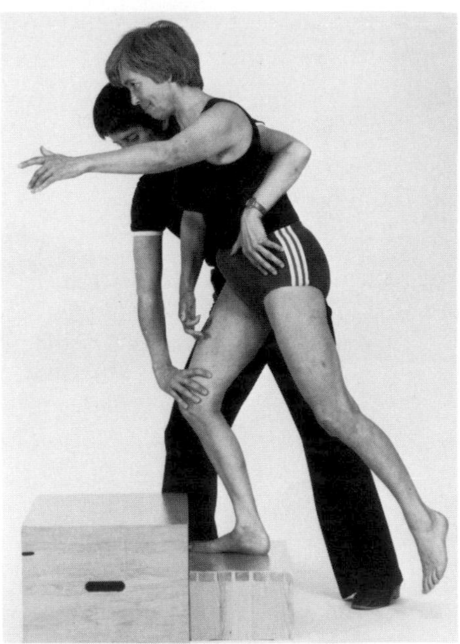

Fig. 6.27. The hemiplegic foot is placed on a step in front of the patient. She practises stepping up with her sound foot and then placing it far back behind her to step down (right hemiplegia)

6.3.4 Stepping up on to a Step with the Hemiplegic Leg

Patients often find it difficult to take weight on their hemiplegic leg without fixing it in a certain position. To give the patient the feeling of mobility during weight-bearing, the affected foot is placed on a step in front of him and he then steps up with the other foot. He steps down placing the sound foot well behind him as slowly as possible. The height of the step can be increased, demanding more activity, as hip ability improves. The therapist helps the patient to place his hemiplegic foot correctly on the step. With her hand over his thigh she draws his knee forwards over his foot and assists the movement up on to the step, with one side of her pelvis facilitating hip extension. With her other hand on his opposite hip she uses her arm and shoulder to bring his trunk forwards over the foot in front (Fig. 6.27). The therapist lessens her support until she is able to stand in front of the patient, perhaps holding his hemiplegic arm forwards in extension while he steps up and down.

6.4 Activities in Standing to Train Selective Movement of the Hemiplegic Leg

Patients have difficulty in taking a step with their hemiplegic leg and often bring it forwards without flexing the hip and knee. They therefore hitch the pelvis up on the affected side, as if they were wearing a full leg brace. Other patients lift the leg actively forwards in the total flexor pattern, with the foot supinated. Many patients are unable to transfer weight correctly, diagonally forwards, on to their unaffected leg, and attempt to move the hemiplegic leg while it is still bearing some of their weight.

6.4.1 Releasing the Hip and Knee

The patient stands with his feet together and lets the hip and knee relax and fall forwards. The pelvis relaxes downwards and forwards at the same time. The therapist, kneeling in front of the patient, facilitates the movement with one hand guiding the pelvis forwards and downwards, and her other hand drawing the knee forwards from the front (Fig. 6.28 a). If her hand pushes behind his knee it might stimulate his pushing against her. The patient carries out the same activity with his hemiplegic foot placed behind him, as in walking. The movement is more difficult in this position, as with the hip in extension extensor spasticity in the whole leg is increased. When the knee and hip fall forward now, the heel must leave the floor, and the therapist helps to prevent the foot pushing into inversion, asking the patient to let the heel fall inwards (Fig. 6.28 b). As the knee flexes, the leg tends to abduct in the total flexor pattern and the patient tries to let the knee relax towards his other knee. Be-

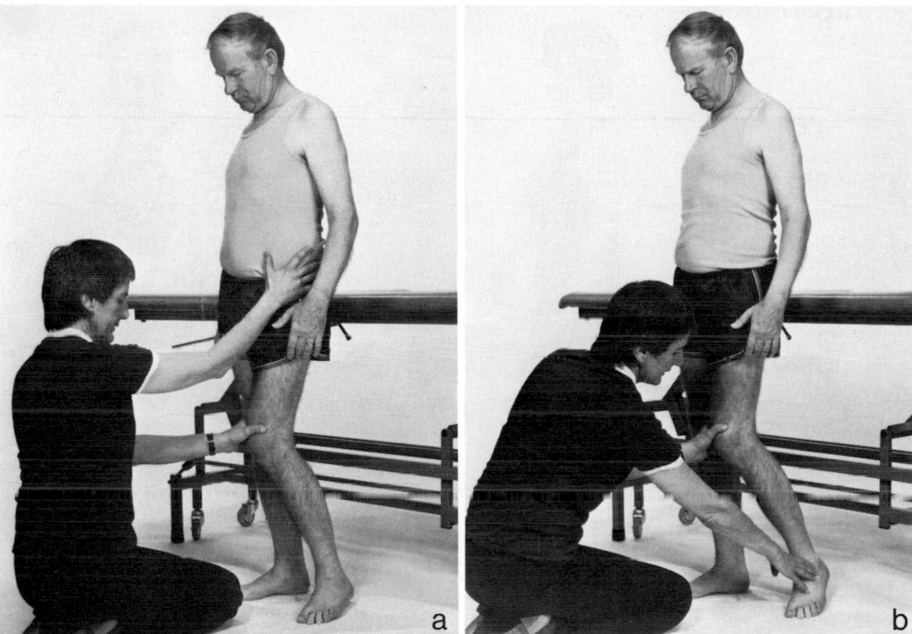

Fig. 6.28 a, b. Standing with the weight on the sound side and relaxing the extensors of the hemiplegic leg (left hemiplegia). **a** With the feet parallel the activity is easier, as there is less extensor hypertonus. **b** With the hemiplegic foot behind, as in walking, extensor spasticity increases in the whole limb. The therapist prevents the foot from pushing into plantar inversion

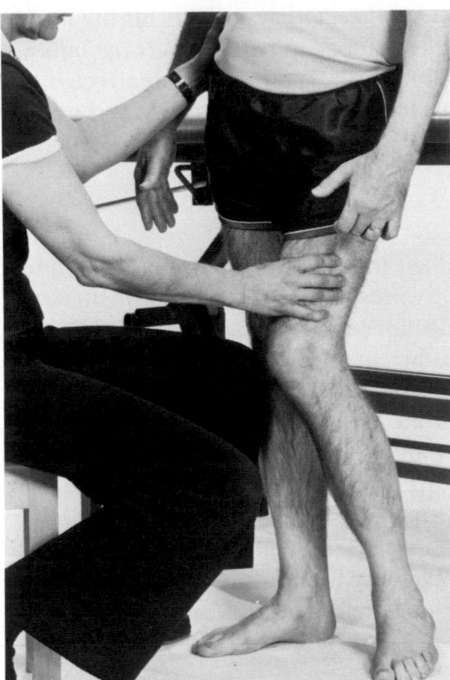

Fig. 6.29. Preventing the sound leg from flexing simultaneously as the hemiplegic leg relaxes (left hemiplegia)

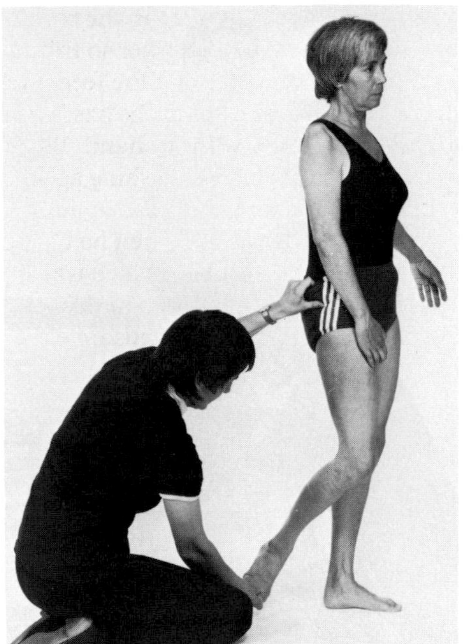

Fig. 6.30. Small steps back with the hemiplegic foot. The patient does not hitch the side of her pelvis up or move it backwards (right hemiplegia)

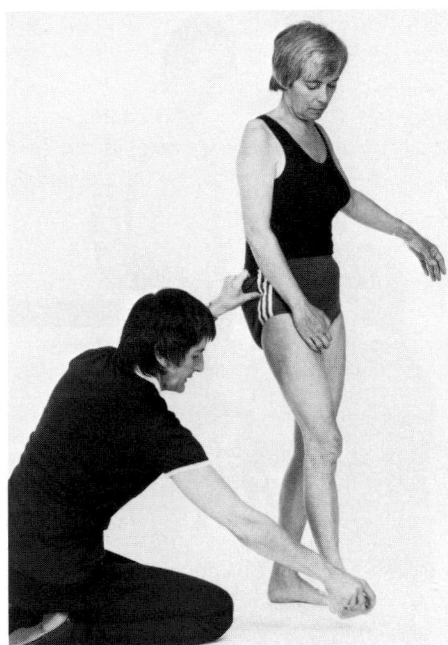

Fig. 6.31. Swinging the hemiplegic foot forwards like a pendulum, without lifting the leg actively (right hemiplegia)

cause the co-ordination is still difficult, most patients bend both knees in order to allow flexion of the hemiplegic knee. If the patient cannot prevent simultaneous flexion the therapist can sit on a stool and block his unaffected knee with her knee, and facilitate the affected leg with her hand (Fig. 6.29). When she feels that his sound leg is remaining in extension, she gradually withdraws the support.

6.4.2 Taking Steps Backwards with the Hemiplegic Leg

The ability to walk backwards is necessary for many functions, for example moving to sit down in a chair. Taking steps backwards is also a part of our protective balance mechanism. Practising the movement enables the patient to move his leg selectively, while transferring his weight fully over the sound leg, and this will also improve the way in which he walks forwards. The patient stands with his weight on the unaffected side and takes a succession of small steps backwards with the hemiplegic leg. The therapist kneels at his hemiplegic side and, with one hand on his iliac crest, prevents him from hitching his pelvis up as he tries to move his leg back in the total extension pattern. With her other hand she holds his toes and foot in dorsiflexion and facilitates the normal action of taking a step backwards, i.e. the knee flexes actively while the hip extends (Fig. 6.30). If the therapist is unable to guide the leg in a normal pattern of movement because of too much resistance, the patient supports himself lightly with his sound hand on the plinth and she asks him to do nothing at all except allow her to move his leg. She then moves the leg in the correct movement pattern, taking very small steps backwards one after the other so that he can feel what should happen. When the resistance stops, she gives him the feedback that the movement is now correct, and asks him to do it with her. Once he has learnt to carry out the activity he also must stop supporting himself with his hand. When the foot is behind him, the patient is asked to leave it there, without pushing against the floor. The therapist then guides the foot forward like a pendulum, as in normal walking (Fig. 6.31). She does not ask the patient to take small steps when he brings the leg forward, as this would encourage active hip and knee flexion, which is not a part of the normal pattern. When the patient can take steps backwards in this way, the therapist can facilitate automatic walking backwards with her hands on either side of his pelvis (see Chap. 9).

6.4.3 Placing the Hemiplegic Leg

In order to take a free normal step forward with his affected leg, the patient needs to be able to stand on his sound leg without the hemiplegic leg participating in maintaining balance. The patient stands with his back to the high plinth and maintains his balance while allowing the therapist to move his hemiplegic leg freely in the air. He then actively holds the leg as she guides it to the floor, until it rests on the floor without taking weight (Fig. 6.32). Placing in the standing position is much more difficult than when lying because the patient has to maintain an upright extended position against gravity, and the extensor tone in the leg is therefore increased.

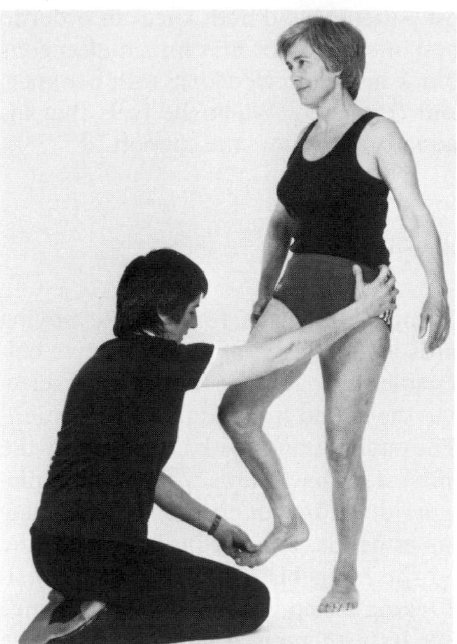

Fig. 6.32. Standing on the sound leg, the patient holds her hemiplegic leg actively throughout range until it rests on the floor (right hemiplegia)

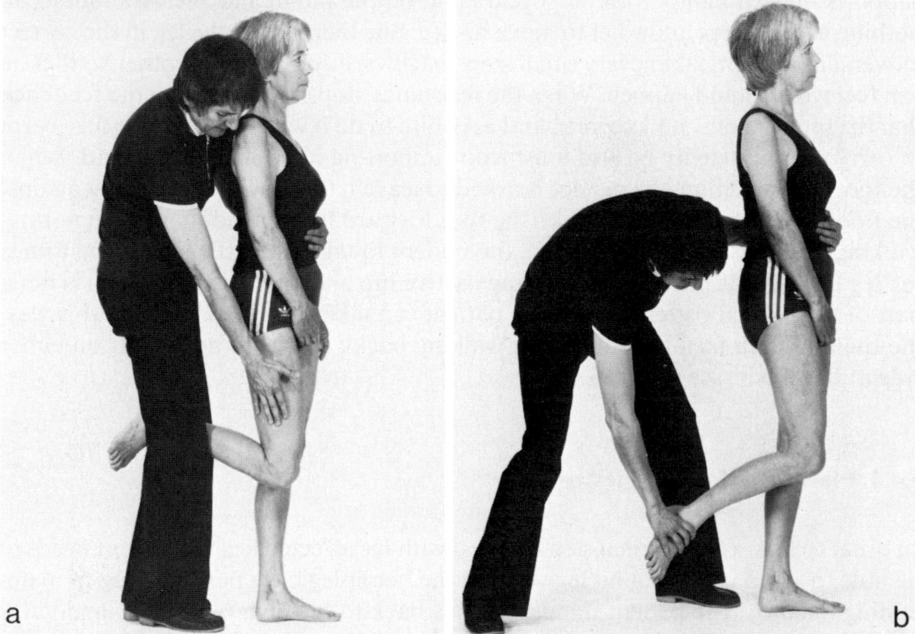

Fig. 6.33 a, b. Inhibition of extensor spasticity with the patient standing on the sound leg (right hemiplegia). **a** Standing behind the patient, the therapist clasps the patient's hemiplegic leg between her knees so that the knee is kept flexed despite hip extension. **b** When the hemiplegic leg is relaxed the therapist lowers the foot slowly to the ground. The patient concentrates on not letting the leg push into extension

Extensor spasticity in the whole leg increases still more when the hip is in extension. To inhibit the spasticity and also to give the patient the ability to stand easily on the sound leg, the therapist flexes his knee by lifting his foot up behind him. She stands behind the patient and holds his lower leg between her knees. She encourages him to keep his pelvis level and to allow the thigh to relax towards the other knee (Fig. 6.33 a). When she feels that the affected leg is no longer pulling into flexion or pushing into extension, she lowers the foot slowly to the floor. The patient concentrates on not pushing, and tries to let his foot just rest on the floor behind him (Fig. 6.33 b).

6.4.4 Allowing the Leg to Be Drawn Forwards Passively

The patient's hemiplegic foot is placed on a broad bandage and, while he tries to inhibit activity in his whole leg, the therapist draws his foot forward with the bandage. The movement is that of the swing phase of walking and improves the release of the hip and knee behind, and the knee extension in front. Because the patient is trying to remain inactive, the foot is not pulled into supination by the over-activity of the anterior tibial muscle as the leg comes forwards. Such relaxation of the leg muscles is necessary for the swing and the patient may need to hold lightly on to the back of a chair for support at first (Fig. 6.34). Later he must be able to maintain the relaxation of the leg without holding on.

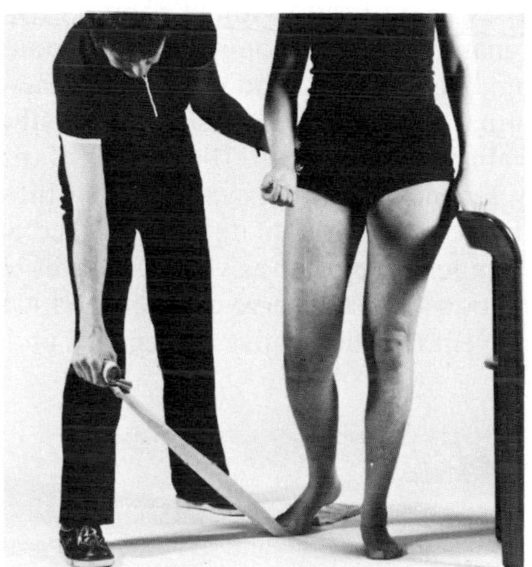

Fig. 6.34. Relaxing the hemiplegic leg and allowing the foot to be drawn forwards on a bandage without resisting the movement (right hemiplegia)

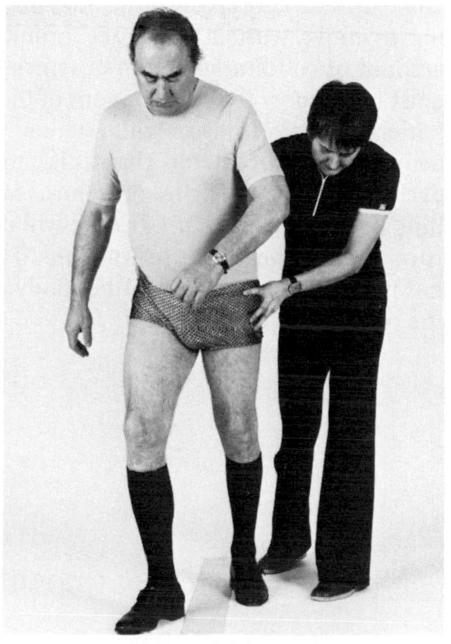

Fig. 6.35. Walking along an unrolled bandage with only the heels touching it (left hemiplegia)

6.4.5 Walking Along a Line with the Legs Outwardly Rotated

The patient has a line or an unrolled bandage in front of him. As he walks forwards, he tries to place only his heels against it (Fig. 6.35). The ensuing external rotation of the sound leg improves the selective extension of the hemiplegic hip during the stance phase. The swing phase also follows more selectively.

6.5 Rolling Over

Rolling is one of the most effective ways of inhibiting spasticity throughout the body when rotation of the trunk is emphasised. The patient can move freely and confidently without having to maintain his balance against gravity, and movement without effort can be facilitated. Head-righting reactions are also stimulated. Therapeutic rolling should only be practised on a wide supporting surface such as a bed, a mat on the floor, a high mat or two plinths pushed together. If the patient is asked to roll on a normal plinth, he will be afraid of falling off it and will not move freely and normally. The facilitation of rolling is described in Chaps. 5 and 11.

6.6 Considerations

When the patient has reached the stage of moving about independently, he will become increasingly spastic if he does not move selectively and without effort. Learning to move without using the primitive mass synergies requires an enormous amount of concentration and exactness from both therapist and patient. The therapist must know the exact pattern of the normal movement before she can help the patient to avoid using only the stereotyped abnormal synergies. The success of the activities described in this chapter is entirely dependent on the exactness with which each is performed. The more enthusiastically the patient tries to do what is asked of him, the greater is the risk that he will use compensatory or evasive mechanisms to carry out the therapist's instructions. The therapist must observe carefully and use her hands and other parts of her body to prevent the substitutive movements until the patient can do so himself.

7 Retraining Balance Reactions in Sitting and Standing

A very important aim of treatment is that the patient may eventually walk in the street again, unafraid and unnoticed by other people. To achieve this aim the patient must be trained to react against gravity in all positions, quickly and automatically. He will also need to regain some form of protective or saving reaction so that he can save himself from falling should he lose his balance.

Adequate balance is necessary not only for walking but also for every activity the patient carries out during his waking hours. The ability to maintain equilibrium in a great variety of positions provides the basis for all the skilled movements that are required for self-care, work and enjoyment. The longer the period of immobilisation in bed after onset of stroke, during which the patient is totally supported and does not have to react to gravity at all, the more will be his fear when he is brought to the upright position later. Therefore, from the earliest opportunity, preferably within the first week, the patient should be helped out of bed and become used to being moved away from the mid-line, in all directions. He must also be taught how to return to the vertical position again. Maximum care must be taken that he does not fall over when he is still incapable of saving himself, because such a frightening experience will certainly increase his anxiety.

7.1 Activities in Sitting

The following activities can be carried out with the patient sitting on the edge of his bed or on a plinth in the physiotherapy department and later in a chair. If balance reactions are retaught in sitting, with the feet unsupported at first, more activity in the head and trunk is stimulated. With the feet on the floor, the sound leg overreacts and prevents or alters normal reactions in other parts of the body. It is necessary, however, to train the reactions with the feet supported on the floor as well, because that is the position in which we normally need to maintain our balance in daily life.

Activities aimed at transferring the weight sideways should be practised towards both sides. Most patients, if untrained, are not able to transfer weight correctly over to their sound side either, and can only do so by supporting themselves with their unaffected hand. The same activities are also carried out with patients in later stages of their rehabilitation when the reactions are still inadequate or too slow. The amount of support given is reduced and the speed increased as the patient's ability improves.

7.1.1 Moving to Elbow Support Sideways

The patient leans over until his elbow is in contact with the plinth, and then brings himself up to sitting again. The therapist facilitates the movement by standing in front of the patient and supporting his uppermost shoulder with her forearm. Her other hand guides the patient's hand or arm (Fig. 7.1 a). By pressing down on his shoulder with her forearm she facilitates the head-righting reaction. When the patient comes up from the sound side, the therapist holds his unaffected hand lightly from above so that he does not push off with it, and his hemiplegic side then has to work actively (Fig. 7.1 b).

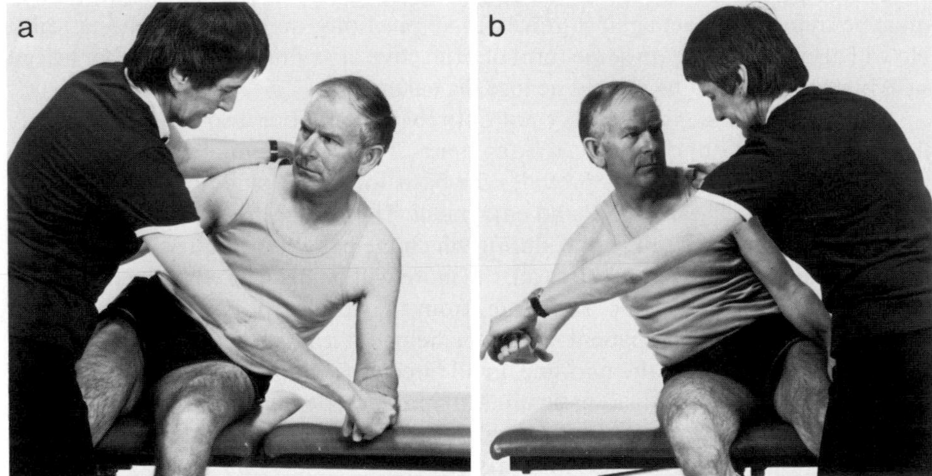

Fig. 7.1 a, b. Sitting, moving to elbow support sideways (left hemiplegia). **a** To the hemiplegic side; **b** to the sound side. The patient does not use his hand to return to the upright position

7.1.2 Transferring the Weight Sideways

The therapist sits on the patient's affected side and brings his weight over towards her. The side of his trunk should lengthen, so her hand in his axilla facilitates this lengthening. Her other hand is over the side flexors on the opposite side to facilitate their shortening as she draws him towards her (Fig. 7.2 a). Before the patient is very adept at the movement, the therapist should never pull on his hemiplegic arm, as the shoulder is easily traumatised in abduction.

The movement is repeated, and the patient starts participating more and more actively. The therapist can ask him to hold the position and stay there while she reduces her support, or to move into the correct position without her assistance. Transferring the weight to the other side requires an active shortening of the hemiplegic side with the head righting to vertical. Using the web of her hand, the therapist applies firm pressure to the trunk side flexors to stimulate their shortening action. With her other hand she presses his shoulder down to facilitate the righting reaction of the head as the patient moves his weight to the sound side (Fig. 7.2 b).

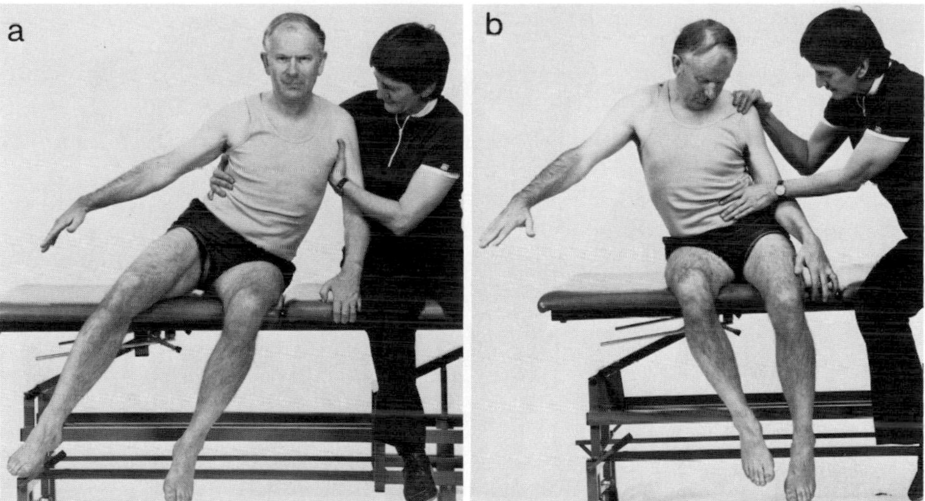

Fig. 7.2 a, b. Facilitating balance reactions in sitting (left hemiplegia). **a** With the weight transferred to the hemiplegic side. The therapist assists the elongation of the side. **b** With the weight transferred to the sound side. The therapist assists the shortening of the side

The therapist asks the patient not to support himself with his sound hand, but to lift it sideways instead.

The therapist gives less and less support until she can stand in front of the patient and he moves freely and easily to both sides, when she merely guides his arm to indicate the direction of the movement.

7.1.3 Sitting with Legs Crossed – Weight Transference Towards the Side of the Underneath Leg

The activity facilitates the outward rotation of the leg over which the weight is being transferred. The patient requires stable balance in this position, as he will use it when putting on his socks and shoes. Standing in front of the patient the therapist places her arm round the back of his shoulder, in such a way that the crook of her elbow can facilitate the head-righting position. Her other hand under the trochanter on the opposite side assists with weight transference and helps him to lift his buttock off the plinth (Fig. 7.3 a). She asks the patient to repeat the movement and to try not to press his head against her arm. She later withdraws her support gradually until he can reproduce the movement correctly on his own. When transferring the weight to the unaffected side the patient crosses his hemiplegic leg over the sound one, to facilitate the normal reaction with lengthening of the weight-bearing side (Fig. 7.3 b).

Weight transference with crossed legs is also practised to both sides, with the foot of the underneath leg placed flat on the floor. If the height of the bed or the plinth is not adjustable, the patient sits on a chair with an additional chair on either

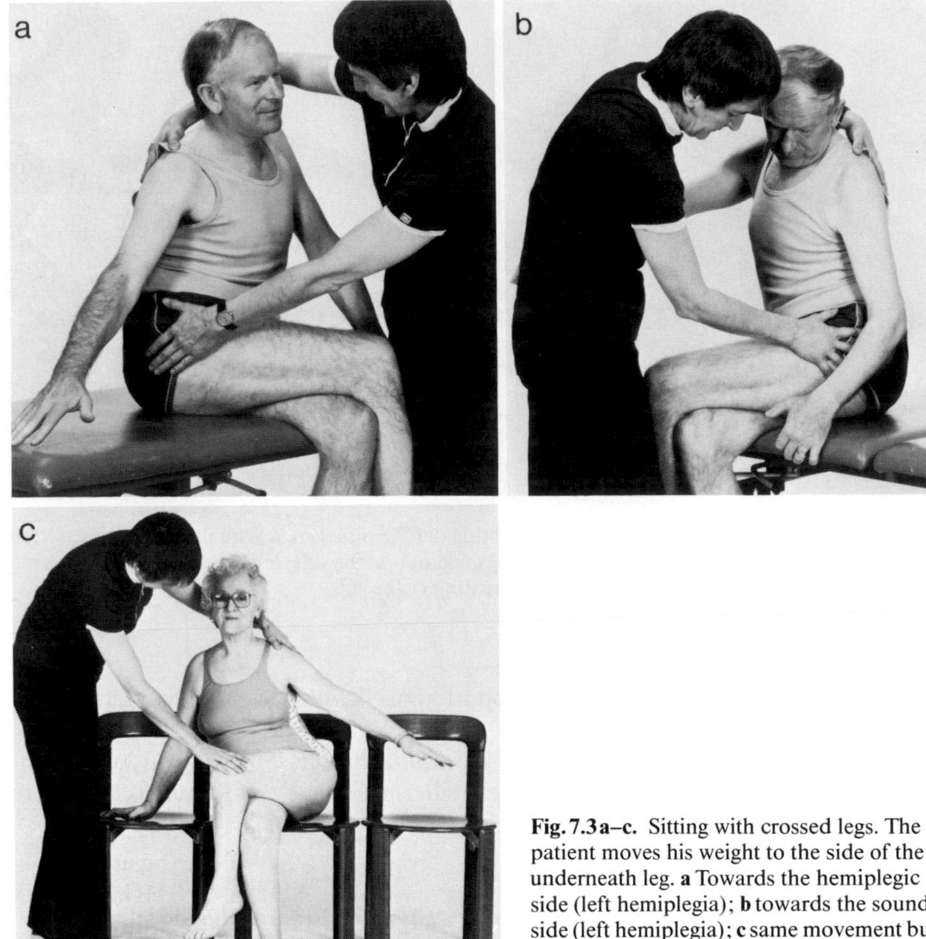

Fig. 7.3 a–c. Sitting with crossed legs. The patient moves his weight to the side of the underneath leg. **a** Towards the hemiplegic side (left hemiplegia); **b** towards the sound side (left hemiplegia); **c** same movement but with the patient's foot on the floor (right hemiplegia)

side of him. The chair at the side gives the patient a feeling of security, and can also be used for activities where weight is taken through the hemiplegic arm (Fig. 7.3 c).

7.1.4 Stimulating Head and Trunk Reactions by Turning Both Flexed Knees to the Side

By using both legs to bring the patient out of balance, more reaction is demanded from the head and trunk, as described in Chap. 2. The therapist sits on a chair or stool in front of the patient and supports his feet on her knees. She then has a hand free to hold the patient's sound hand lightly as a safety precaution. If he should lose his balance, she can save him from falling (Fig. 7.4). With her other hand she turns his knees, slowly at first, to one side so that all his weight is over that side. She re-

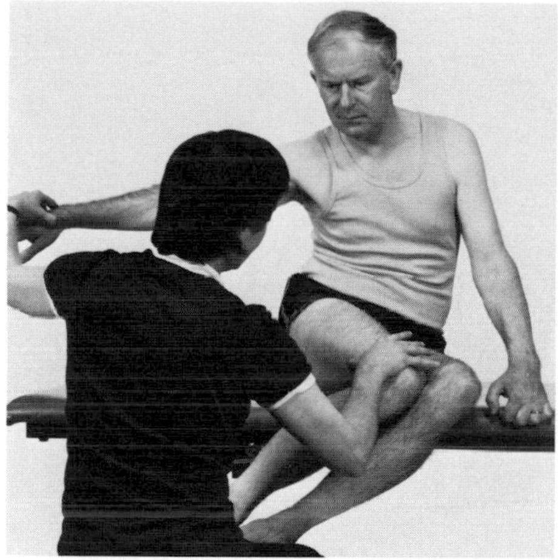

Fig. 7.4. Stimulating head and trunk reactions. The therapist holds the sound hand as a safety measure (left hemiplegia)

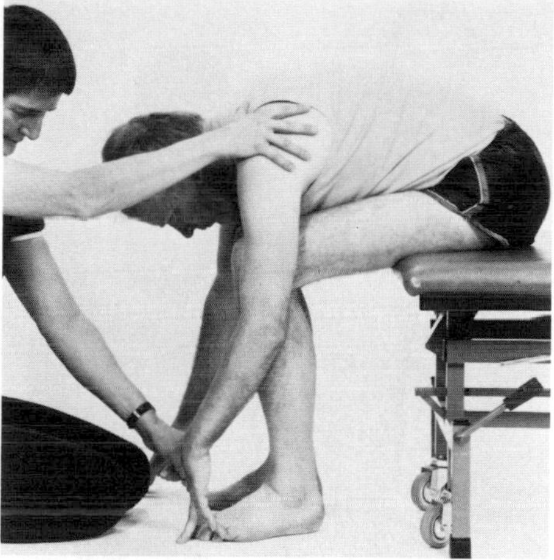

Fig. 7.5. The patient touches his toes with both feet remaining flat on the floor (left hemiplegia)

peats the movement to the other side, and later can increase the speed and change the direction unexpectedly, as the patient's reactions improve.

7.1.5 Reaching Forward to Touch the Floor

The therapist kneels in front of the patient, whose feet are supported on the floor. She guides his hands forward to touch his toes, making him aware that his hemiplegic hand must arrive first (Fig. 7.5). Both the patient's feet should stay flat on the floor without pushing, and it may require a careful progression, coming at first only so far forward that he is able to return to sitting upright without his heels coming off the floor. The patient can also practise reaching down to his feet with his hands clasped.

7.1.6 Reaching Forward with Clasped Hands

The patient stretches his clasped hands forward and in all directions, while the feet remain flat on the floor, with the therapist supporting the hemiplegic knee at first. Interest and automatic reactions can be stimulated by letting him push a ball away in various directions or by hitting a balloon to another person.

7.2 Activities in Standing with the Weight on Both Legs

7.2.1 Both Knees Flexed – Weight Transference Sideways

From the starting position the patient transfers his weight from side to side with his hips slightly flexed, and rotating as if he were skiing. His arms swing relaxed at his

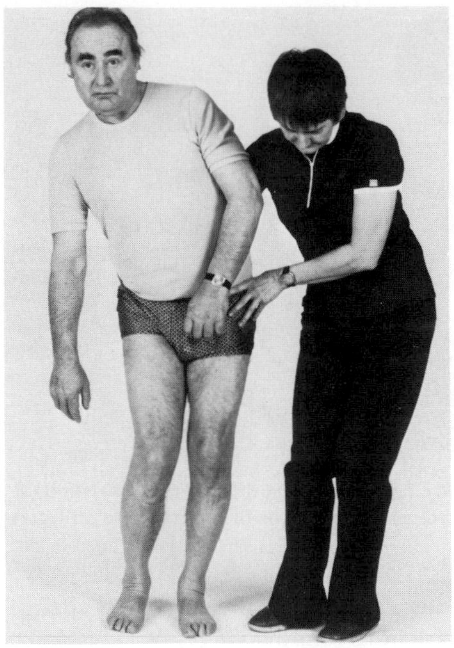

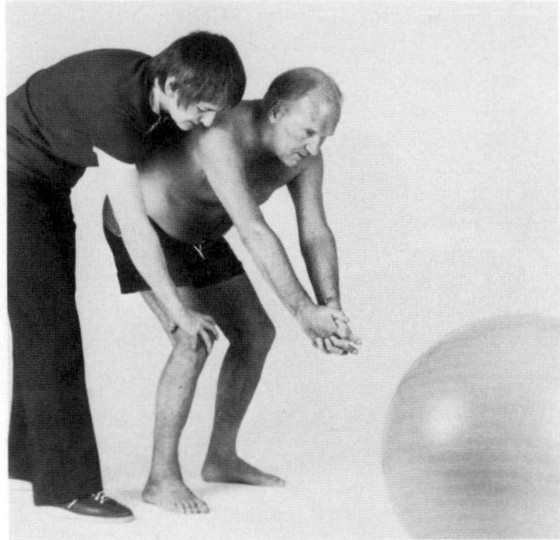

Fig. 7.7. Pushing a ball helps to overcome the patient's fear of leaning forwards while standing (right hemiplegia)

◁ **Fig. 7.6.** Transferring weight over the hemiplegic side in standing. Both knees are flexed (left hemiplegia)

side. The therapist facilitates the movement with her hands on either side of his pelvis, keeping his hips forward and assisting the rotation (Fig. 7.6).

7.2.2 Pushing a Ball Away with Clasped Hands

Patients are often afraid of bringing their weight forward, but when concentrating on an activity such as pushing a ball away, they do so spontaneously. The therapist facilitates the movement with her hands on either side of the pelvis, steadying the patient while keeping his weight over both legs (Fig. 7.7). The activity can also be practised while walk-standing, to encourage the weight coming forward over one leg.

7.2.3 Playing with a Balloon

The patient plays with a balloon, hitting it away or tapping it repeatedly into the air with his clasped hands. As balance and the ability to take steps improves, he can be encouraged to step forwards while he keeps the balloon up in the air (see Fig. 8.11 a).

7.2.4 Being Tipped Backwards

When being tipped backwards, the patient must relearn the normal balance reactions. At first the therapist gives him total support, and guides the forwards move-

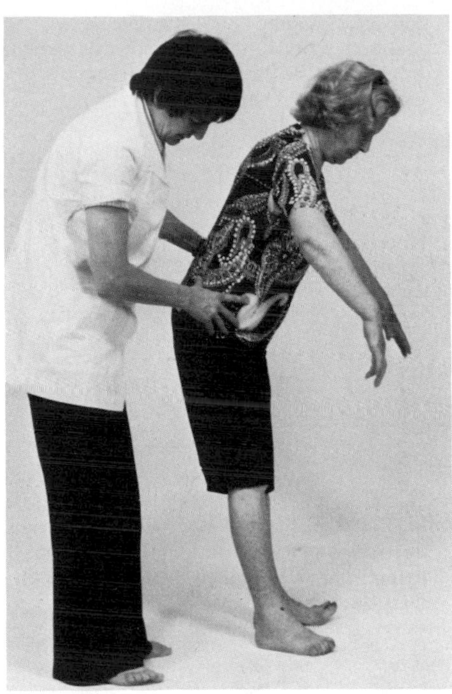

Fig. 7.8. Training balance reactions by tipping the patient backwards while she is standing (right hemiplegia)

ment of the trunk and arms. The patient tends to remain extended at the hips and fall over backwards if the correct reaction is not carefully trained. The movement is carried out slowly with the patient voluntarily correcting the position of his head, trunk and arms. The speed is later increased until the reaction occurs automatically even when the therapist suddenly shifts the patient backwards from the pelvis, without giving him any warning (Fig. 7.8). Because dorsal extension of the feet is a normal part of the balance reaction, the movement is also useful for stimulating activity in the hemiplegic foot.

7.3 Activities in Standing with the Weight on the Hemiplegic Leg

If the patient is to walk confidently without support, he needs to be able to bear weight on the hemiplegic leg without fear of losing his balance. Taking weight through the leg makes him aware of it, improves sensation and normalises tone. The hip should remain extended and at no time should the affected knee hyperextend.

Hyperextension of the knee is caused by the retraction of the pelvis on the hemiplegic side, and the inadequate active hip extension. The leg becomes a rigid pillar as a result, usually with the foot pushing into plantar flexion in the total pattern of extension. Because the support is then static, it makes normal dynamic balance reactions impossible, and to take a quick step with that leg to regain balance is difficult if not impossible.

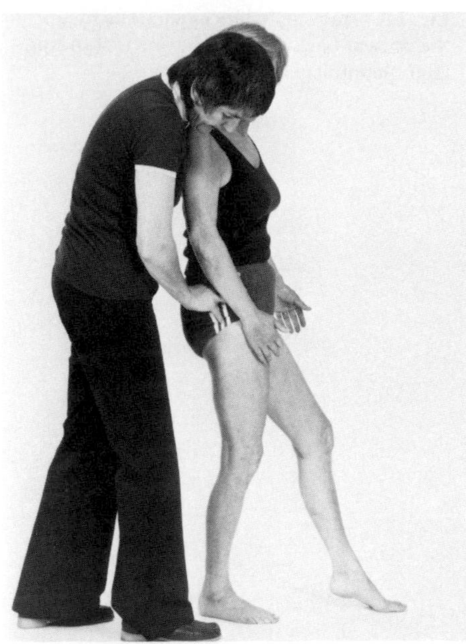

Fig. 7.9. Standing on the hemiplegic leg, taking steps forwards and backwards with the other foot. The therapist assists the hip extension (right hemiplegia)

Fig. 7.10 a, b. Stainding on the hemiplegic leg the patient places his foot on a step (right hemiplegia). **a** With the step in front; **b** with the step at the side

▽

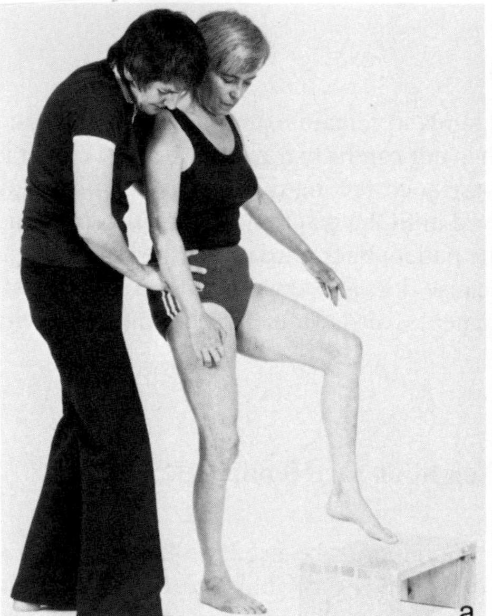

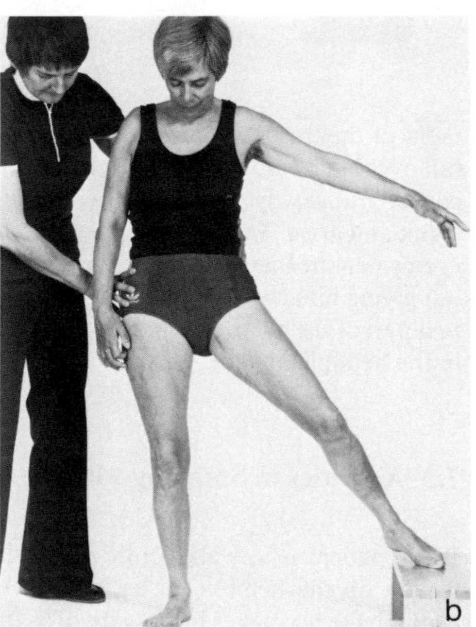

During weight-bearing activities, the therapist helps the patient to prevent the knee from hyperextending by tilting his pelvis posteriorly, i.e. by assisting hip extension.

1. Standing with his weight over the hemiplegic leg, the patient takes small steps forwards and backwards with his other foot, and also to the side. He does not trans-

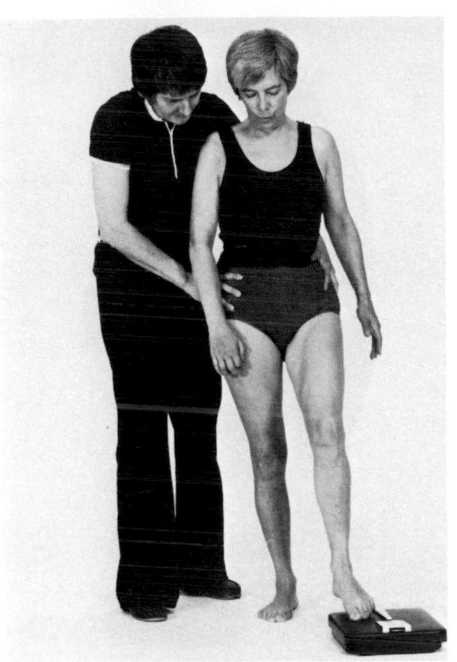

Fig. 7.11. Standing on the hemiplegic leg, placing the sound foot gently on a scale (right hemiplegia)

fer his weight immediately on to the sound leg, but remains steadily on the hemiplegic leg (Fig. 7.9).

2. The patient places his sound foot on a small step in front of him. He puts it slowly and carefully on the step, without rushing or banging it down (Fig. 7.10a). While balancing on the hemiplegic leg he can tap the sound foot lightly and rhythmically on the step, later tapping his foot first to one side and then the other as his control improves. If the step is placed to the side of the patient, control of extension of the hemiplegic hip with abduction will be stimulated. He places his foot on the step without transferring his weight away from the affected leg (Fig. 7.10b).
3. Standing with his weight over the hemiplegic leg, the patient moves or kicks a football with his other foot. He kicks the ball against a wall or to another person but only so vigorously that he is still able to control the hemiplegic leg and prevent it from pushing into the total extension pattern.
4. The patient places his sound foot on a scale, which can be placed in different positions in front or to the side of him. He tries to reduce the registered weight until he can achieve zero from the moment his foot touches the scale (Fig. 7.11).

   Both the activities with the ball and the scale are valuable because they encourage the patient to balance on his hemiplegic leg without holding his head in a fixed position to stabilise himself. He automatically looks at the ball to kick it, or at the scale to read the figures.
5. Standing with his back to a high plinth, the patient places his unaffected foot gently on the knee of the therapist, who is kneeling in front of him (Fig. 7.12). He then puts his foot behind him while still maintaining all his weight forward over the hemiplegic leg. The advantage of the therapist being in this position is that she

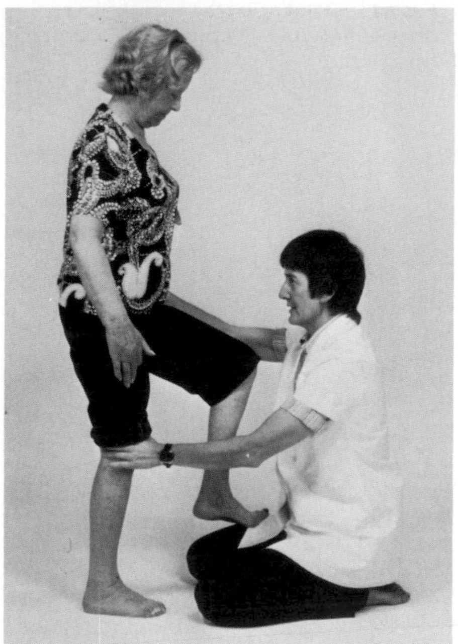

Fig. 7.12. Standing on the hemiplegic leg and placing the sound foot on the therapist's knee. The patient's knee does not hyperextend (right hemiplegia)

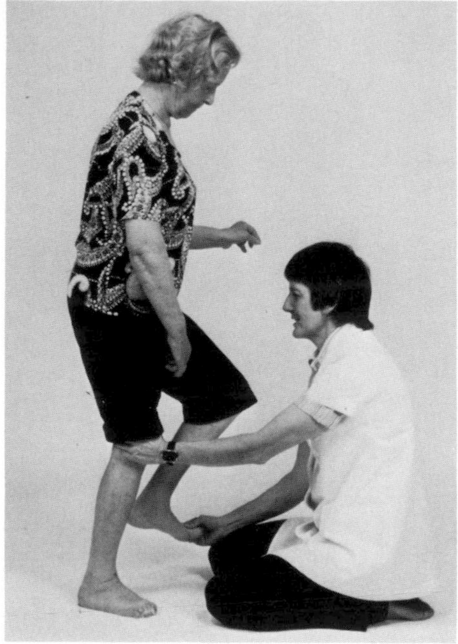

Fig. 7.13. The therapist moves the patient's sound foot in different directions (right hemiplegia)

can facilitate his hip and knee to encourage dynamic weight-bearing as he extends and flexes his knee. She can also place her fingers under the toes of the hemiplegic foot, to prevent them from clawing and to facilitate balance reactions in the foot.

As the patient's ability to balance on his hemiplegic leg improves, the therapist can hold his sound foot with one hand and move it slowly into different positions while the patient adapts accordingly (Fig. 7.13). During the whole activity the patient's hands are left free, not clasped, as spontaneous movements may occur while he balances on one leg.

7.4 Activities Where the Weight Is on Alternate Legs

7.4.1 Going up and down Stairs

Climbing stairs brings an automatic transference of weight, first over one leg and then over the other. It is a familiar activity for adults and often produces a very normal pattern of movement for the patients. The activity can be used with patients who may still not be able to walk unaided, and their walking improves as a result. The ability to negotiate stairs easily is also an important part of full rehabilitation, as we come across stairs frequently in our daily life. Right from the beginning the patient is helped to go up and down stairs in a normal way i. e. forwards, one foot after the other, and not with both feet coming on to the same step.

The procedure for going up stairs is as follows:

1. The patient holds on to the bannister with his sound hand if he or the therapist feel uncertain in any way. He should be encouraged to hold as lightly as possible and not support his whole forearm on the bannister. The patient transfers his weight over his hemiplegic leg and places his other foot on the first step (Fig. 7.14a).
2. As he transfers his weight well forward over the sound foot in front, the therapist slides one hand down over his other knee to the shin, and with a circular motion places that foot up on to the second step (Fig. 7.14b). Most patients require such help at first because, with the hip in extension, extensor tonus throughout the leg is increased and sufficient active flexion of the hip and knee is not possible. The therapist places her other hand round to the opposite side of the pelvis, using her arm and hand to steady the patient while his hemiplegic leg is lifted.
3. Immediately the affected foot is in place, the therapist moves her hand on to the patient's thigh, pressing downwards and forwards to draw his knee forward over the foot as he steps up with the sound leg. At no time does either knee fully extend, but instead a rhythmical cycling-type movement takes place as in the normal pattern.

As the patient's ability and confidence improve the activity is carried out with his hands clasped together in front of him (Fig. 7.14c) or with his arms free (Fig. 7.14d). The therapist feels when the patient is actively controlling the movement of his legs, and moves her hands so that she only gives support to either side of the pelvis. The amount of support is gradually reduced until finally he can manage alone.

For most patients, going down stairs is more difficult than climbing up stairs, particularly when stepping down with the hemiplegic leg. As the leg is brought forward, it pulls strongly into adduction across in front of the other leg, and the foot inverts in the total pattern of extension. The patient is unable to place the foot flat on the next step, or has difficulty in doing so. He may also feel apprehensive looking down the flight of stairs. The procedure is as follows:

1. The patient holds the handrail lightly and the therapist, standing at his hemiplegic side, asks him to step down first with his sound leg. With one hand placed just above his affected knee she draws the knee forward into sufficient flexion to allow the other foot to reach the step below (Fig. 7.15a). Her other hand is placed on the far side of his pelvis, and her arm around his back helps to bring his hips forward over the foot in front.
2. The hand on the hemiplegic leg remains in the same position, as the patient brings his leg forward. When the leg starts to adduct, the therapist guides it outwards, and once again uses her other arm from behind to bring his pelvis forwards (Fig. 7.15b).
3. When the patient's foot is correctly placed on the step below, the therapist draws his knee forward to prevent the leg pushing into total extension as he starts to bear weight on it (Fig. 7.15c). He then steps forwards with the sound leg.

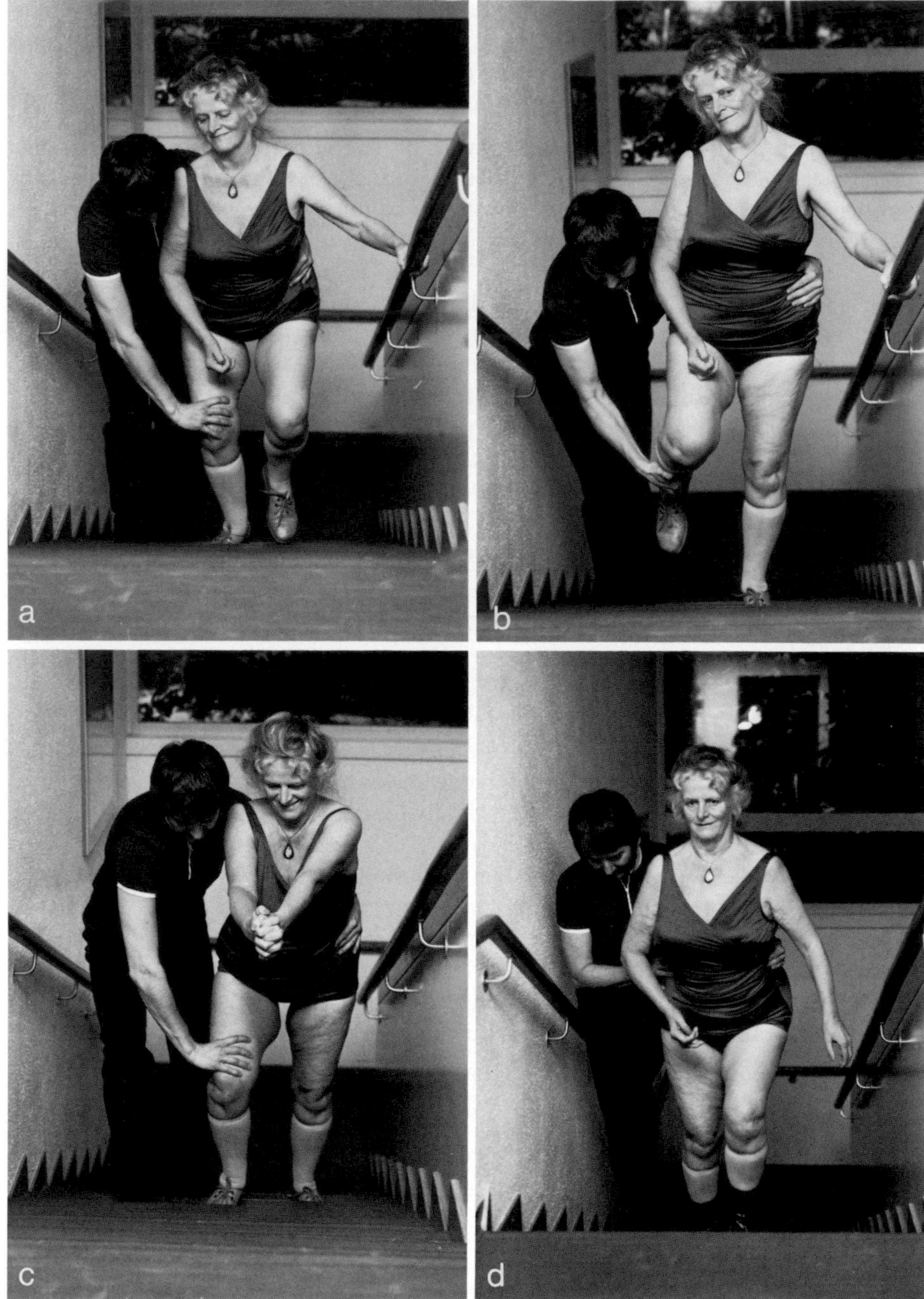

Fig. 7.14 a–d. Going upstairs (right hemiplegia). **a** With the weight on the hemiplegic leg, the patient brings her sound foot to the step above. **b** The therapist slides her hand down over the shin and with a circular motion helps to place the hemiplegic foot on the next step. **c** The therapist draws the patient's knee forwards as she steps up with her sound foot. Feeling more confident, the patient clasps her hands. **d** The patient no longer needs to hold on to the bannister, and the therapist has reduced her support

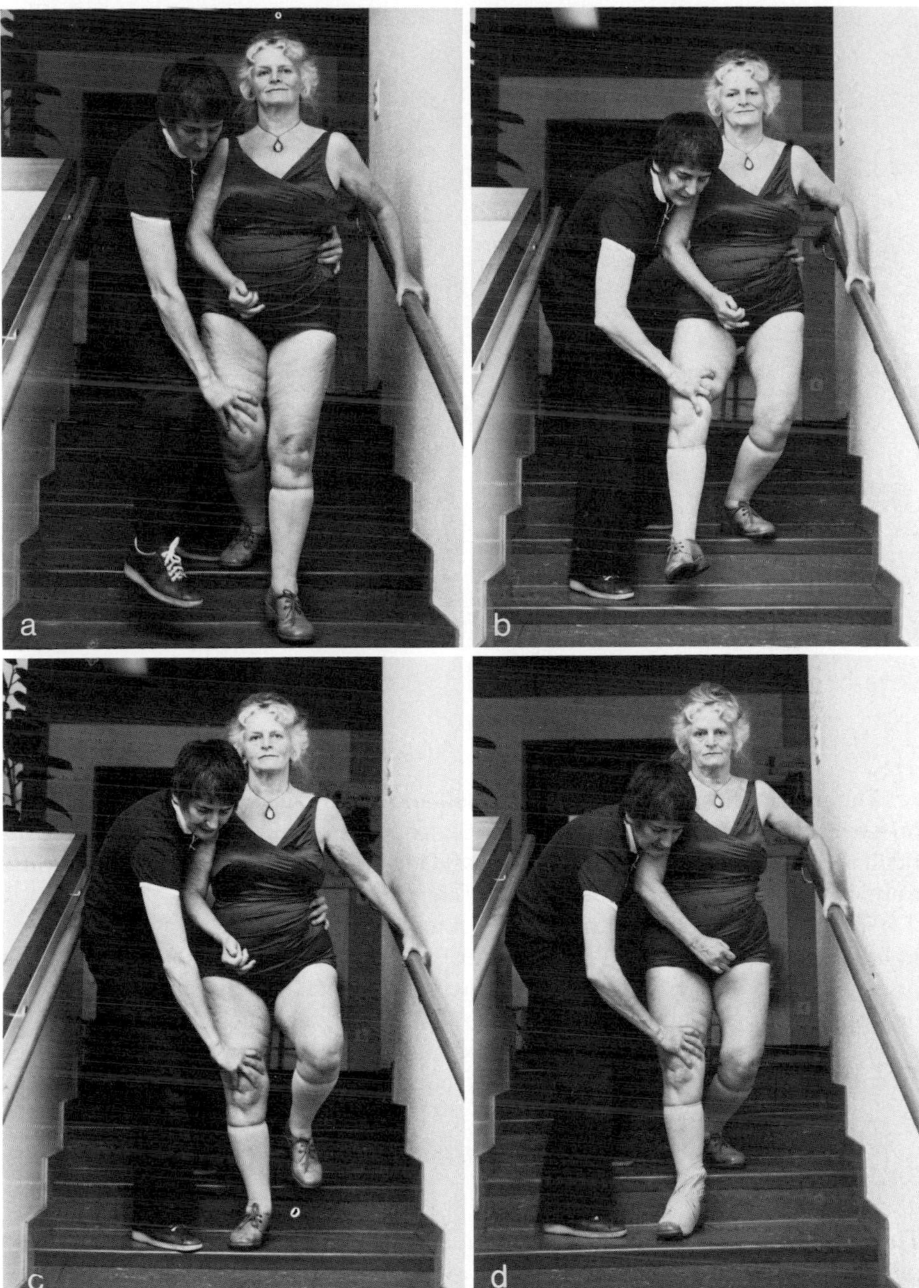

Fig. 7.15 a–e. Going downstairs (right hemiplegia). **a** The patient steps down first with her sound foot. The therapist draws the hemiplegic knee forwards. **b** As the patient steps down with her hemiplegic foot the therapist prevents adduction. **c** When the hemiplegic foot is in place the therapist helps the patient to bring her weight forwards without hyperextending the knee. **d** A bandage prevents supination of the foot during early training. **e** The patient steadies herself with the sound hand on the wall as she no longer needs to hold the handrail

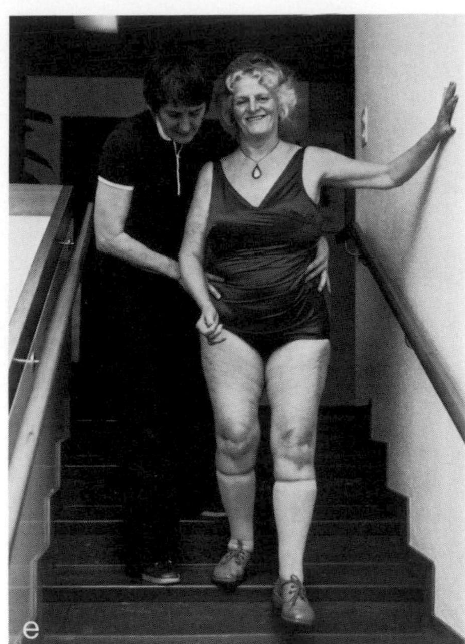

Fig. 7.15e (caption see page 111)

The patient must be carefully instructed and encouraged to place only one foot on each step right from the first attempt. Should the inversion of the foot be too difficult to control at first, the foot can be bandaged firmly for protection during early training to give patient and therapist confidence (Fig. 7.15 d).

When the patient has learnt the correct movement sequence he no longer needs to hold on to the handrail. As an intermediate stage he steadies himself by placing his sound hand on the wall at his side (Fig. 7.15 e). When he feels sufficiently secure he stops using the hand for support, and the therapist facilitates balance and movement from the pelvis. Once again she gradually withdraws her support until he can go confidently up or down stairs without requiring help at all (see Chap. 9).

7.4.2 Moving on the Tilt-Board

The tilt-board can be useful when retraining balance reactions in standing. Even patients who are not yet able to walk without assistance learn to transfer their weight correctly as they feel and see the movement of the board, and the controls are very clear. The board tilts sideways or forwards until it meets the absolute resistance of the floor. To avoid any anxiety for the patient, the therapist can give him complete support at first by placing both her arms around him, if necessary, and drawing him towards her until he feels more confident. She then gradually withdraws the assistance.

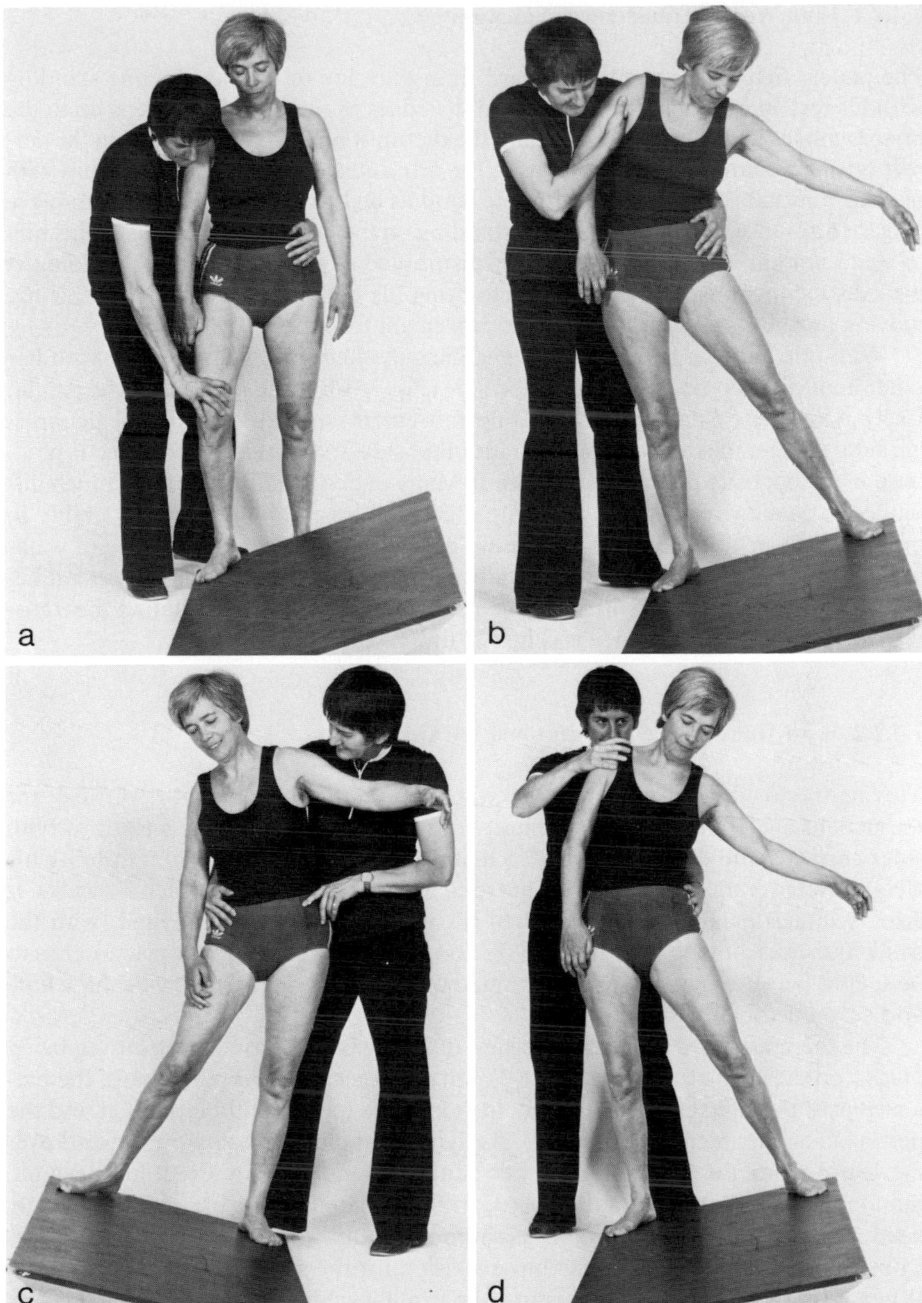

Fig. 7.16a–d. Moving the tilt-board sideways (right hemiplegia). **a** Stepping on to the board with the hemiplegic foot first. The therapist guides the knee forwards. **b** Transferring weight to the hemiplegic side. The therapist lengthens the side of the trunk, and her hip maintains extension of the patient's hip. **c** Transferring the weight to the sound leg. The therapist has changed her position so that the patient moves towards her. **d** The therapist reduces the amount of support

7.4.2.1 With Weight Transference Sideways

The patient first learns to tilt the board from one side to the other while standing with his feet apart and placed parallel to the edges of the board. He steps on to the board with his hemiplegic foot first and the therapist helps him to place it in the correct position. Standing close to him on the affected side she supports his hip with her hip, and stabilises his knee with one hand as he brings his other foot into place (Fig. 7.16 a). Once the patient is safely standing on the board, the therapist helps him to stand upright with his weight evenly distributed over both legs. Still standing at his side, the therapist asks the patient to bring his weight towards her with his hip moving first, and facilitates the correct movement for him.

With one hand in his axilla she lengthens the hemiplegic side, while with her other hand she shortens the unaffected side (Fig. 7.16 b). The patient's arms remain freely at his sides. When he can repeat the movement correctly towards the hemiplegic side, the therapist moves round to his other side and the same sequence is practised in the opposite direction (Fig. 7.16 c). Many patients will have just as much difficulty in coming correctly over the unaffected side, and will need this ability in order to take an easy step with the hemiplegic leg during the swing phase of walking. When the movement to both sides becomes easier, the therapist can stand behind the patient making small adjustments to his posture, and facilitating the transference of weight from his pelvis (Fig. 7.16 d).

7.4.2.2 With Transference Forwards and Backwards

Moving the weight forwards and backwards on the tilt-board is more difficult for the patient and should not be attempted until he can transfer his weight to both sides correctly and confidently. The activity is useful as it teaches him to bring his weight well over the supporting leg in front, as he will need to do when he walks. It also facilitates balance reactions when his weight is on the leg behind, with the trunk and arms moving forward with flexion at the hips. The correct reaction has to be taught because patients tend to come backwards in one piece, with the whole body extended.

The therapist helps the patient to step on to the board, his hemiplegic leg being placed on the edge of the board first. When the other foot is on the board, the patient places his affected foot carefully in front. The feet should be parallel and the pelvis facing symmetrically forwards. As the patient moves his weight forward over the leg in front, the therapist uses her hands as required to correct his position. Standing on the floor next to the board, and at his hemiplegic side, she will usually need to place one hand flat on his sternum while the other hand guides his pelvis from behind to achieve adequate hip extension for the supporting leg (Fig. 7.17 a). When he moves his weight backwards, she facilitates hip flexion and the necessary forward inclination of his trunk (Fig. 7.17 b).

The same activity is also practised with the hemiplegic leg behind, which is more difficult as extension must be maintained despite the considerable dorsiflexion at the ankle and the possibly disturbed sensation in the leg which he can no longer see.

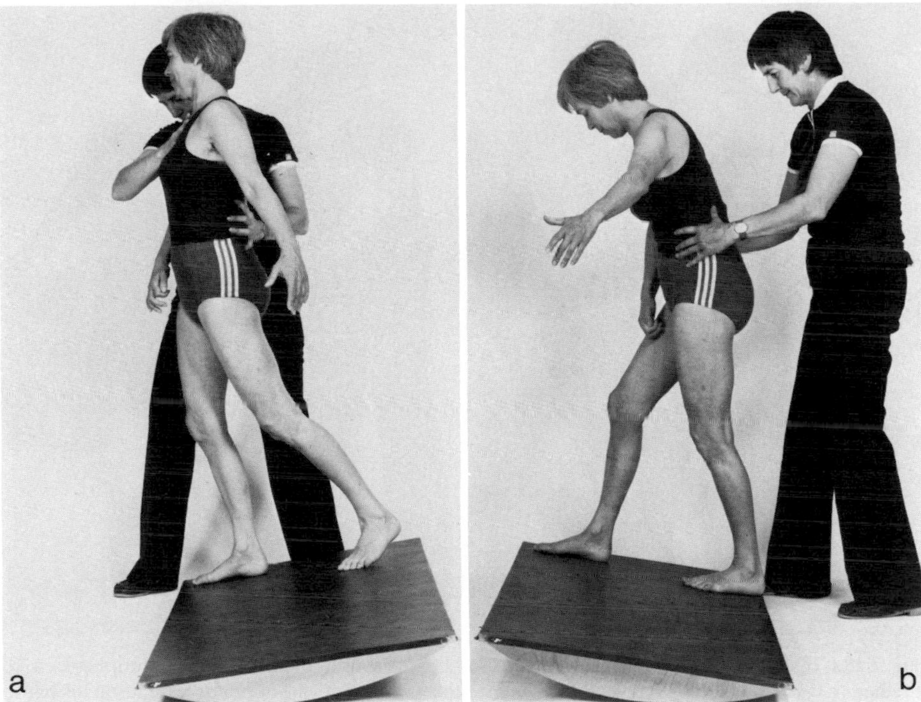

Fig. 7.17a, b. Moving the tilt-board forwards and backwards (right hemiplegia). **a** With the weight transferred over the leg in front. The therapist uses her hands as required to facilitate the correct movement. **b** With the weight transferred to the leg behind. The therapist facilitates the forward inclination of the trunk

7.4.3 Stepping Sideways with One Leg Crossing over in Front of the Other

The ability to take steps sideways is an important part of our balance and saving mechanism. The activity also teaches the patient to transfer his weight over alternate sides. It is first carried out slowly and correctly with facilitation, and is practised until the patient can take rapid automatic steps when he is displaced sideways to either side.

7.4.3.1 Moving Towards the Hemiplegic Side

The patient brings his weight over the affected leg, and steps across in front with the other leg, taking care that his knee does not snap back into hyperextension as he does so. The therapist facilitates the movement with her hands on either side of his pelvis, helping to prevent retraction on the affected side. The movement requires considerable adduction of the supporting leg and elongation of the hemiplegic side. If necessary, the therapist elongates the side with one hand in the patient's axilla as he brings his weight well over the affected leg (Fig. 7.18a).

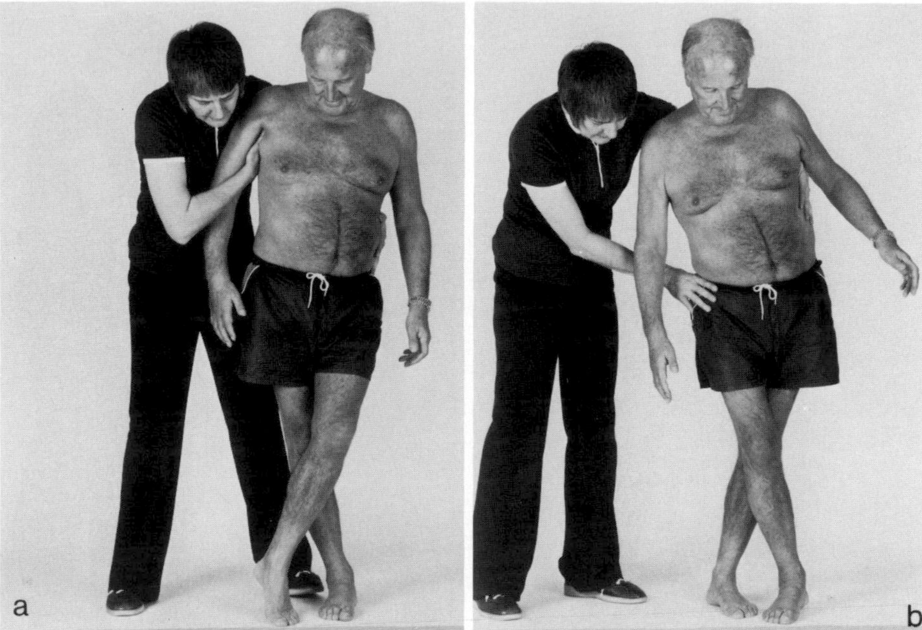

Fig. 7.18 a, b. Walking sideways with one leg crossing in front of the other (right hemiplegia). **a** To the hemiplegic side. The patient steps across with the sound foot without hyperextending his hemiplegic knee. The therapist facilitates the elongation of the side. **b** To the sound side. The therapist assists the forward and downward movement of the pelvis

7.4.3.2 Moving Towards the Sound Side

The normal movement sequence is the same, but because of the patient's difficulties the facilitation required is different. When taking a step across sideways with his hemiplegic leg he needs help to adduct it, and to release the whole side in order to place the foot flat on the floor. The therapist assists by pressing firmly down on the iliac crest, and by helping to transfer his weight over the leg (Fig. 7.18 b). She also helps him to maintain hip extension as he takes the next step sideways with the sound leg.

Walking sideways behind a line on the floor increases the degree of control and difficulty. The patient otherwise compensates by walking sideways along a diagonal path. An unrolled bandage can be used to indicate the line.

7.5 Activities in Standing with the Weight on the Sound Leg

The patient must be able to stand effortlessly on the sound foot with the hemiplegic leg relaxed as a prerequisite for the normal swing phase of walking. To practise the ability the therapist kneels in front of the patient and lifts his affected foot into the air, with increasing rapidity and with less and less warning or preparation. Finally, the patient should be able to allow his foot to be lowered right to the floor without its pushing down at all (Fig. 7.19).

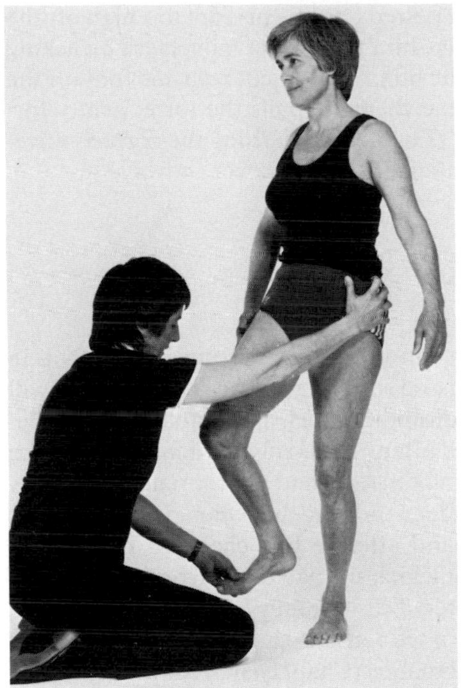

Fig. 7.19. Standing on the sound leg, the patient controls the hemiplegic leg through range without it pushing into extension (right hemiplegia)

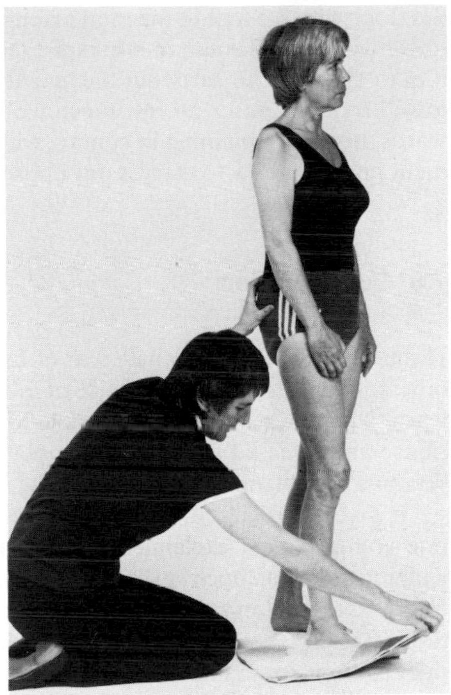

Fig. 7.20. The hemiplegic foot is drawn forwards on a towel while the patient concentrates on giving no resistance to the movement (right hemiplegia)

For the many patients who have difficulty transferring their weight adequately over the sound side in order to leave the hemiplegic leg free to swing forward, activities in which the hemiplegic foot moves an actual object will often enable him to transfer his weight spontaneously.

7.5.1 Kicking a Football with the Affected Foot

The ball is placed in front of the patient in such a position that he can step forwards first with his sound leg and then swing his hemiplegic leg forwards to kick the ball. Alternatively, the therapist can help him to place his foot behind him prior to the kick. He should not attempt to kick when his feet are next to each other, as he will then flex his leg actively to do so, instead of swinging it forwards as in walking. Kicking a ball is a familiar movement, learnt in childhood, and it is amazing how it enables a patient to produce a normal movement, even though he may be unable to move his leg on command. Patients of all ages enjoy the activity enormously.

7.5.2 Sliding a Towel or Piece of Paper Forward with the Affected Foot

With his foot placed on a towel the patient slides it forward and is helped to bring it back again. If the movement is difficult for him at first because he pushes against the floor with his foot in the total extension pattern, or lifts his foot too high off the towel with total flexion, the therapist teaches him the correct movement by asking him to allow her to carry out the activity for him. The patient rests his foot on the towel, trying to offer no resistance while the therapist pulls the towel gently forwards, his foot remaining in contact with it (Fig. 7.20). By feeling the correct movement he learns how to carry it out himself, and slowly takes over actively.

7.6 Considerations

Human beings have an innate fear of falling, more marked in some people than in others. Through actual experience of falling and suffering pain as a result, some will learn to fear even more. Many people with disabilities such as hemiplegia will experience an increased fear for which they are often mistakenly admonished or even sent to a psychiatrist, although the fear is quite natural and appropriate.

It is very difficult for the therapist to understand why the patient is so afraid. As one young patient exclaimed to her husband after he had chastised her for not walking across an open space similar to that which she had crossed only the day before, "But you don't know what I see and feel!" It is perhaps easier to understand the fear experienced by hemiplegic patients if we consider that usually all or most of the reactions for maintaining or regaining balance (Chap. 2) are reduced if not absent altogether, unless they are carefully retrained.

To summarize:

1. The head is held in a fixed position by hypertonus, by over-activity on the unaffected side or by a posture which the patient adapts to stabilize himself, and so it cannot move freely to help him to balance.
2. The trunk fails to shorten and lengthen appropriately due to hypertonus or hypotonus and over-activity of the unaffected side.
3. The legs fail to abduct to serve as a counterweight, and the patient is unable to take quick steps to save himself. The hemiplegic leg reacts too slowly due to spasticity, and he is often unable to take a quick step with the sound leg because to do so would entail weight-bearing on the hemiplegic leg.
4. The hemiplegic arm is not able to react either in extension and abduction or in protective extension. Hypertonus pulls it against the patient's side, or hypotonus renders it incapable of springing into action. The untrained patient is therefore left with only his unaffected hand to help him to maintain his balance, either by holding on to something or pushing against a supporting surface. When he is standing or walking this means leaning on a stick, and even then he is not protected against falling to the hemiplegic side or backwards. Only a small movement away from the mid-line would be sufficient to cause him to lose his balance, as the stick will leave the floor.

If the patient is to move freely without fear and walk without a walking-stick, his balance reactions must be re-established and some form of protective mechanism made possible. For all the tasks in his daily life he needs to be able to use his unaffected hand functionally, and he cannot do so when he is totally dependent on it for maintaining his balance. The restoration of balance reactions therefore plays an important role in successful rehabiliatation. Even patients who show little return of voluntary muscle activity in the arm and leg can relearn the balance reactions remarkably well and recover the ability to take quick steps to regain balance when standing or walking. Only when balance is adequate will fear disappear.

8 Encouraging the Return of Activity in the Arm and Hand and Minimising Associated Reactions

Because rehabilitation strives to teach the patient to walk again and to be independent in the activities of daily living, his arm and hand tend to be neglected. The patient becomes more and more skilled in managing all activities with one hand, and the full potential in the affected hand may never be fully developed. Even if no activity appears in the arm and hand it is important to treat them, as each part of the body effects the other parts. If the arm shows a marked associated reaction, pulling strongly in the spastic pattern of flexion, it will influence how the patient walks, hamper balance reactions and interfere with the activities of his daily life. Cosmetically, he will be distressed by the constant pulling up of the arm.

From the onset of the illness, the patient's arm must be kept fully mobile and the spastic flexion pattern inhibited. As many of the following activities as possible should be carried out carefully even when the arm is still hypotonic. The full inhibition of spasticity in the arm and trunk and the facilitation of any active movement possible is an integral part of the treatment during all stages of the rehabilitation. The following sequences, with the patient lying, sitting and standing, show how the spasticity in the arm can be reduced by proximal and distal inhibition, and how active movement can be stimulated. If any of the movements is limited by painful shortening of the various muscle groups, the therapist must work carefully but determinedly to regain the lost extensibility. Pain or contracture will inhibit the return of active movement, or prevent the patient from being able to use what movement he has.

8.1 Activities in Supine Lying

1. Before moving the arm, the therapist reduces the spasticity in the trunk to allow the scapula to move freely. She elongates the side and brings the pelvis forward, placing the leg in a flexed position with the knee leaning across the other leg (Fig. 8.1 a). The therapist works until the pelvis remains forward on the affected side and the leg lies without having to be held in the required position. If the tone is really reduced, the leg and pelvis will stay in place without the patient having to hold the position actively, or the therapist placing a sandbag or pillow to stabilise the buttock or foot. Should the leg push into extension or the knee fall sideways during the arm activities, the therapist must then repeat the inhibition of the side before continuing. The passive maintenance of the position of the leg is her indication that the tone is not increasing, and the leg must therefore not be held in place mechanically.

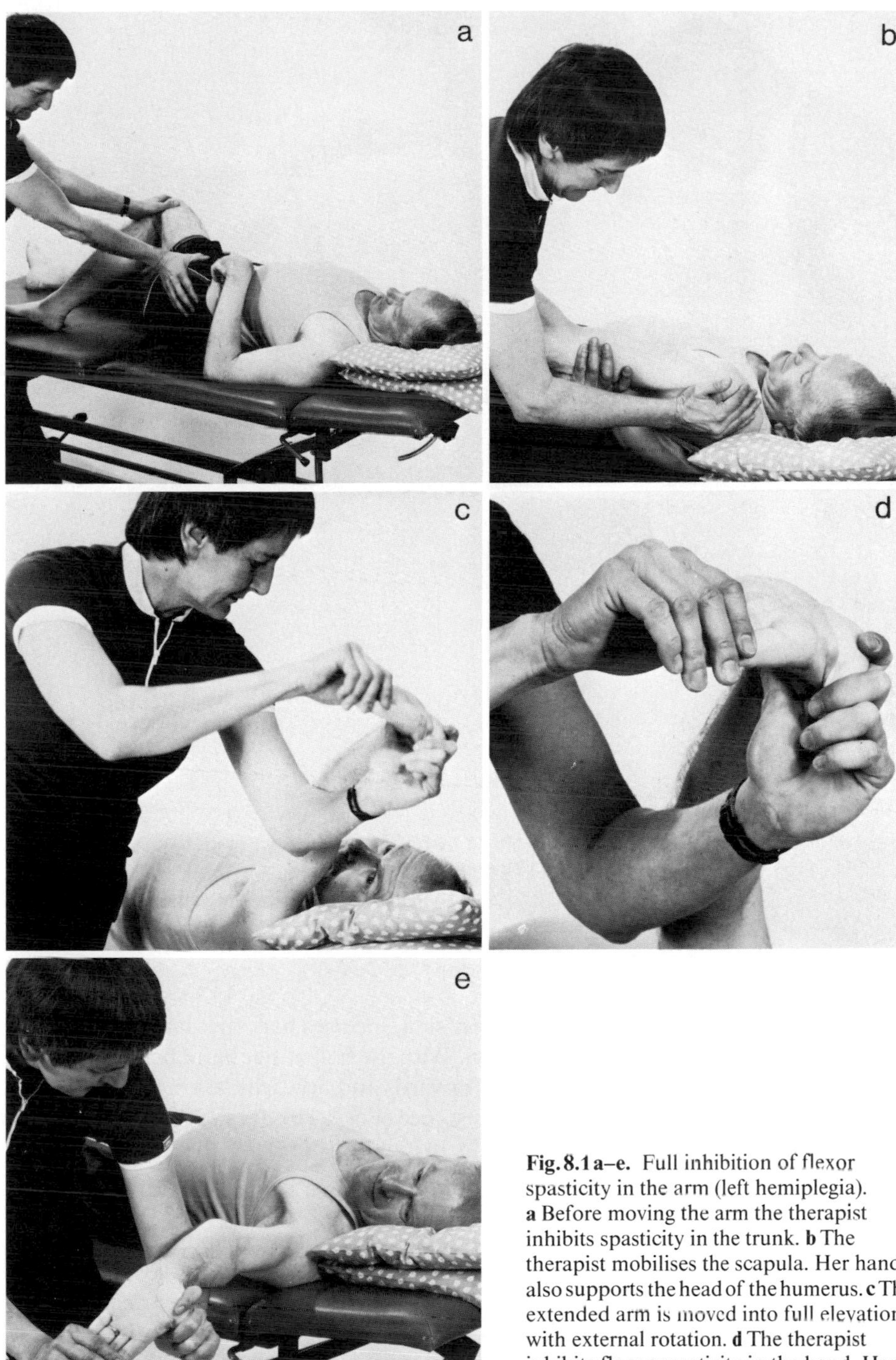

Fig. 8.1 a–e. Full inhibition of flexor spasticity in the arm (left hemiplegia). **a** Before moving the arm the therapist inhibits spasticity in the trunk. **b** The therapist mobilises the scapula. Her hand also supports the head of the humerus. **c** The extended arm is moved into full elevation with external rotation. **d** The therapist inhibits flexor spasticity in the hand. Her thumb on the dorsum of the wrist gives counter-pressure. **e** The arm is taken into abduction at an angle of 90° to the body.

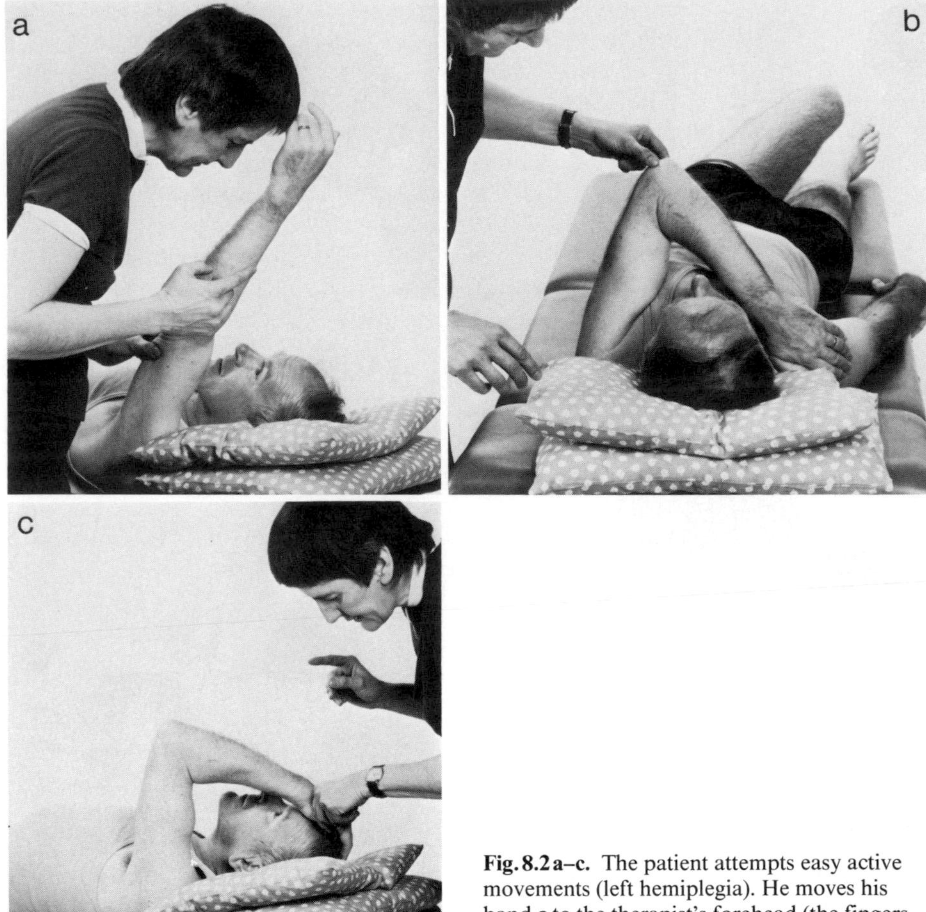

Fig. 8.2 a–c. The patient attempts easy active movements (left hemiplegia). He moves his hand **a** to the therapist's forehead (the fingers remain relaxed), **b** to his opposite shoulder and **c** to rest on his own head

2. Cradling the hemiplegic arm against her side, she uses her other hand to move his scapula into elevation with protraction. With the ball of her hand below the spine of the scapula she moves the scapula forwards and upwards, asking the patient to try to allow the movement without resistance (Fig. 8.1 b). As she moves the scapula the spasticity is reduced both proximally and distally, and the therapist brings the arm slowly into outward rotation.
3. Once the scapula is moving easily the therapist brings the arm forwards and upwards into elevation while maintaining protraction of the scapula and extension at the elbow. She then opens the hand by drawing the thumb out of the palm and dorsally extending the wrist and fingers fully (Fig. 8.1 c). The therapist's thumb against the dorsal aspect of the wrist provides a pivot enabling her to overcome the resistance offered by the flexors of the wrist and fingers (Fig. 8.1 d).
4. When full elevation of the extended arm has been achieved, the therapist should also move the arm into horizontal abduction with supination of the forearm.

With her elbow beneath the patient's elbow she holds it in extension and at the same time prevents the shoulder from pulling into retraction (Fig. 8.1 c). The movement ensures the maintenance of full extensibility of the flexor muscles acting on the shoulder and of the internal rotators.

5. When the spasticity in the arm has been inhibited and passive movement is possible without resistance, the patient can attempt to move his arm actively, but without effort. The therapist asks him to let his hand remain against her forehead (Fig. 8.2 a). He can then take his hand to his other shoulder, with the appropriate amount of assistance, and try to let it stay there without the arm pulling into the total pattern of flexion (Fig. 8.2 b). Similarly, he can move his hand to his own head and let it rest there (Fig. 8.2 c) and then move it again to the therapist's forehead.
6. More difficult for the patient is the attempt to let the arm remain in different positions, with the hand free, i.e. placing (Fig. 8.3 a). He must learn to grade movement in this way if he is to use the arm and hand for different functions. The degree of difficulty is increased by placing the arm in more and more complex positions, i.e. those positions which are more influenced by the spastic patterns or mass synergies. For example, the patient slowly lowers the arm to his side without the elbow flexing or the hand clenching (Fig. 8.3 b).

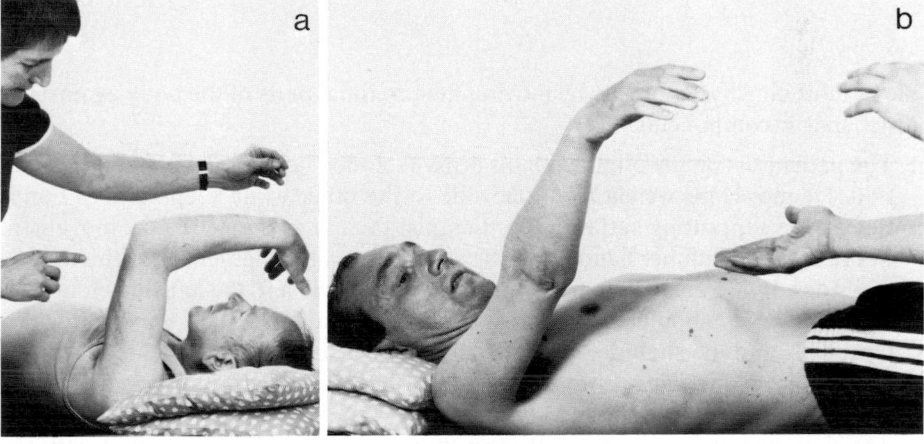

Fig. 8.3 a, b. Placing the arm with the hand free. **a** In different degrees of flexion (left hemiplegia); **b** lowering it to his side with the elbow extended and the fingers relaxed (right hemiplegia)

8.2 Activities in Sitting

In our daily life we use our hands mainly when we are sitting or standing; we get dressed, eat, write, work and play in these positions. The patient is therefore preferably treated in the sitting and standing positions when attempting to move actively with facilitation. These positions also enable the therapist to use the valuable princi-

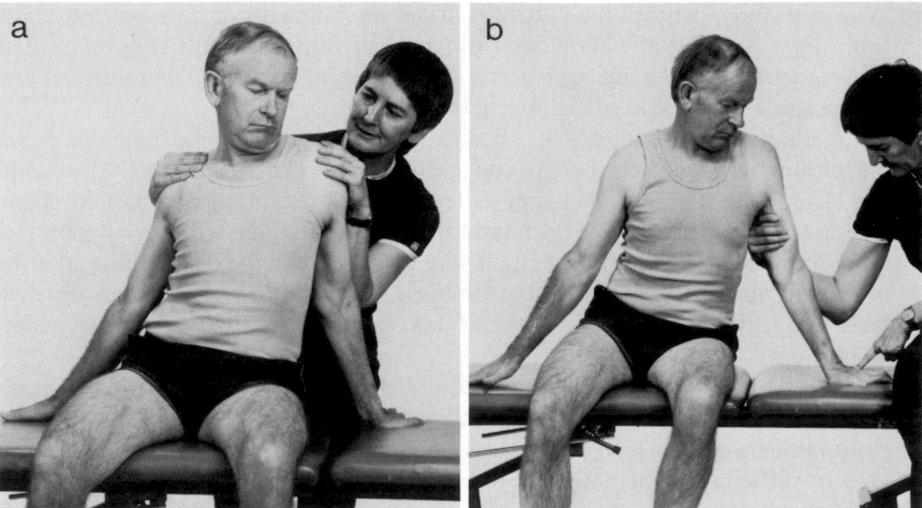

Fig. 8.4 a, b. Inhibiting hypertonus in the arm by moving the body proximally against the distal spastic components (left hemiplegia). **a** With arms extended and his hands flat on the table behind him the patient moves from side to side. **b** With the hemiplegic arm supported beside him in extension, the patient brings his weight towards the arm. The scapula elevates and the hand remains extended

ple of inhibiting hypertonicity by moving the proximal parts of the body against the distal spastic components.

1. The patient sits on the plinth with his arms extended behind him in outward rotation. He moves his weight from one side to the other while keeping both hands flat on the supporting surface. The therapist facilitates the necessary movement of the scapula with her hands, and the shortening and lengthening of the respective sides. When the patient transfers his weight to the left, the left side elongates, allowing the left shoulder girdle and scapula to elevate. The right side shortens reciprocally and the shoulder girdle is depressed. The therapist uses her elbows to keep those of the patient in extension until he can maintain the position alone (Fig. 8.4 a).
2. The therapist places the patient's arm at his side, in outward rotation with the fingers extended. Using her forearm to support his elbow in extension and her hand to keep his shoulder forward, she helps him to bring his weight over that side (Fig. 8.4 b). Once again, the scapula must elevate and the side elongate. He transfers his weight from side to side, moving proximally against the spastic arm. When the spasticity has been inhibited the therapist withdraws her support, and can then ask the patient to flex and extend his elbow selectively, i. e. without moving his trunk to produce flexion and extension at the elbow, and without using inward rotation of the shoulder to reinforce the extension attempt.
3. Because the scapula is very often the key to the spasticity in the whole upper extremity, the therapist must pay particular attention to the inhibition of hypertonicity in that area.

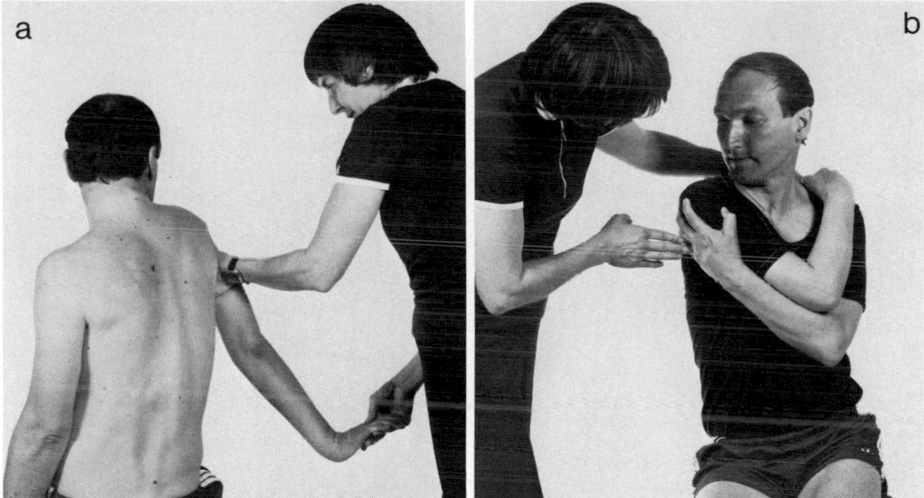

Fig. 8.5 a, b. Inhibition of retraction and depression of the scapula (right hemiplegia). **a** With the arm in extension and external rotation the point of the shoulder is moved towards the nose. **b** With arms crossed the patient rotates his trunk to the sound side. His sound hand brings the hemiplegic shoulder forwards

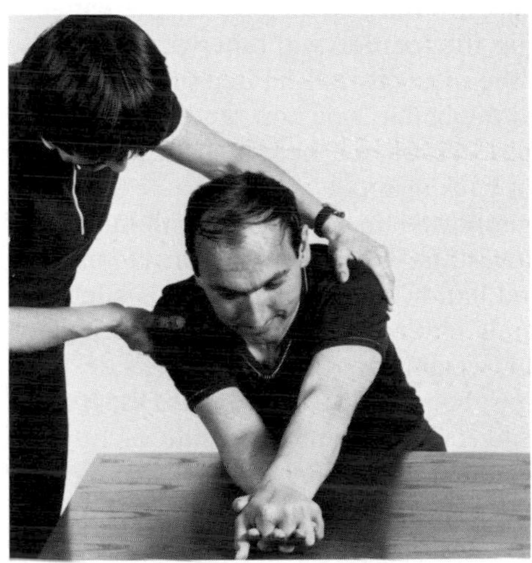

Fig. 8.6. Inhibition of pronation of the forearm. The patient moves his weight from one side to the other (right hemiplegia)

a) She moves the point of the patient's shoulder in the direction of his nose, forwards and upwards, so working against the spastic pattern. She asks the patient to try not to resist the movement, and when she feels that there is no longer a resistance, he can assist actively. The therapist keeps the patient's hand in full dorsiflexion with finger extension, while he moves actively (Fig. 8.5 a).
b) With both arms flexed across his chest, the patient uses his sound hand to draw the affected scapula forward into protraction. The affected hand remains relaxed on the opposite shoulder as he rotates the trunk in a smooth continuous

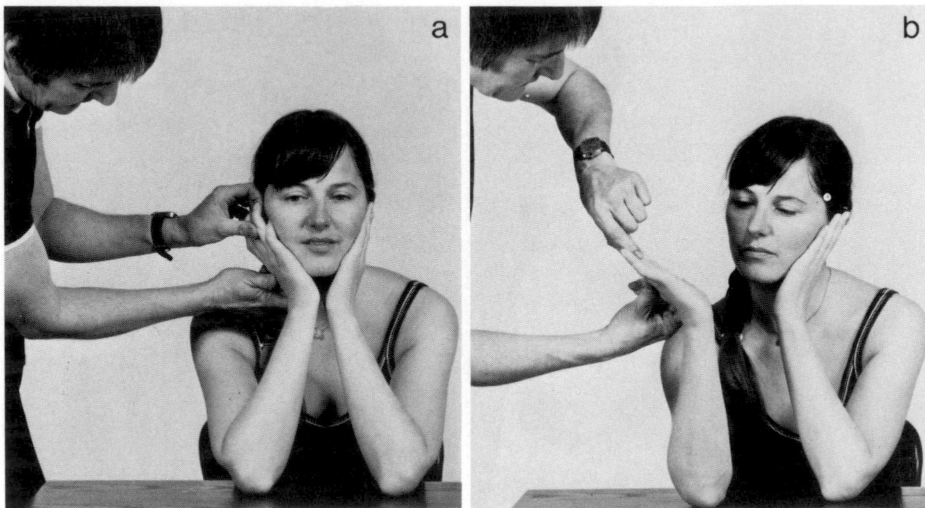

Fig. 8.7 a, b. Selective flexion of the elbow with supination (right hemiplegia). **a** The patient rests her chin on her hands. The fingers remain relaxed. **b** The therapist moves the hemiplegic hand away and the patient brings it back to her face

movement, back and forth (Fig. 8.5 b). Care must be taken that the patient's knees remain in the starting position, as the rotation will otherwise take place in the hips instead of the trunk. When the spasticity is inhibited sufficiently, the patient gradually gives less support to the hemiplegic arm, until it can finally remain in place itself. With the therapist's assistance, he brings the hemiplegic hand away from his shoulder and then back again.

4. The patient sits with his clasped hands supported on a table or plinth in front of him. Keeping his elbows extended he moves first to one side and then to the other, to inhibit the spasticity in the arm and hand (Fig. 8.6). Pushing his hands far over to the sound side will bring the scapula into protraction. Pushing then along the table towards the other side brings his weight over the hemiplegic side. With the elbows remaining in place, the therapist helps the patient to place the balls of his hands under his chin, letting the fingers rest against the side of his face (Fig. 8.7 a). When she feels that the fingers are relaxed, she brings his hemiplegic hand away from his face and then asks him to replace it gently (Fig. 8.7 b). The movement encourages selective flexion of the elbow in supination without the fingers flexing. If the hand remains relaxed, the patient is asked to bring it further into extension before placing it under his chin again.
5. To help the patient to move smoothly and without over-activity, the therapist places his extended hand on her hand and asks him to follow her hand as she moves (Fig. 8.8 a). By increasing the speed of the movement and by changing the direction, the therapist can increase the degree of complexity according to the patient's ability. If he places both his hands on her hands and she asks him to follow the movement of both simultaneously, the activity becomes more difficult but has the advantage of preventing over-activity of the sound arm, as it must follow appropriately (Fig. 8.8 b).

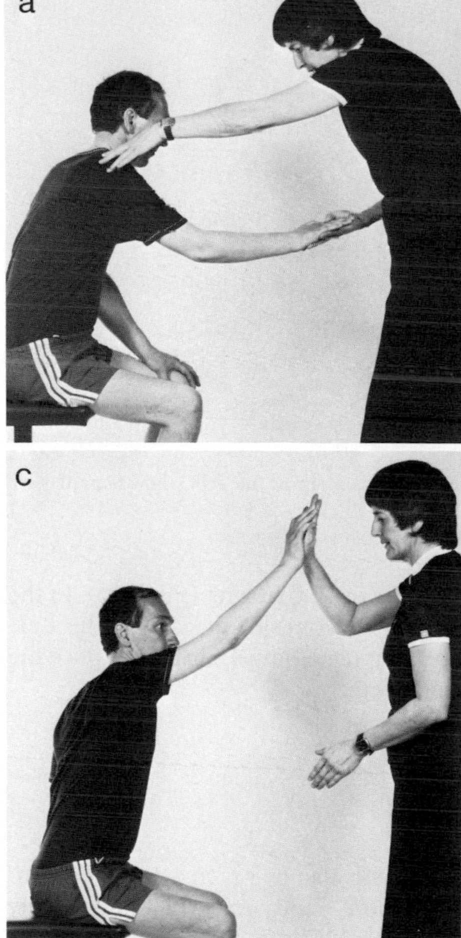

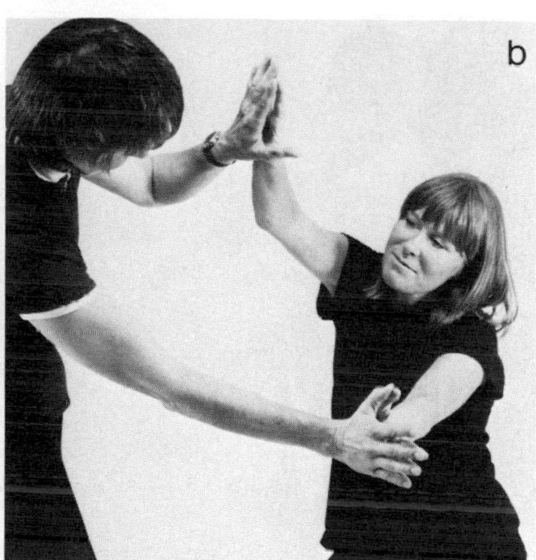

Fig. 8.8 a–c. Moving without effort (right hemiplegia). **a** With his hemiplegic hand resting on the therapist's hand the patient follows her movements. **b** With both of her hands against those of the therapist, the patient follows more complex movements. **c** The patient follows the therapist's hand forwards and upwards. The therapist gives quick repeated approximation through the ball of his hand

6. The patient follows the therapist's hand forwards and upwards, and she facilitates the movement with short quick approximating impulses through the ball of his hand (Fig. 8.8 c).
7. A ball will often facilitate activity for the patient because its movement is so familiar to him. The ball also adds interest to the treatment.
   a) The patient places his clasped hands on the ball and pushes it as far forwards as he can (Fig. 8.9 a). He can also push it far over to the sound side, so bringing his shoulder forward. The activity inhibits spasticity and also encourages the patient to bring his weight forward. Not only the arm is being treated, but other movements are being retrained simultaneously. Bringing the ball towards his hemiplegic side will facilitate weight-bearing spontaneously.
   b) When the hypertonus is reduced, activity can be stimulated in the affected limb by helping the patient to move the ball with one hand. Selective movement is

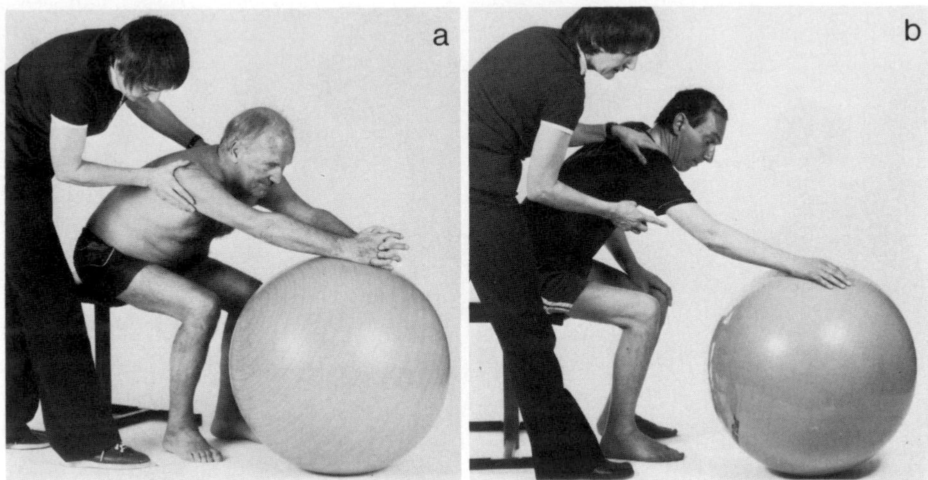

Fig. 8.9 a, b. Sitting, moving a ball to facilitate selective movement in the arm (right hemiplegia). **a** With both hands clasped; **b** with the hemiplegic hand

trained by his controlling the ball without the fingers flexing (Fig. 8.9 b). In the same starting position he can also move the ball from side to side, but this time stabilising his shoulder and moving only from the elbow. He can also push the ball away with the dorsum of his hand and fingers.

8.3 Activities in Standing

Pushing the ball away with the back of his hand can also be practised with the patient standing. He is then able to swing his arm more freely, and will automatically bring his weight forwards without fear (Fig. 8.10 a). The therapist facilitates the movement and also helps to prevent abnormal movements from occurring, e.g. adduction of the hip or retraction of the shoulder.

The patient can also drop and catch the ball using both hands, guided by the therapist who holds his thumb and fingers in the required extension during the activity (Fig. 8.10 b, c).
The patient may bounce the ball with the hemiplegic hand or with alternate hands. The therapist guides his affected hand to ensure a smooth, even rhythm (Fig. 8.10 d) and allows him to continue on his own if possible (Fig. 8.10 e). Both dropping and catching the ball and bouncing the ball are useful when combined with walking. Walking is more automatic and the patient looks at the ball instead of fixing his eyes on the ground.

A balloon will often stimulate extensor activity without exaggerated effort, and hand-eye co-ordination will occur spontaneously. The patient hits the balloon into the air with his clasped hands (Fig. 8.11 a) or with the hemiplegic hand alone (Fig. 8.11 b). He should swing his arm forward together with the whole side of his

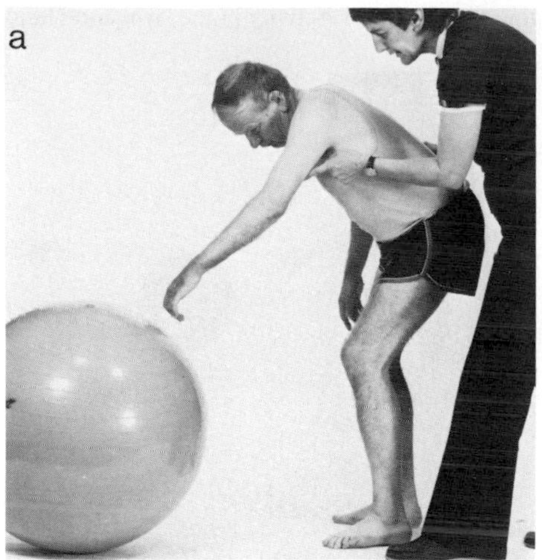

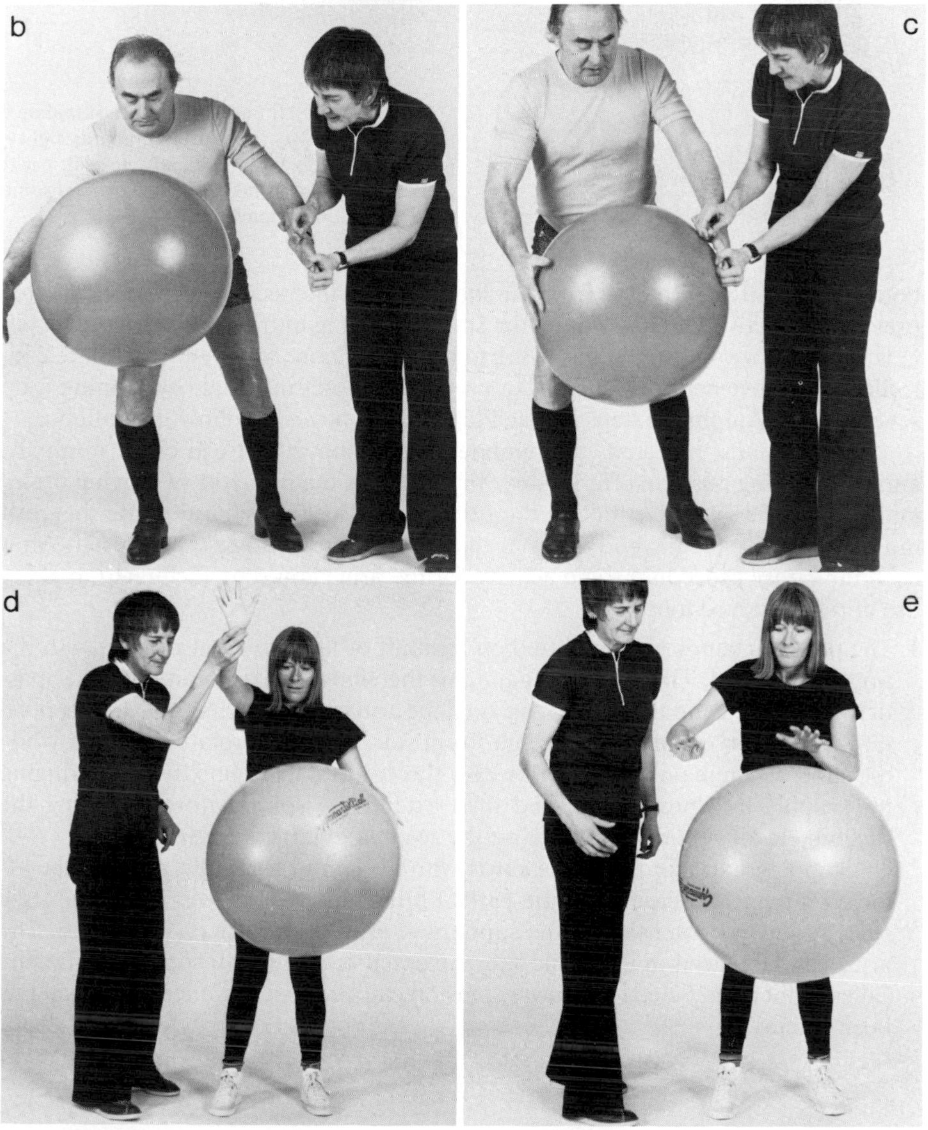

Fig. 8.10 a–e. Standing, using a ball to stimulate activity in the arm. **a** Pushing the ball away with the back of the hand (left hemiplegia). **b, c** Dropping and catching the ball. The therapist guides the patient's hemiplegic hand (left hemiplegia). **d, e** Bouncing a ball with alternate hands. The therapist first guides the hemiplegic hand until the patient can continue on her own

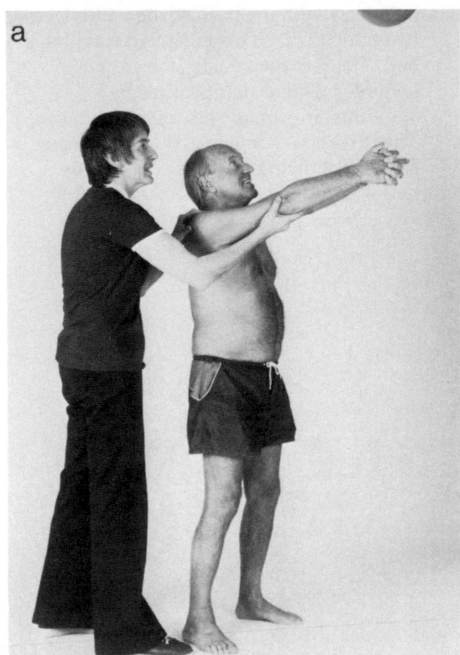

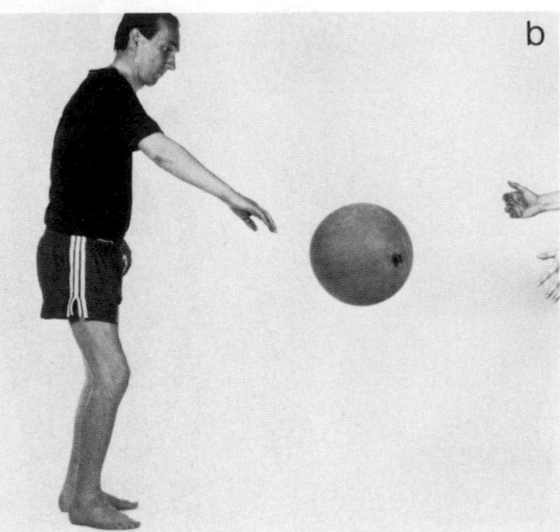

Fig. 8.11 a, b. Hitting a balloon to stimulate extensor activity in the arm and hand (right hemiplegia). **a** With the hands clasped; **b** with the hemiplegic hand, when the arm has some return of active movement

body and not attempt to lift it from the shoulder. It is interesting to notice how often previously inactive muscles around the shoulder spring into action when the scapula is brought forward during the swing to hit the balloon. A patient with more controlled arm movement can attempt to keep the balloon in the air by tapping it up several times. Automatic steps are facilitated as he moves to follow the balloon.

Spasticity must repeatedly be inhibited before movement can occur normally, and the standing position offers many ways of using the principle of moving proximally to reduce excessive tone in the extremities. For full inhibition the therapist must move the patient's body further than he can move it actively himself. After each inhibitory procedure some activity for the arm should be facilitated, making use of the improved tone.

1. The patient's hands are supported on a plinth or table in front of him, with the fingers extended. The therapist maintains the elbow in extension until the spasticity is reduced and the patient can keep the arm in position himself. In this position the patient can move his weight from side to side, or rotate his trunk while the shoulders remain fixed. He can also flex his thoracic spine fully, so bringing his scapula into protraction, and then extend the spine before repeating the flexion. He moves his thorax against the scapula to inhibit the spasticity.

   Stepping backwards and forwards with his sound leg while keeping the affected hip against the plinth, the patient brings his weight over the hemiplegic side, and active extension in the supporting arm is stimulated (Fig. 8.12 a). The arms can be placed in more and more external rotation with supination for the fullest inhibition. Selective elbow extension can be practised once inhibition has been achieved.

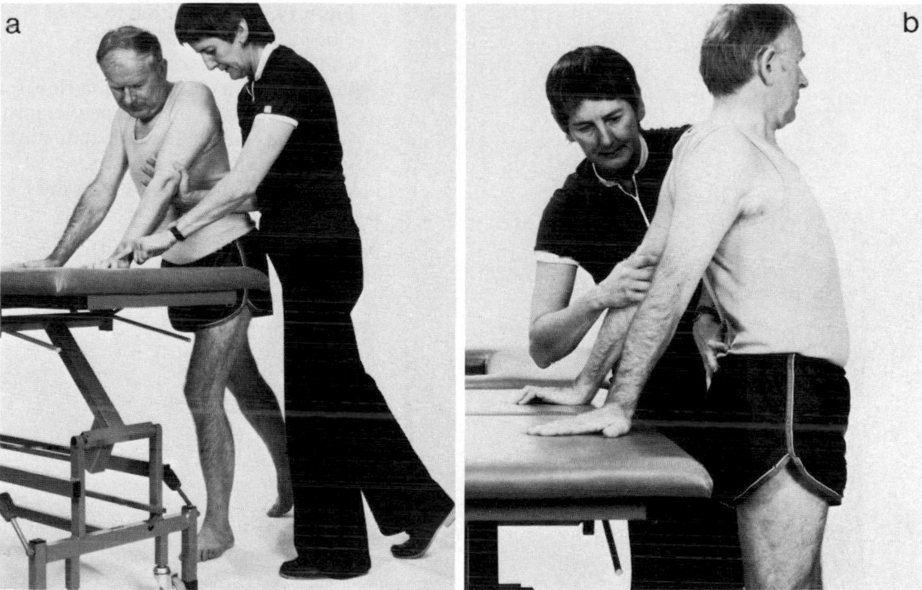

Fig. 8.12 a, b. Inhibiting spasticity in standing with weight taken through the extended arms (left hemiplegia). **a** With the hands supported on a plinth in front of him, the patient takes a step backwards with his sound leg while the therapist helps to maintain elbow extension. **b** With the hands supported on a plinth behind him, the patient brings his hips as far forwards as possible and extends his whole spine

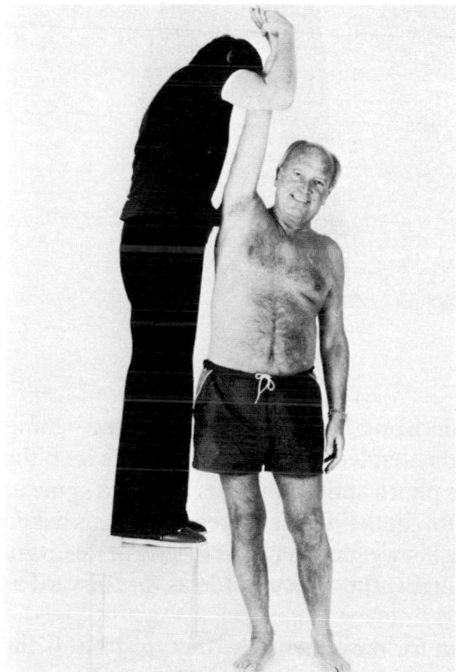

Fig. 8.13. Inhibiting flexor spasticity in the arm by elongating the side of the trunk. The therapist holds the extended arm in full elevation with external rotation. The patient moves his weight over to the hemiplegic leg (right hemiplegia)

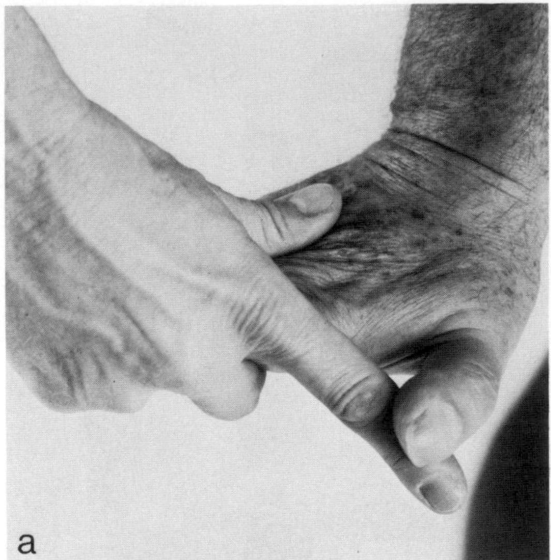

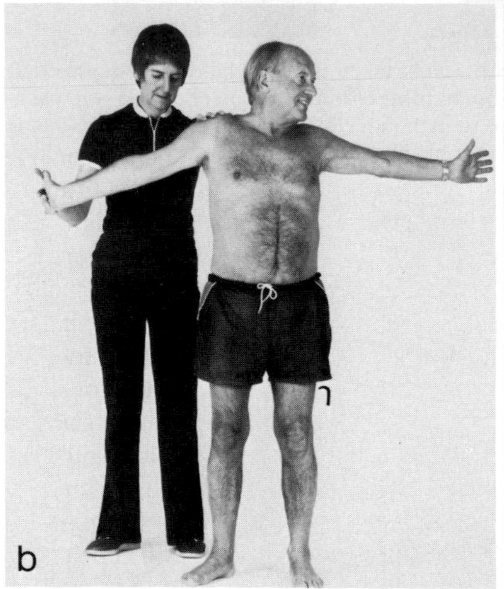

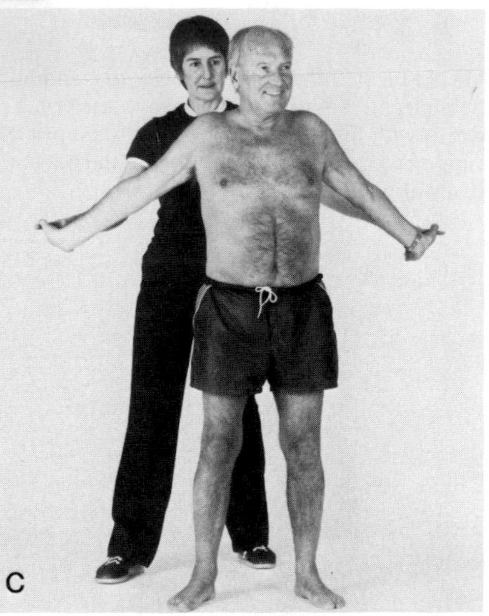

Fig. 8.14 a–c. Inhibition to allow elbow extension during active abduction of the arm (right hemiplegia). **a** Grip to inhibit flexor spasticity in the hand. **b** The therapist holds the extended arm in abduction while the patient turns away. **c** Abducting the arms without the elbow flexing

2. The patient stands with his back to the plinth and his hands are supported behind him with the arms outwardly rotated and extended. With the therapist's help the patient brings his buttocks away from the plinth and extends his hips and spine as fully as possible (Fig. 8.12 b). The extension in the hips is increased if he is asked to straighten his knees. He can also move his weight from side to side in this position, or rotate his pelvis, emphasising bringing the affected side as far forward as possible.
3. To elongate the side and free the scapula for movement, the therapist holds the patient's arm in full elevation with outward rotation. With one hand she main-

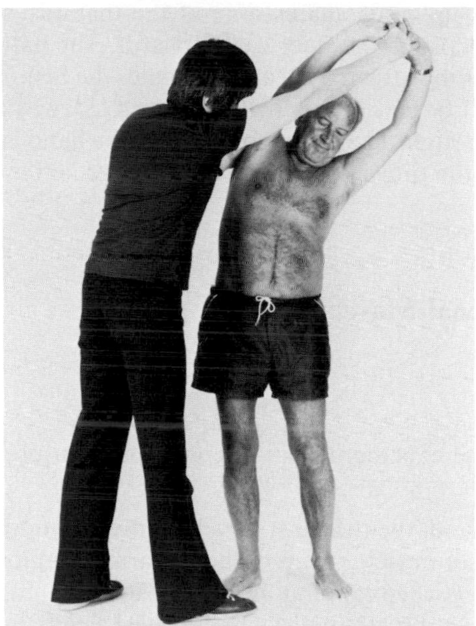

Fig. 8.15. Inhibiting flexor spasticity in the arm and hand (right hemiplegia). The patient's clasped hands are turned so that the palms face upwards. He leans them towards his sound side

tains full inhibition of the patient's hand and with her other hand she keeps his shoulder forward and outwardly rotated. She will probably need to stand on a stool for the necessary height (Fig. 8.13). The patient then moves his weight over the hemiplegic leg and back again, to increase the elongation and inhibition. The spasticity in the whole arm is reduced by the proximal inhibition.

4. Patients have difficulty in maintaining extension at the elbow when abducting the arm. To inhibit fully the strong pull of the flexor muscles, the therapist stands behind the patient. With one hand she holds the wrist and fingers in full dorsal extension with the thumb abducted (Fig. 8.14a), and with her other hand she prevents compensatory movement of the shoulder. While the arm is held in outward rotation and extension, the patient turns away with his other arm outstretched, as far as he possibly can (Fig. 8.14b). He then brings the hand round forwards towards his affected hand. He tries to go further back each time he repeats the movement as the spasticity releases.
5. Holding both the patient's hands in the same position the therapist brings his arms sideways and upwards, and the patient tries to assist actively (Fig. 8.14c). He also concentrates on not allowing the elbow to pull into flexion as the degree of abduction is gradually increased. As soon as the therapist feels that the elbows are about to flex, she lowers the hands again. If the therapist cannot reach both the patient's hands, he can be asked to move his sound arm correctly himself. The therapist can then assist or stimulate elbow extension with her free hand.
6. The patient first claps his hands together and then turns them over so that the palms face away from him. He pushes then against the therapist's chest while she helps him to protract the scapula and extend the elbows. With the hands in this position, they are brought above the patient's head until the shoulders are fully

elevated. The patient pushes his hands upwards against one of the therapist's hands, while with her other hand she keeps his shoulder well forwards. The patient then moves his weight sideways over the affected leg and elongates the hemiplegic side as much as possible (Fig. 8.15). He repeats the movement sideways and each time tries to elongate the side further. The flexor spasticity in the hand is dramatically reduced, and extension of the fingers can often be stimulated afterwards.

8.4 Stimulation of Active and Functional Movement

8.4.1 By Applying an Excitatory Stimulus

To activate the finger extensors or increase existing activity the therapist can use three useful methods of stimulation.

1. Supporting the patient's arm with one hand, the therapist uses her other hand to sweep firmly and briskly over the extensor muscle group of the forearm, from its origin above the elbow to the fingertips (sweep-tapping, Bobath) (Fig. 8.16a, b). The sweeping movement is performed with the therapist's fingers held firmly in extension. As she passes the wrist, she gives pressure downwards on the dorsum of the hand, quickly sweeping upwards again over the fingers. After a few sweeps, the patient may spontaneously extend the fingers, or otherwise can be asked to attempt the movement gently.

   When re-educating finger extension, it is most important to avoid dorsal extension of the wrist until the patient can maintain active finger extension while extending his wrist. If he is encouraged to extend the wrist before he can extend his fingers, the tenodesis action reinforces their flexor spasticity and the hand cannot be opened or used functionally. After stimulation, the therapist should therefore ask the patient to try to lift just his fingertips, so that finger extension preceeds wrist extension.
2. Placing the patient's hand in a mixture of crushed ice and water causes a reflex relaxation of the flexor spasticity of the fingers and wrist (Fig. 8.17a, b). In many instances there is absolutely no resistance to passive dorsal extension immediately following the immersion in ice, and the patient may be able to extend his fingers afterwards. Some patients without marked spasticity in the hand also seem to react well to the intense stimulation, and movement may be elicited as a result. The ice and water ratio must be correct for the best results, that is only so much water as to allow the patient's affected hand to glide into the mixture without difficulty. The therapist holds the patient's hand in the ice mixture to estimate how long it should stay immersed. It has been found that three immersions, each of about 3 seconds duration and following one after the other with only a few seconds' interval, are necessary before total inhibition of the spasticity is achieved.
3. The therapist, supporting the patient's arm forwards in extension, draws a bottlebrush through his hand. She asks the patient to hold the brush very gently and then pulls it out of his hand and asks him to grasp it again. Often he is able to extend the fingers enough to do so (Fig. 8.18).

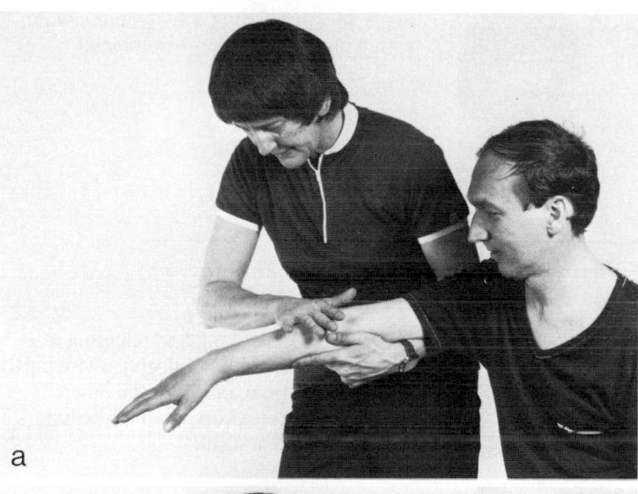

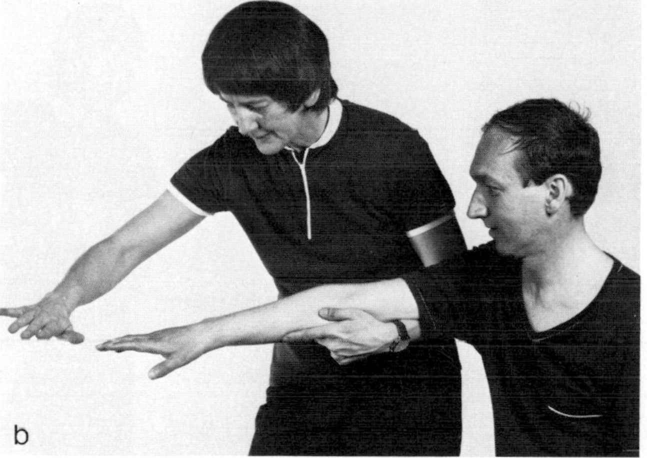

Fig. 8.16 a, b. Sweep-tapping to stimulate finger extension (right hemiplegia)

Fig. 8.17 a, b. Inhibiting flexor spasticity in the hand using ice (left hemiplegia). **a** The hand before inhibition; **b** the hand immediately following immersion in ice

▽

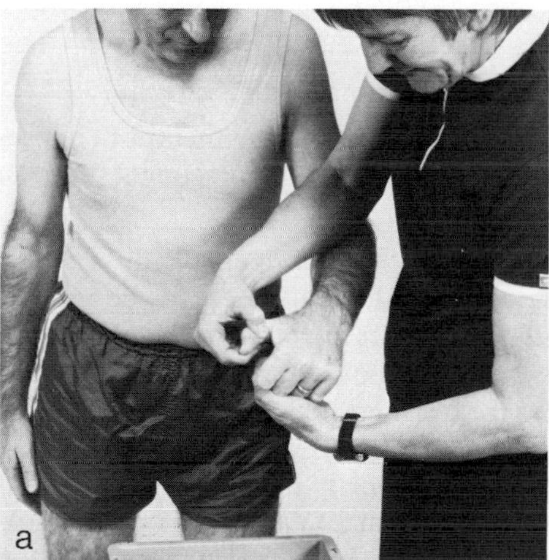

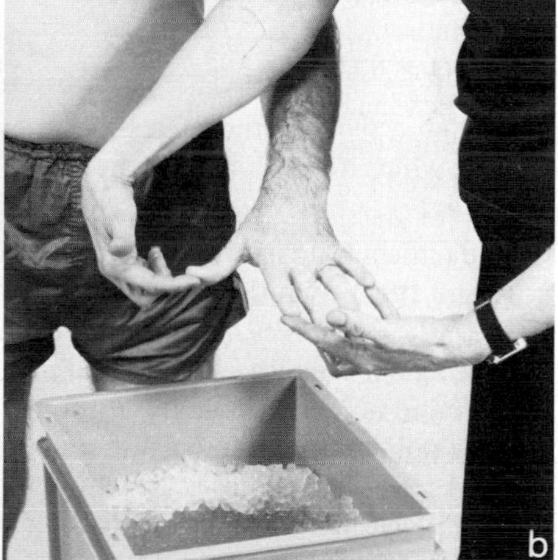

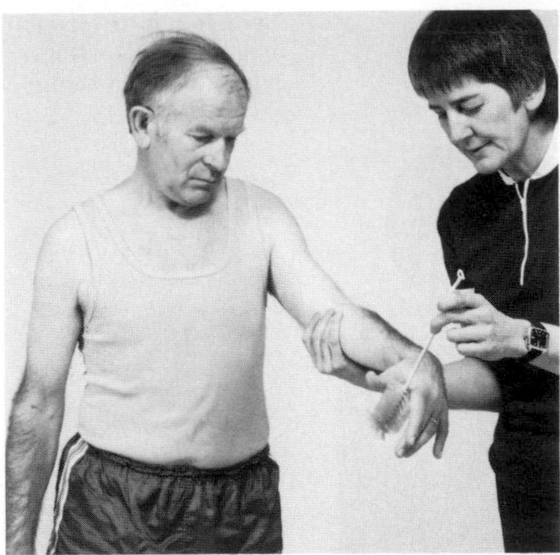

Fig. 8.18. Stimulating activity in the hand with a bottle-brush (left hemiplegia)

Fig. 8.19 a, b. Grasping and releasing a wooden pole (right hemiplegia). **a** Moving the hands up the pole, one after the other. **b** Letting the pole drop down a fraction before catching it again
▽

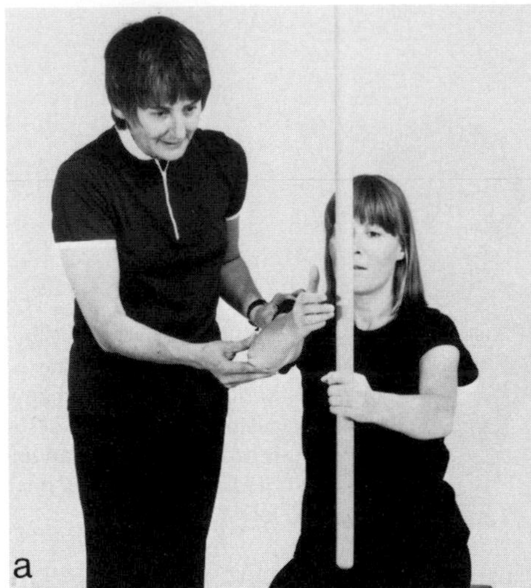

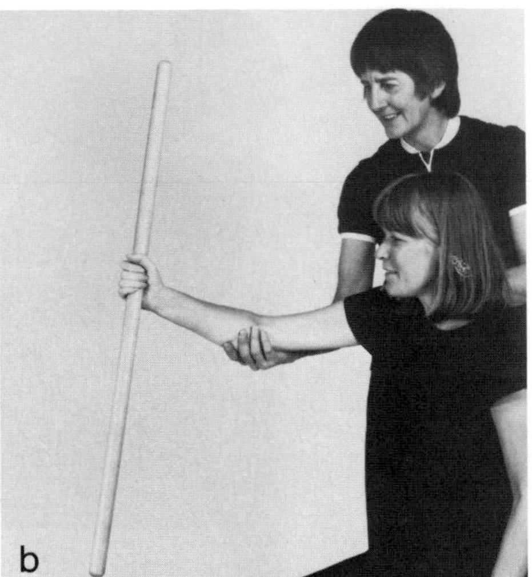

When activity in the fingers occurs with the stimulation, the therapist chooses objects which help to produce the re-appearing movements in a functional way. For example:

1. The patient holds a wooden pole in front of him, either horizontally or vertically (Fig. 8.19 a). With the therapist assisting where and when necessary, he releases the pole and moves his hemiplegic hand up and over the other hand to grasp the pole again. Then the sound hand makes a similar movement, while the hemiplegic hand holds the pole in position. The therapist ensures that the affected arm does not pull into flexion, and the patient keeps his elbows extended.

   As his skill increases, he can hold the pole vertically in front of him with his hemiplegic hand and, after releasing it slightly so that it falls, catch it again quickly (Fig. 8.19 b). The patient measures his improving ability by counting the num-

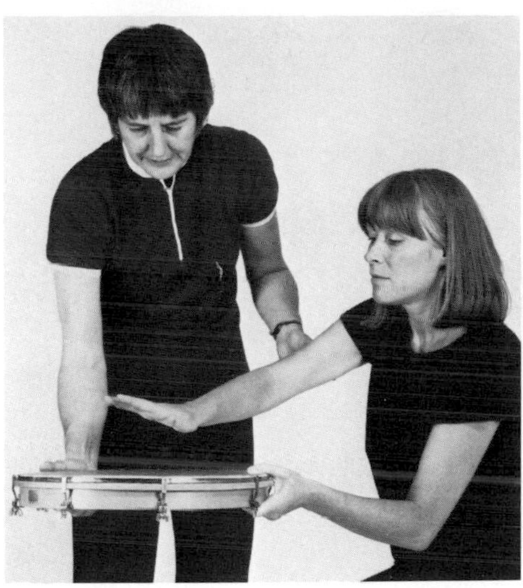

Fig. 8.20. Playing the tambourine (right hemiplegia)

ber of times he can release and catch the pole before his hand reaches the top end.

2. A tambourine provides many opportunities for using the hand in different ways, with an acoustic feedback. The patient can beat it with his hand flat, stroke it with a circular movement and then beat it, or tap it with alternate fingers (Fig. 8.20). By changing the position of the tambourine, supination and pronation of the forearm and lifting the extended arm are encouraged without the fingers flexing. Using a drumstick to play the tambourine requires still finer control of the wrist and fingers.

8.4.2 By Using the Protective Extension Reaction

When overbalancing towards the hemiplegic side, most patients will be unable to save themselves with their affected arm. The so-called parachute reaction fails because of insufficient extensor activity, particularly when flexor tonus increases due to fear of falling. With patients who have some active movement in the upper limb, protective extension can be facilitated. It is useful not only for protection, but also for stimulating extensor activity and speeding up existing motor function.

8.4.2.1 In Sitting

To prepare for the protective extension reaction in the arm, the patient is asked to lean towards his hemiplegic side and help to support himself with his arm. The therapist gives a gentle pull to bring him off balance and then pushes quickly up through the ball of his hand. In doing so she approximates the joints of the upper extremity, causing a stabilising contraction of the supporting muscles. At first she supports the elbow in extension with one hand (Fig. 8.21 a), and then as the activity increases she withdraws her support and reminds him only to keep his shoulder forwards (Fig. 8.21 b).

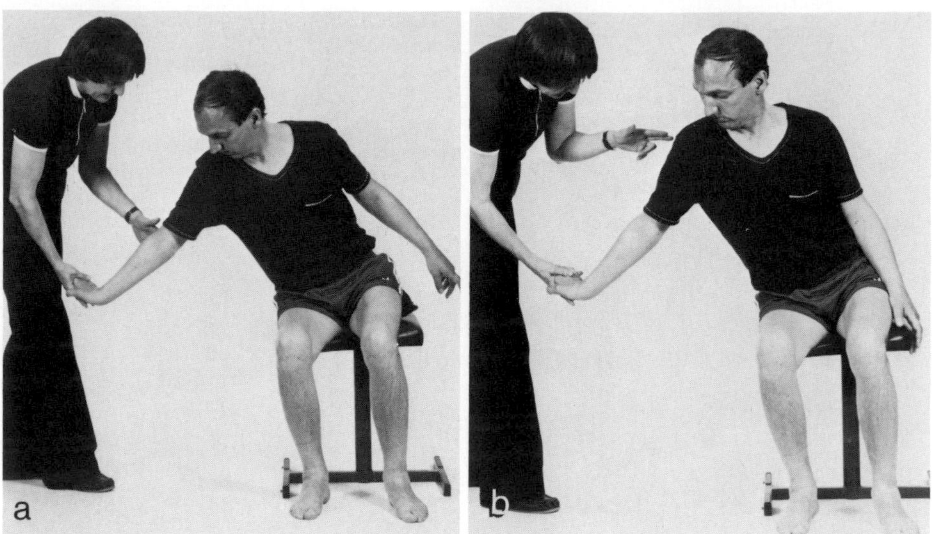

Fig. 8.21 a, b. Protective extension reaction stimulates active extension (right hemiplegia). **a** The therapist assists elbow extension. **b** The patient maintains elbow extension

Later, with the patient sitting on a plinth she draws him further and further to the side and then lets go of his hand, allowing it to rest quickly on the plinth. The activity can be carried out in various directions, and also in a standing position as the patient's ability increases.

8.4.2.2 In Standing and While Walking

The therapist holds the patient's sound arm and pushes him forwards or sideways in the direction of the plinth, a table or a wall. The patient saves himself with his extended hemiplegic arm, and the therapist controls the speed and prevents him from falling by guiding from his sound arm.

8.4.2.3 In a Kneeling Position

Protective extension can also be practised on the mat. Kneeling has the advantage that it is very easy to bring the patient off balance, to stimulate the activity. When the patient is kneeling the therapist can also control finger and wrist extension if she kneels in front of him and holds his hemiplegic hand open. He inhibits the reaction in his sound arm voluntarily, as it will otherwise dominate and reach the floor more quickly than the other.

8.4.3 By Using the Hand for Simple Tasks

As described in Chap. 1, the patient can be helped to regain lost abilities by learning to move in appropriate familiar activities. The actual objects and events confronting him assist the retrieval of movement patterns from his storage systems or memory.

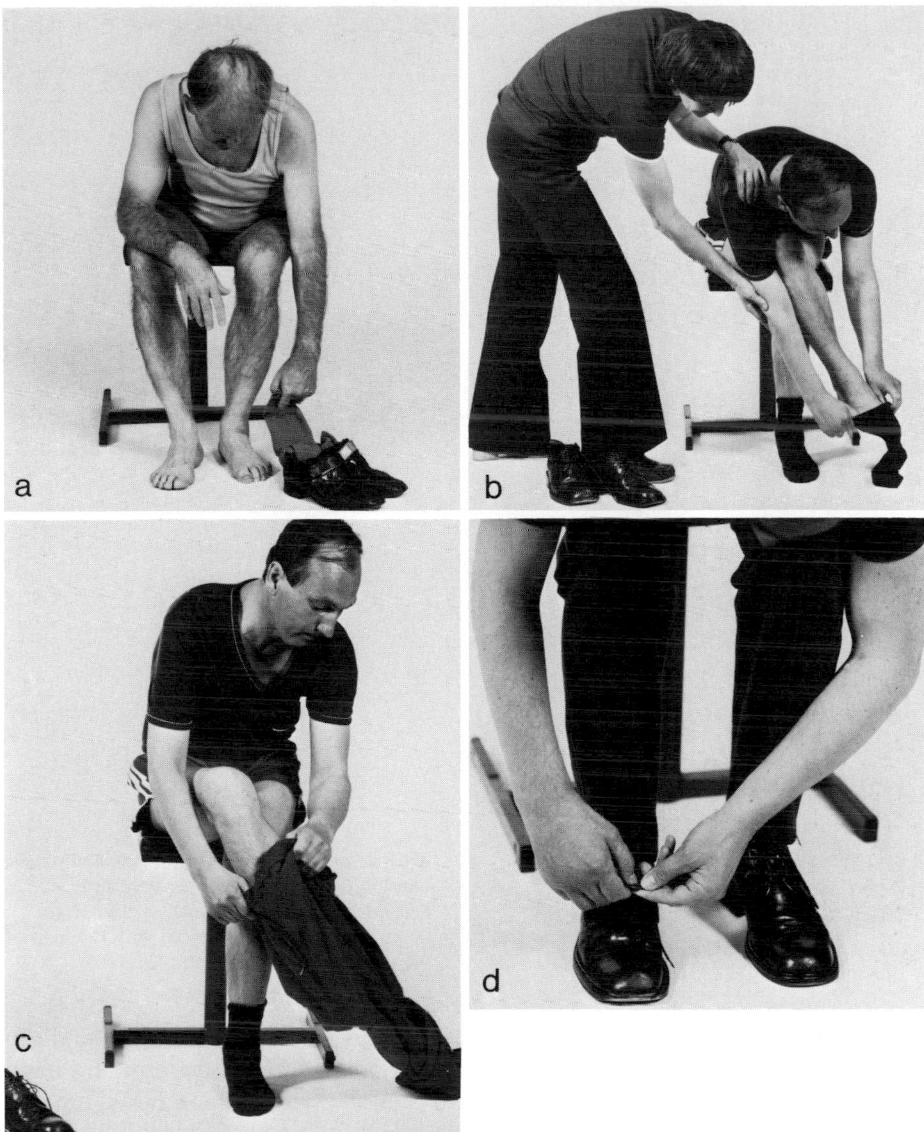

Fig. 8.22 a–d. Simple activities for the hemiplegic hand while the patient is getting dressed. **a** Picking up a sock; **b** putting on a sock with both hands; **c** pulling up a pair of trousers with both hands; **d** helping to tie shoe-laces

When some active movement has returned in the hemiplegic arm or hand, the patient should be helped to use it as often as possible, during treatment and in his daily life. Even where active movement is absent, the hand should be guided during activities as a therapy. The sensation and awareness of the hemiplegic side can be improved in this way, and the return of potential active movement will be stimulated.

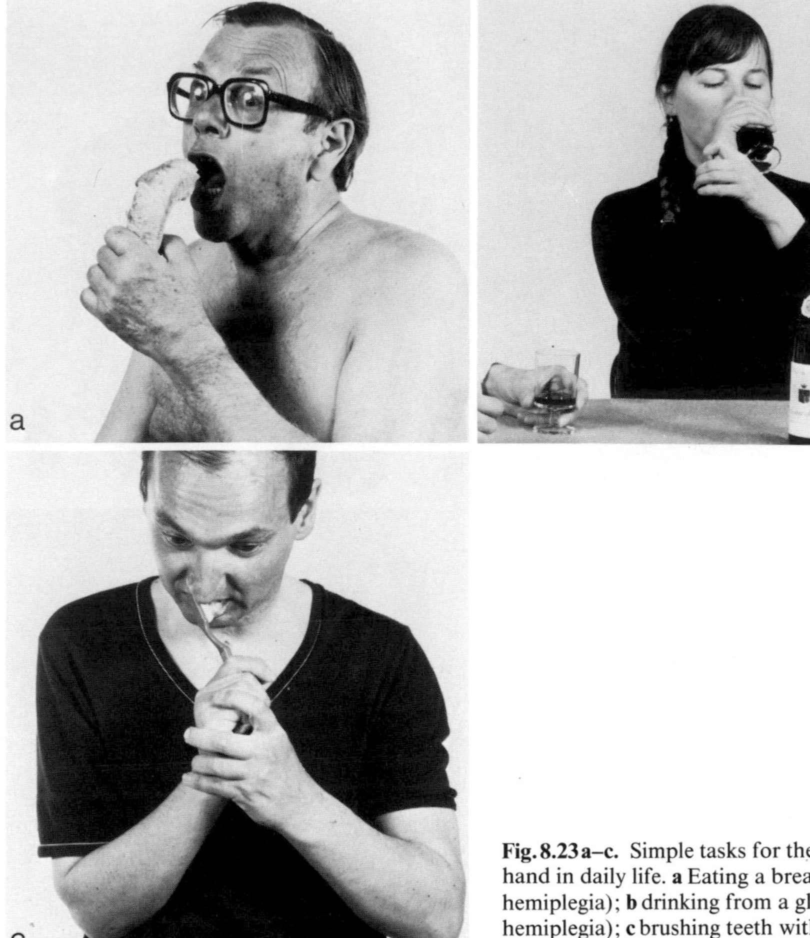

Fig. 8.23 a–c. Simple tasks for the hemiplegic hand in daily life. **a** Eating a bread roll (left hemiplegia); **b** drinking from a glass (right hemiplegia); **c** brushing teeth with the help of the sound hand (right hemiplegia)

The following are examples of activities during which the hemiplegic hand can be used, even if only slight active movement is present. Using the arm and hand even for very simple tasks is the best way to prevent associated reactions from occurring, as they do when the patient struggles to perform an activity with his sound hand alone.

1. Dressing provides several comparatively simple activities for the affected arm, i. e. activities where little stabilisation of the shoulder is required.
   a) The patient picks his sock up with his hemiplegic hand (Fig. 8.22 a) and then puts it on with his sound hand.
   b) If at all feasible, the patient puts on his socks using both his hands, as the therapist assists minimally (Fig. 8.22 b).
   c) The patient uses both hands to put on his trousers (Fig. 8.22 c).
   d) With very little activity in the fingers and thumb, the patient can tie his shoelaces, using the affected hand merely to hold one end of the lace (Fig. 8.22 d).

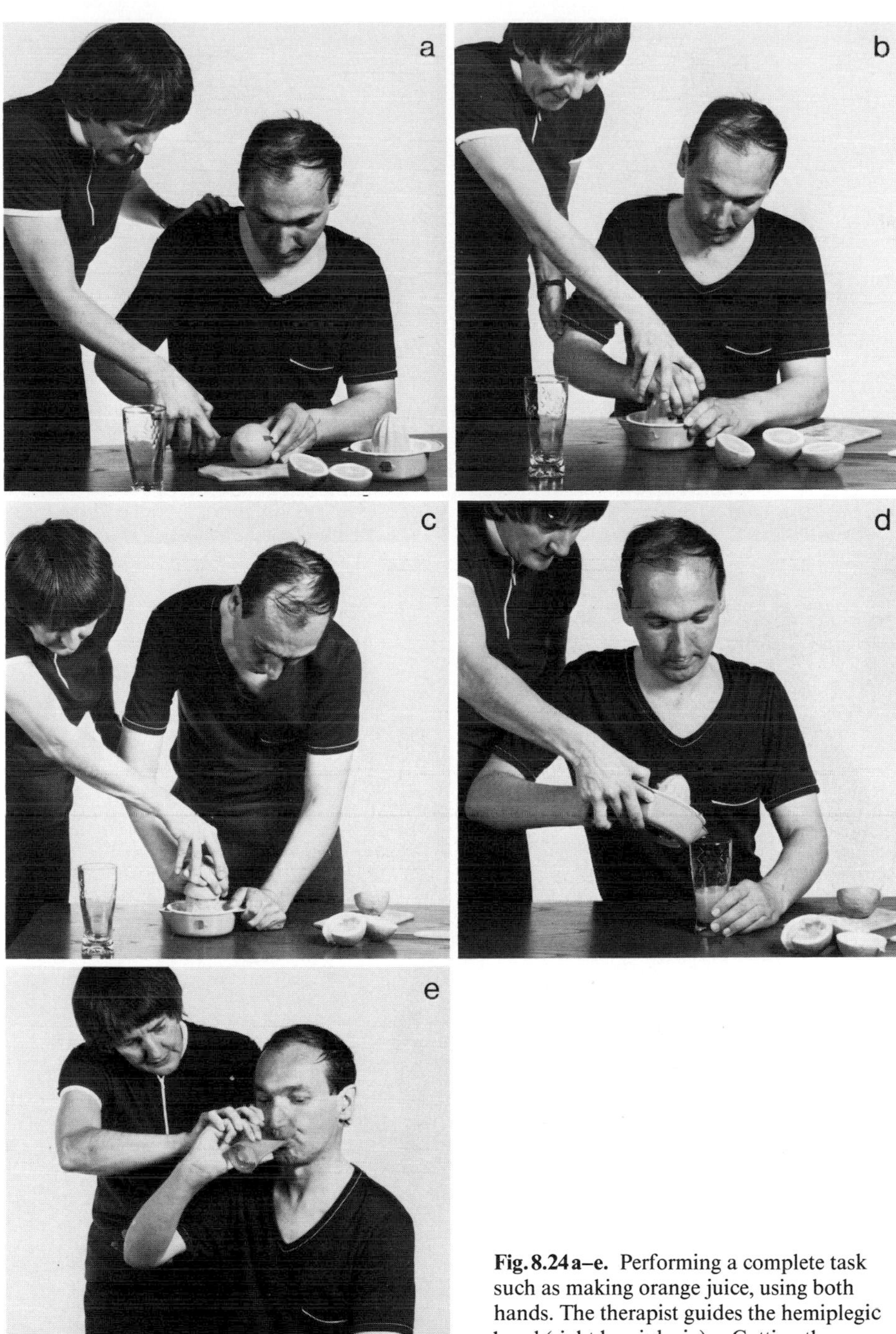

Fig. 8.24 a–e. Performing a complete task such as making orange juice, using both hands. The therapist guides the hemiplegic hand (right hemiplegia). **a** Cutting the oranges in half; **b** squeezing an orange; **c** standing to squeeze an orange (automatic standing improves balance); **d** pouring the juice into a glass; **e** having a drink of juice

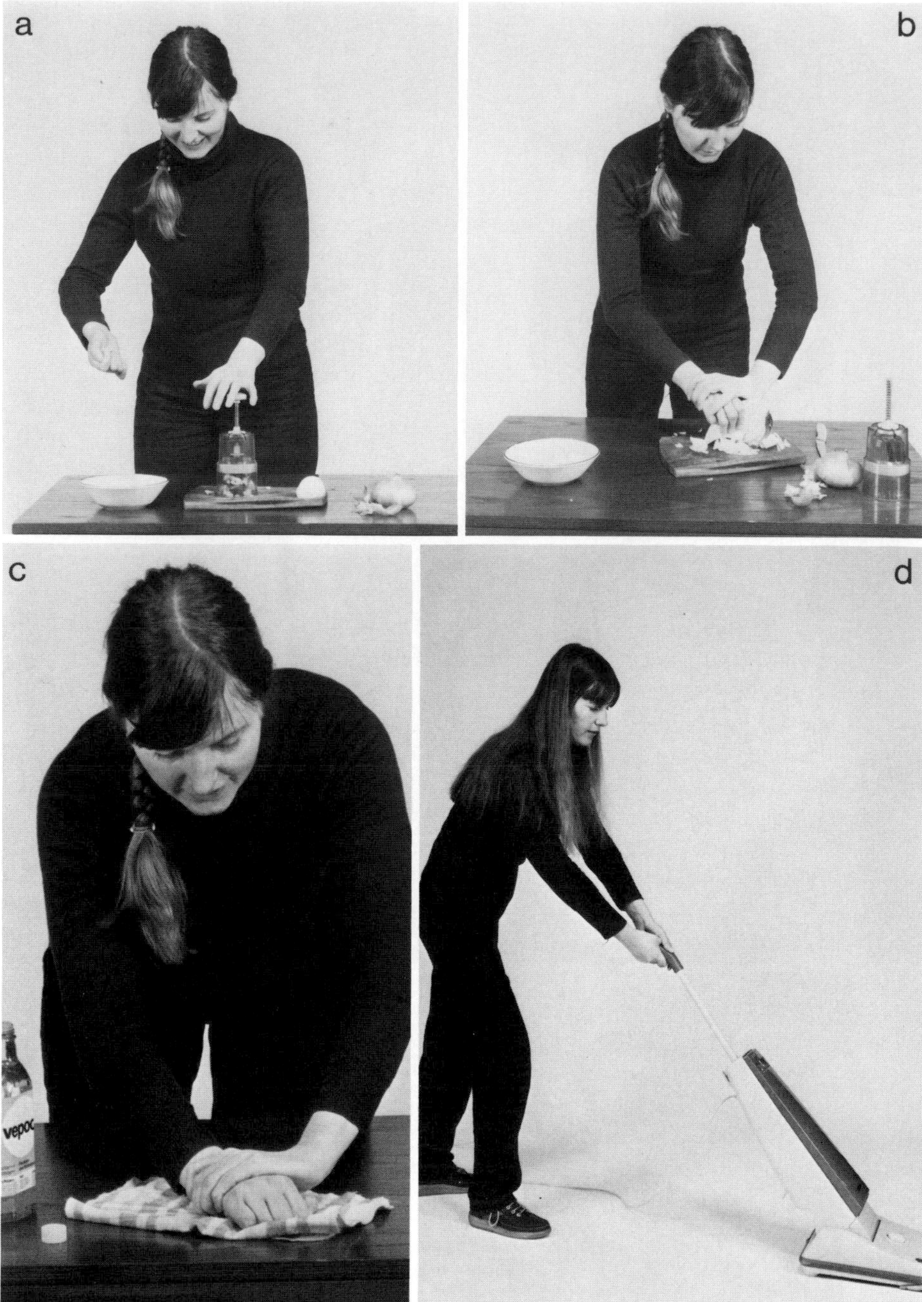

Fig. 8.25 a–d. Preventing associated reactions and stimulating recovery by using both hands (right hemiplegia). **a** Chopping up onions using only the sound hand causes the hemiplegic arm to pull into flexion. **b** Chopping onions using both hands, the arm takes part in the movement. **c** Polishing furniture. **d** Vacuum-cleaning

2. Other activities in his daily life provide opportunities for using the hemiplegic hand for easy tasks, such as:
   a) Eating toast or a bread roll (Fig. 8.23 a).
   b) Drinking from a glass (Fig. 8.23 b).
   c) Putting toothpaste on the tooth-brush and brushing the teeth (Fig. 8.23 c).

   At first, the patient may need to assist the hemiplegic hand with his sound hand, until he feels he can manage and gradually withdraws the help.
3. While the patient carries out a more complex task which consists of several steps and requires the use of both hands, the therapist guides his hemiplegic hand to perform all the necessary movements in a normal manner (see Chap. 1).

   An example is cutting oranges in half (Fig. 8.24 a), pressing out the juice (Fig. 8.24 b, c), pouring the juice into a glass (Fig. 8.24 d) and then drinking it (Fig. 8.24 e). Clearing up afterwards and washing and drying the utensils are also a part of the whole event.
4. Using two hands to carry out an activity which could be done with only one hand prevents associated reactions in the hemiplegic arm, and encourages the return of active control. The incorporation of the hemiplegic hand is therefore most important even before active movement has returned in the affected upper limb. For example:
   a) Chopping up onions. If the patient uses only the sound hand, his hemiplegic arm pulls immediately into flexion (Fig. 8.25 a). Using perhaps another type of implement both hands are used, the sound hand holding the hemiplegic hand in place. The associated reaction is prevented; the whole body becomes more symmetrical and the movement more normal (Fig. 8.25 b).
   b) Dusting or polishing furniture. The patient can use his clasped hands to dust or polish furniture or his motor car. If possible the hemiplegic hand lies flat on the duster and the other hand is placed over it (Fig. 8.25 c).

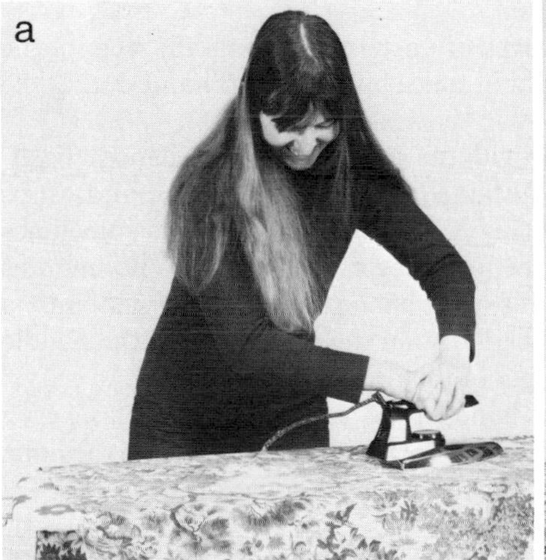

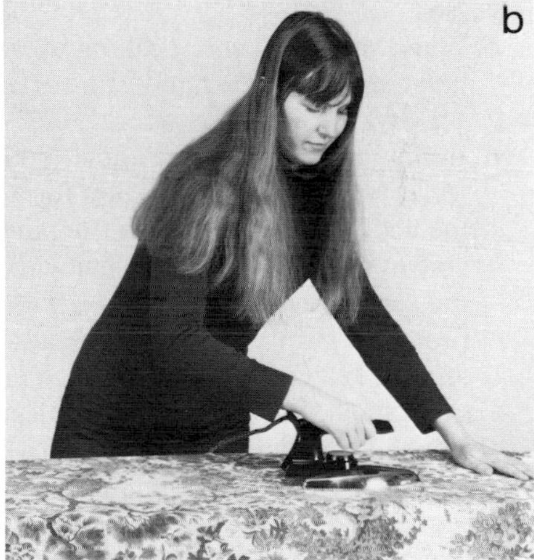

Fig. 8.26 a, b. Stimulating active movement by using both hands (right hemiplegia). **a** Ironing with both hands. **b** The hemiplegic hand continues alone for a short time

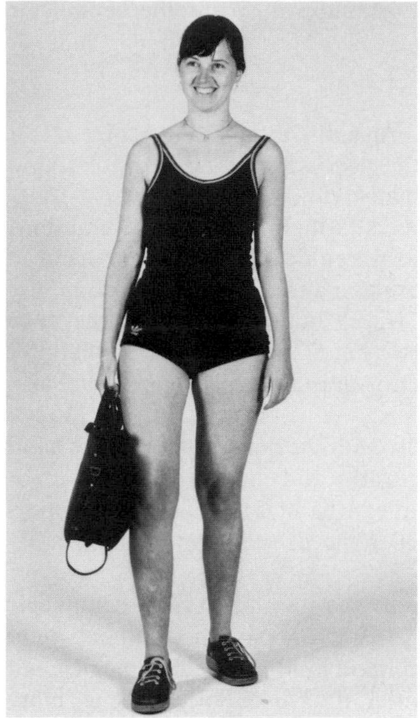

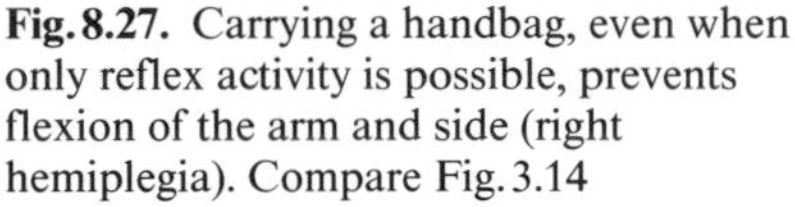

Fig. 8.27. Carrying a handbag, even when only reflex activity is possible, prevents flexion of the arm and side (right hemiplegia). Compare Fig. 3.14

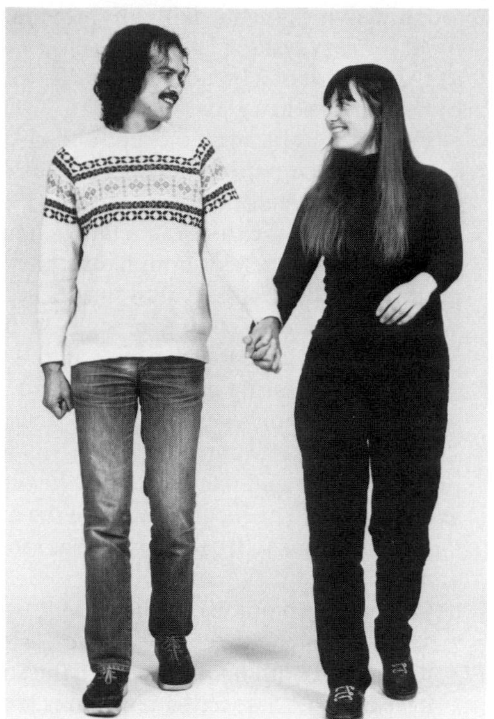

Fig. 8.28. Holding hands when walking prevents associated reactions in the arm

c) When shovelling snow, raking up leaves or vacuum-cleaning, the hemiplegic hand also holds the handle and is held in place by the sound hand during the activity (Fig. 8.25 d).

d) Ironing takes a long time and, if done with the sound hand only, causes the affected arm to pull into flexion for a sustained period. Using both hands turns the activity into a beneficial therapy (Fig. 8.26 a) and the patient is sometimes able to continue the movement with the hemiplegic hand alone, as he smooths the garment in front of the iron with his other hand (Fig. 8.26 b). If necessary a protective strip of wood can be attached around the iron between the handle and the heated part, to avoid the danger of the fingers being burned.

5. Carrying something with the hemiplegic hand, e.g. a handbag or brief-case, even if only reflex activity is possible, helps to focus the patient's attention on the limb. Associated reactions are diminished and, in addition, the patient is free to use his other hand for more skilled activities (Fig. 8.27).
6. While walking, associated reactions can be inhibited by the patient holding his affected hand behind his back with outward rotation of the shoulder, using his sound hand to maintain the position (see Fig. 9.10). When out of doors with a

close friend or relative, the patient holds hands with the other person, ensuring a natural appearance and a good arm swing without the arm pulling into flexion (Fig. 8.28).

8.5 Considerations

If the arm and hand are not incorporated in movement and in the activities of daily life, they will have almost no experience or input at all. The sensation is not stimulated and active movements may remain dormant. The hand becomes discarded as a useless tool, unlike the lower extremity, which has to be activated with every step the patient takes. It could be postulated that this is the reason why the sensation in the leg tends to improve, while that in the hand remains more impaired.

The patient should make a personal rule always to use the hemiplegic hand when it is possible for it to be used for a certain function, even though it may be easier and quicker to use the sound hand on its own.

"Of course some patients may not regain any function regardless of what is done, but it seems a shame to consign the arm to oblivion from the start before giving it a chance" (Semans 1965).

9 The Re-education of Functional Walking

"The ability to walk upright on two legs has played a key role in human life-style for more than 3 million years" (Sagan 1979). The ability has broadened our lives and enabled us to acquire countless skills which would otherwise not have been possible. Because of our relatively small base in the upright posture, we require highly complex reactions to maintain our balance when walking. These balance reactions are dependent upon normal postural tone and the capacity to perform selective movements, as described in Chaps. 2 and 3.

For every patient who has suffered a hemiplegia, the restoration of walking plays a prime role in his rehabilitation. To be able to walk again is his greatest hope and expectation, an aim which he can fully understand. Some studies have estimated that 60%–75% (Lehmann et al. 1975; Marquardsen 1969; Satterfield 1982) of the patients disabled with hemiplegia following non-fatal strokes were able to walk unaided after hospitalisation; others put the figure even higher at 85% (Shilbeck et al. 1983; Moskowitz et al. 1972). With improved training not only should a higher figure be possible, but also a more normal and economic walking pattern achieved.

In order to be truly functional, walking must be:

Safe, so that the patient is not afraid and in constant danger of injuring himself through falling.

Relatively effortless, so that not all the patient's available energy is required for moving from place to place.

Cosmetically pleasing, so that the patient can walk amongst other people without being constantly stared at.

Possible without the use of a stick, so that the patient can use his sound hand to carry out tasks.

Carried out at an automatic level to enable the patient to concentrate on other activities.

If these goals are to be achieved, the separate components of gait must be understood and taught, and the patient enabled to achieve the most normal walking pattern possible for him. None of the aims is met if the patient is allowed or encouraged to walk in a typical hemiplegic pattern, leaning on a stick for support.

It is most important that walking be included early in the treatment programme. A patient who is kept sitting in a wheelchair too long will be afraid of the new height when he starts moving in the upright position again. Prolonged sitting in a wheelchair also increases flexion throughout the body, making it more difficult for the patient to extend against gravity later. As soon as the patient can take weight on his affected leg, albeit with help, and does not require excessive support when moving, walking can be facilitated.

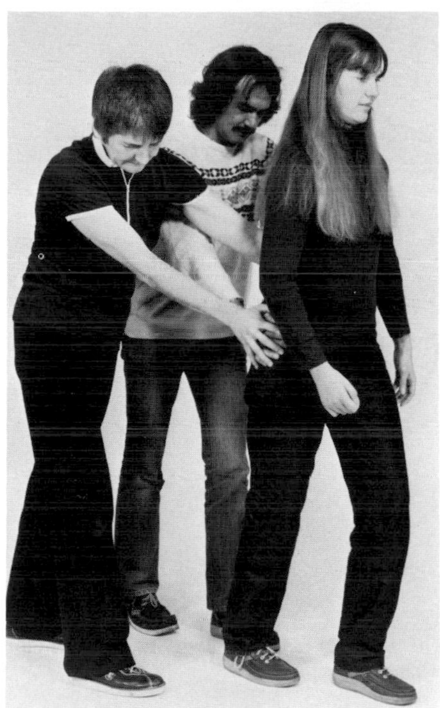

Fig. 9.1. A patient's husband learns to facilitate walking (right hemiplegia)

Nursing staff and relatives should be carefully taught how to walk with the patient so that bad habits are avoided. They will otherwise automatically walk on the patient's sound side, allowing him to hold on with his sound hand and lean towards them. Instruction must include practical experience for the nursing staff or relatives. The best way of teaching the correct facilitation is to let the assistant feel the therapist's hands on his own body first, so that he knows in which direction she is giving pressure. When he walks with the patient, the therapist places her hands over his hands and asks him to let his hands be passive and feel what her hands are doing (Fig. 9.1). The patient does not need to use a stick for support when someone is assisting him, as the person walking with him can maintain balance for him and ensure the correct weight transference.

The patient should wear sturdy shoes with a leather sole and low rubber heels right from the beginning. They give better support and he can be asked to listen to the rhythm of his own walking, the sound of his shoes on the floor. Slippers encourage a shuffling gait and provide no support for the feet. We all tend to walk differently when wearing slippers!

9.1 Important Considerations Before Facilitating Walking

1. The ability to stand up and sit down easily and safely constitutes an integral part of normal functional walking. A correct upright posture has been described as the

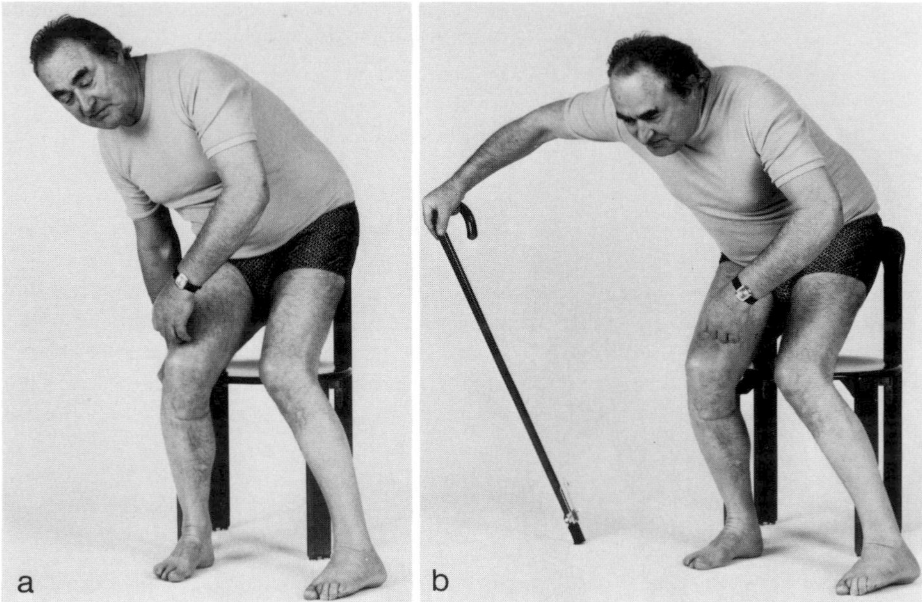

Fig. 9.2. a, b. Patient standing up asymmetrically (left hemiplegia). **a** Assisting with his sound hand; **b** using a stick

state of readiness to walk and therefore as potential walking (Klein-Vogelbach 1976).

Common difficulties: Patients who stand up asymmetrically and without bringing their weight sufficiently far forward will have an incorrect posture on achieving the upright position. The walking pattern will be adversely affected from the very first step (Fig. 9.2 a, b).

2. The initiation of walking from a stance posture was shown by Carslöö (1966) to result from "the body losing its balance as a result of cessation of activity in postural muscles (including erector spinae and certain thigh and leg muscles)". "The various torques of the body weight displace the line of gravity, first laterally and dorsally, and then ventrally, to a position in which the propulsive muscles are able to contribute to and complete the first step" (Basmajian 1979).

The steps that follow are caused by a continuous shifting forwards of the centre of gravity (Klein-Vogelbach 1976). "The force that produces forward progression in gait is the potential energy obtained as the body falls ahead of the supporting foot. Kinetic energy is gained in this fall and then used to regain potential energy when the body is lifted up over the contralateral foot in the next support phase" (Knuttson 1981). Houtz and Fischer (1961) showed that "a movement of the torso and hip region, that shifts their position over the feet, initiates the movement of each foot during walking. Movements initiated in the trunk lead automatically to changes in the position of the leg and foot."

The movement direction of the two femoral trochanters is never backwards in normal walking. Both hip joints move continually forwards through space along a wave-shaped path (Klein-Vogelbach 1976).

Common difficulties: Most hemiplegic patients walk with their centre of gravity well behind the normal line. They have difficulty in bringing their weight forward over the standing leg due to the forces of the spastic extensor muscles and the loss of selective movement patterns. Many are afraid of falling forwards, as the protective mechanisms are not adequate, and patients therefore feel safer when their weight is kept further back than in normal walking. The first step must therefore be an active placing of the foot forward, as the pendulum action is not produced spontaneously through the weight transference forward, or the body falling ahead of the supporting foot.

The distortion of the trunk- and hip-initiated movements causes the steps that follow to be abnormal too. Even the sound foot does not adopt a normal position, but tends to be turned inwards toward the mid-line, and is placed flat on the ground without a primary heel contact phase. The knee remains flexed at heel-strike. Without weight being transferred fully forward over the sound leg the hemiplegic leg has to be lifted actively, either in a total flexion pattern or with the knee stiffly extended.

The hips do not always move forwards as in normal walking, but the direction of movement varies and often the hip joint actually moves backwards in the opposite direction to that in which the patient is walking.

3. Normal gait is symmetrical with respect both to time and distance. The support times for right and left sides are equal, as are right and left step lengths. "The most comfortable walking speed lies close to 3.00 feet per second (0.91 m per second) to minimise 'energy consumption' and permit a reasonable propulsion speed" (Basmajian 1979).

An economically ideal walking speed is that which requires the minimum of effort for the relatively longest distance covered in a unit of time. The economic walking speed described by Klein-Vogelbach (1976) has approximately 120 steps a minute. "An increase in velocity can be achieved by decreasing stride time (increasing cadence) or increasing stride length and is normally achieved by a combination of both" (Wall and Ashburn 1979). If the walking speed decreases to fewer than 70 steps per minute the rotation of the pelvis is almost entirely absent, and the arms will therefore no longer swing alternately (Klein-Vogelbach 1976).

Common difficulties: The hemiplegic patient walks asymmetrically with respect both to time and distance. He takes a short quick step with the sound leg to avoid standing and balancing on the affected leg, and also to avoid the extension pattern of spasticity being provoked by the ensuing hip extension when the hemiplegic foot is behind. The patient also walks slowly and carefully and requires more balance and energy as a result. Because of the reduced walking speed and the hypertonus in the muscles of the trunk, the rotation of the pelvis ceases and arm swing no longer occurs. The spasticity in the arm itself also prevents the arm from swinging freely.

4. "The swing phase of a normal gait is a low-energy phase. Once initiated the weight of the leg swings forward like a pendulum, but its course is regulated by several muscles of the thigh and leg" (Basmajian 1979). "The hip is laterally rotating during the entire swing phase due to pelvic rotation in conjunction with the leg's forward controlled momentum" (Basmajian 1979). Klein-Vogelbach (1984) states

that the movement of the leg is always one of outward rotation at the hip throughout its swing phase.

In order for the toes to clear the ground during the swing phase, the foot needs to be actively dorsiflexed. It is important to note that dorsiflexion of the ankle is achieved by tibialis anterior with the assistance of extensor digitorum longus and extensor hallucis. The peroneii are inactive during dorsiflexion. “At mid-swing the tibialis anterior becomes inactive for a period to allow the foot to evert and remain everted during mid-swing. This allows for adequate clearance, while the inactivity of the invertor fits the concept of reciprocal inhibition of antagonists” (Basmajian 1979).

The popular concept that supination of the foot is due to peroneal weakness should therefore be reconsidered. The peroneii are only active and important during the stance phase to prevent excessive inversion of the foot, and thus maintain appropriate contact with the ground. The peroneus longus helps to stabilise the leg and foot during mid-stance, and Walmsley (1977) found peroneus brevis to act synchronously with peroneus longus during ordinary walking.

Common difficulties: Patients with hemiplegia have difficulty in achieving a normal swing phase when walking. There is a great variety in the degree of difficulty, but classically the problems are caused by three factors.

a) *The spastic pattern of extension.* After a step forwards with the sound leg, the affected leg behind has a marked hypertonus in all the extensor muscle groups. The extension at the hip increases extensor spasticity throughout the leg in the total pattern of extension (Fig. 9.3 a). With flexion at hip, knee and ankle difficult if not impossible (Fig. 9.3 b), the patient hitches up the side of his pelvis and brings the extended leg forwards through circumduction in order to clear the floor (Fig. 9.3 c).
   Dimitrijevic et al. (1981) state that “the observed paralysis of the foot in hemiplegic patients seems to be, in the majority of cases, an ‘active’ paralysis due to the pull of the hypertonic triceps surae muscles.”
   The foot is placed flat on the floor at the end of the swing phase, and often the ball of the foot makes contact with the ground first. The foot often remains outwardly rotated as the pelvis is retracted on that side. Some patients may succeed in bringing the whole side of the trunk forward, and the leg is then rotated towards the mid-line when it reaches the floor in front.
b) *Loss of selective movement with disturbed reciprocal inhibition.* Where this problem predominates, the patient lifts his hemiplegic leg to take a step forwards, and in the mass pattern of flexion the side of the pelvis is lifted, the hip flexed in abduction and outward rotation, the knee flexed and the ankle and foot dorsiflexed and supinated with the toes in flexion. The continuous activity of tibialis anterior without reciprocal inhibition causes the foot to remain supinated throughout the movement forward (Fig. 9.4). The leg is brought forward without the knee extending before the foot makes contact with the ground.
c) *Inability to transfer weight adequately over the sound leg and free the affected leg for the swing.* Most patients who have difficulty with the swing phase of gait will have difficulty in transferring their weight correctly over the sound leg, while at

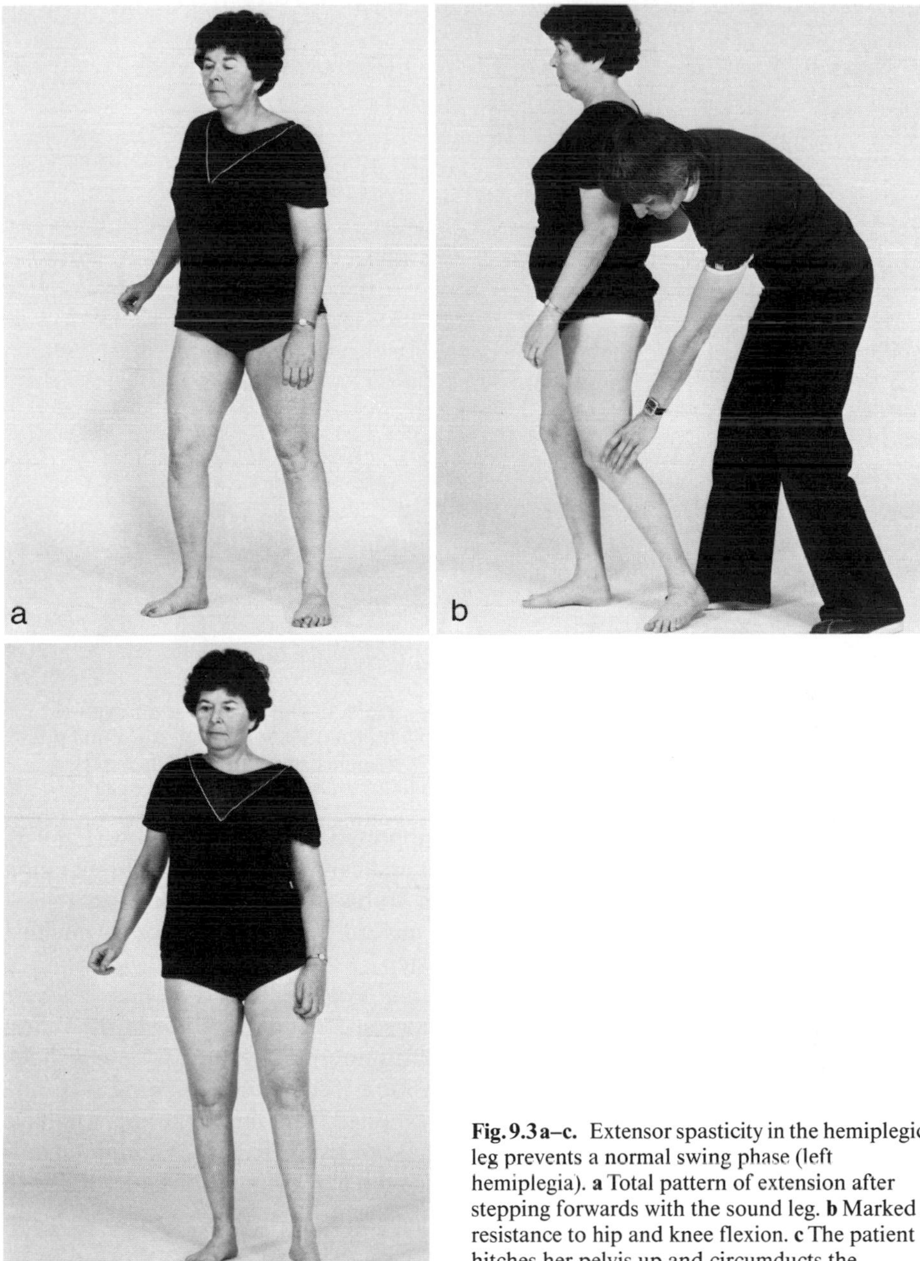

Fig. 9.3 a–c. Extensor spasticity in the hemiplegic leg prevents a normal swing phase (left hemiplegia). **a** Total pattern of extension after stepping forwards with the sound leg. **b** Marked resistance to hip and knee flexion. **c** The patient hitches her pelvis up and circumducts the extended leg to clear the floor

the same time supporting the contralateral side of the pelvis from the trunk musculature above. In order for the leg to swing freely forward its weight has to be suspended from above, requiring an appropriate activity in the ventral muscles of the trunk. When such activity is inadequate, too much weight remains over the

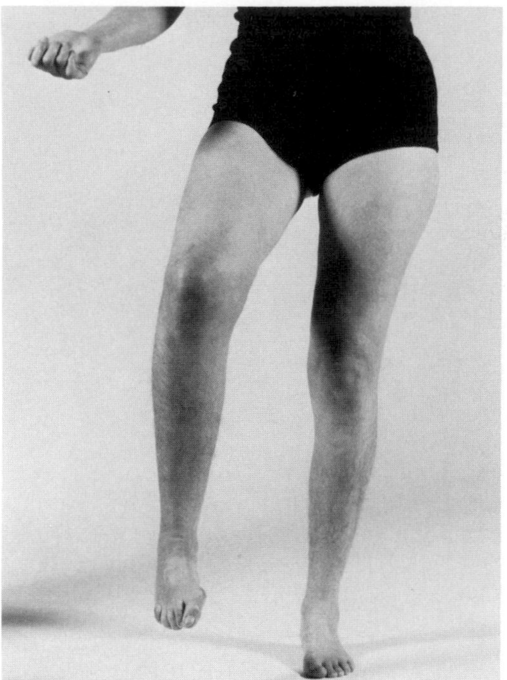

Fig. 9.4. Supination of the foot during the swing phase due to uninhibited activity in the tibials anterior (right hemiplegia)

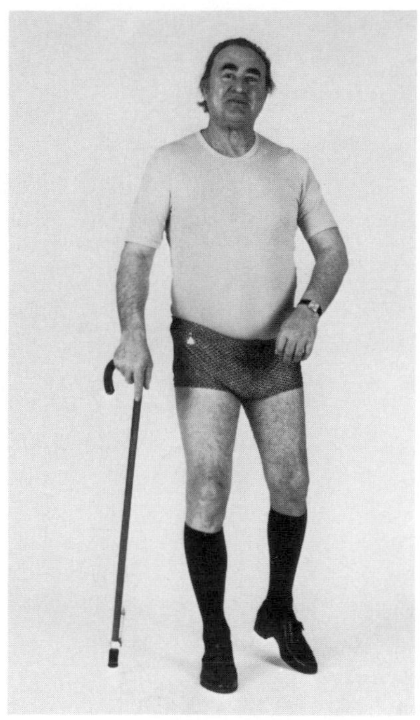

Fig. 9.5. The patient has difficulty in transferring weight over the sound side, despite using a stick (left hemiplegia)

hemiplegic leg, as the side of the pelvis is supported instead from below (Fig. 9.5). The foot continues to push against the floor and cannot be relaxed in preparation for the swing phase. The patient has then to lift his leg actively with effort, releasing the weight either by leaning sideways toward the sound side or by hitching up the side of his pelvis, before taking the step.

d) *The knee is never fully extended during normal walking.* In certain phases where extension can be observed, it is always between 5° and 10° short of the fullest possible range. The maintenance of this small amount of flexion serves as a shock absorber and permits a smooth, easy transition from stance to swing phase. A large percentage of patients, if not correctly trained from the beginning, will have a hyperextended knee during the stance phase of gait (Fig. 9.6). Without the necessary amount of knee flexion during stance the leg will not move forward with momentum for the swing phase that follows.

The hyperextended or "locked" knee occurs because:

- Active selective hip extension is not possible for the patient and he is therefore unable to bring his weight forward over the hemiplegic foot. He steps forward with the sound leg and the hemiplegic hip moves backwards, its continuous forward movement being interrupted. Because the femur is sloping backwards the knee hyperextends, and the weight hangs on the ligaments and soft tissue structures of the hip and knee.

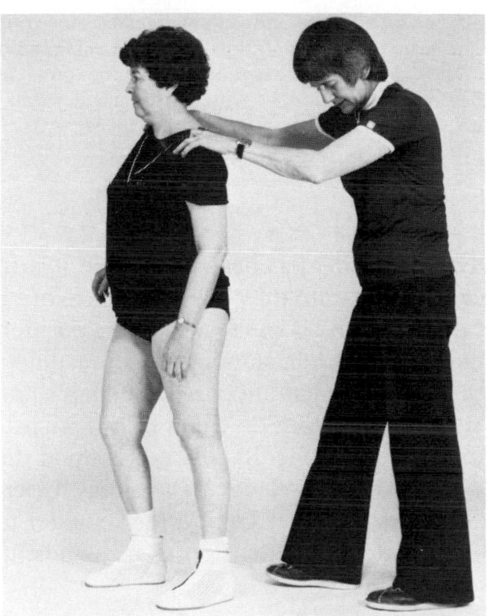

Fig. 9.6. The hemiplegic knee hyperextended during the stance phase. The hip has moved backwards (left hemiplegia)

- In the attempt to extend the hip and knee for weight-bearing, the whole lower limb extends in a mass pattern, including plantar flexion of the ankle. The foot pushes down against the floor, and the resulting backward movement of the tibia produces hyperextension of the knee.
  Knuttson (1981) has shown that during hemiplegic gait "the triceps surae activity may occur prematurely, starting immediately or shortly after foot-floor contact, since the contact is often made with the foot flat on the floor, or with low toe elevation." The early activation of the triceps surae muscle usually leads to a tension increase sufficiently large to shorten the muscles before the body has passed ahead of the foot.
  Bobath (1978) describes how the heel of the hemiplegic leg is placed down after the toes have touched the ground. "The spastic resistance of the calf muscles makes full dorsiflexion in weight-bearing and weight transfer forward impossible. The patient therefore leans forward at the hip and bends it in order to transfer his weight over the standing leg. This results in hyperextension of the knee." Bobath also states that if the patient is made to extend his hip and bring it well forward, his knee also extends but without hyperextension.

9.2 Facilitation

To facilitate walking the therapist uses her hands to prevent all the observed difficulties from occurring. Her hands either assist the selective movement pattern or inhibit and prevent the unwanted activity. As Bobath (1978) so rightly says, however, "all the various phases of walking can be prepared for in standing". And:

In order to prepare for a reasonably normal gait, balance, stance and weight transfer should be practised. For the swing-phase the patient needs release of spasticity at hip, knee and ankle to lift his leg and make a step. He also needs control of the extending leg when putting his foot down to the ground. If all this is first practised while in the standing position, he will develop a better walking pattern than if he is made to walk immediately without the necessary control of his leg.

9.2.1 Standing up and Sitting down

The preparation for standing up correctly from sitting has been described fully in Chap. 6. The activities should be practised carefully until the patient is able to bring his weight forwards over his feet without difficulty and come to a standing position without having to use his sound hand for support. When standing up in readiness for walking, the patient should be given the necessary amount of help to enable him to do so in a normal pattern. The therapist places her hands on either side of the patient's pelvis, and as he comes to the upright position she tilts the pelvis up at the front. By so doing she helps the patient to extend his hip selectively, avoiding hyperextension of the knee. If necessary, she uses her shoulder behind his shoulder to prevent him from pushing back in the total pattern of extension as he stands up (Fig. 9.7).

9.2.2 Walking

When the individual components of the action have been practised and experienced in standing, walking can be facilitated by the therapist. Facilitation would imply that the patient is enabled to bear weight on the hemiplegic leg without hyperextending his knee and to swing his leg forward without hitching up his pelvis or circumducting his leg, and that the step lengths are more similar both in time and space. Facilitation should make walking less effortful and more rhythmic. Any form of facilitation which helps the patient to walk easily and rhythmically is appropriate when treating, but generally the following methods have proved to be the most useful:

9.2.2.1 With Assistance Given to Either Side of the Pelvis to Facilitate Hip Extension and Weight Transference

For the patient who still requires assistance to extend his hip and so avoid hyperextending his knee, the therapist places her hands on each side of the pelvis. She uses her thumbs or the ball of her hand over the gluteal muscles to facilitate hip extension, tilting the pelvis up at the front (Fig. 9.8 a, b).

The patient should take the first step with his sound leg, as he will otherwise flex his hemiplegic leg too actively, instead of letting the foot swing forward. The therapist controls and organises the walking completely at first, until the patient has learnt the sequence and pattern of movement.

The patient brings his weight over his hemiplegic foot, without his knee pushing back into full extension. The therapist, standing on the patient's hemiplegic side, uses her hands to ensure hip extension and weight transference (Fig. 9.9 a).

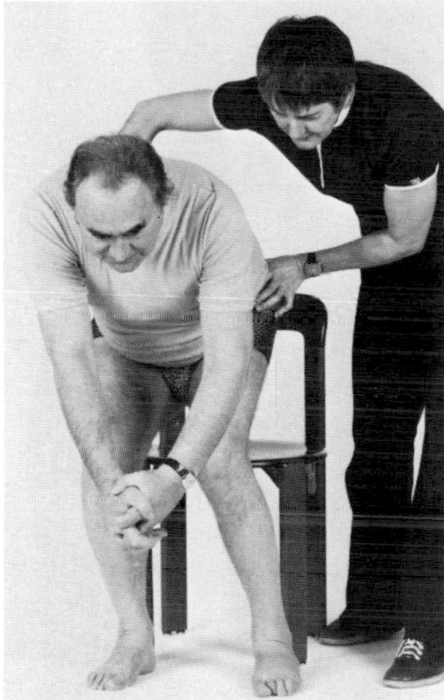

Fig. 9.7. Standing up from a sitting postion without using the hand for support (left hemiplegia)

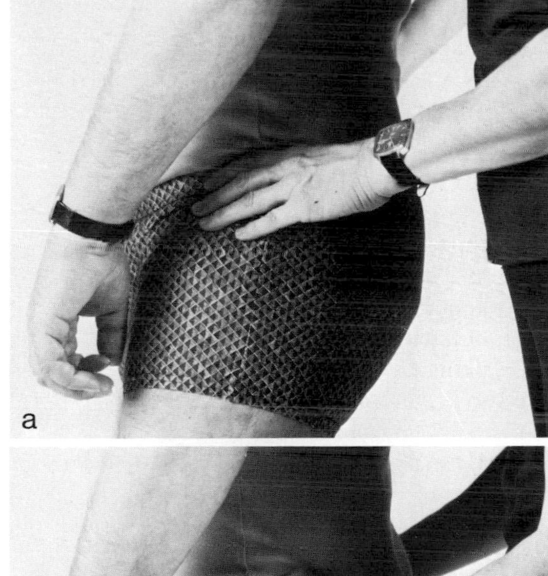

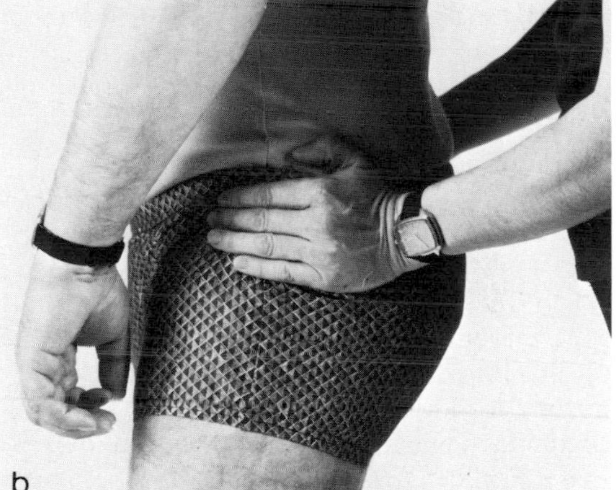

Fig. 9.8 a, b. The therapist places her hands on either side of the pelvis to facilitate walking (left hemiplegia). **a** With her thumbs over the gluteal region; **b** with the balls of her hands over the gluteal region

The patient takes a step forward with his sound leg, being told to place his heel on the ground in front and turn the foot slightly outwards. The therapist helps to transfer the weight forward while preventing hyperextension of the knee, and lengthens the weight-bearing phase.
The weight is then brought diagonally forwards over the extended sound limb, until the hemiplegic leg is free to start the swing phase.
The patient releases his hip and knee and lets his heel fall inwards, i.e. in outward rotation of the hip, in preparation for the swing. The therapist presses downwards and forwards on the pelvis, along the line of the femur as the hip and knee flex (Fig. 9.9 b). She prevents the patient from hitching up the side of the pelvis, and helps its forward rotation.
As the patient's foot reaches the ground in front, the therapist guides the weight forwards over that leg, to avoid the push into the total pattern of extension (Fig. 9.9 c).

The sequence is then repeated, starting with the swing phase of the sound leg. The walking movements are carried out slowly and exactly at first, and the patient is giv-

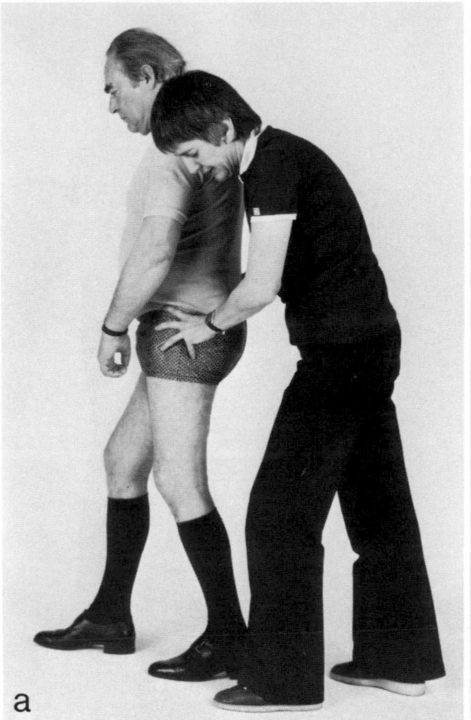

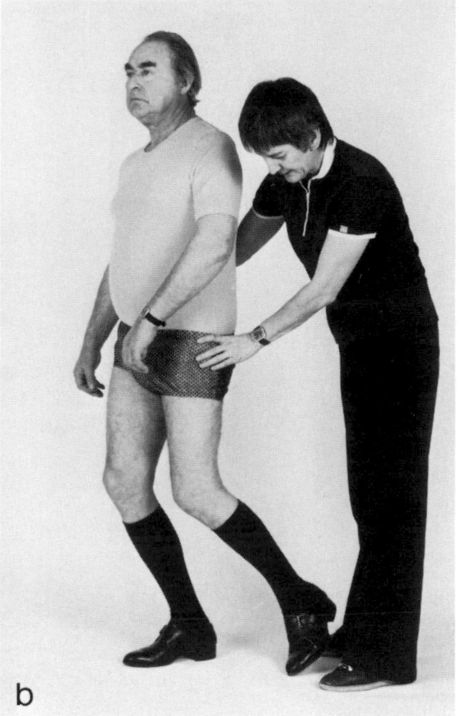

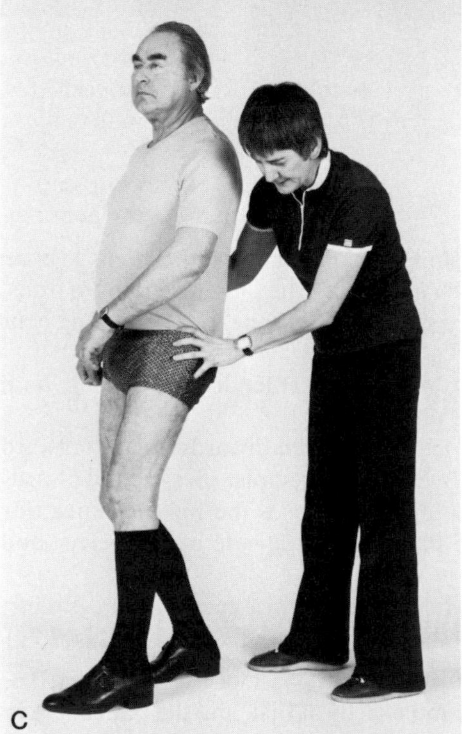

Fig. 9.9 a–c. Facilitation of walking (left hemiplegia). **a** Assisted hip extension prevents the knee from locking during the stance phase. **b** The therapist presses downwards and forwards to initiate the swing phase. (The patient has difficulty in keeping his sound knee extended while flexing the hemiplegic leg.) **c** Guiding the weight forwards over the hemiplegic leg and preventing the hip from moving backwards

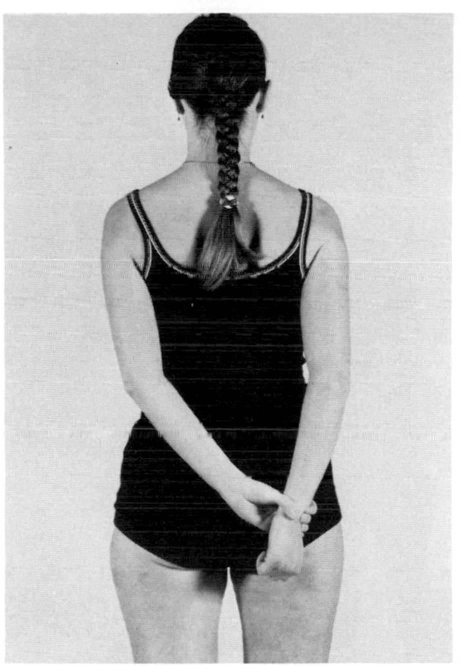
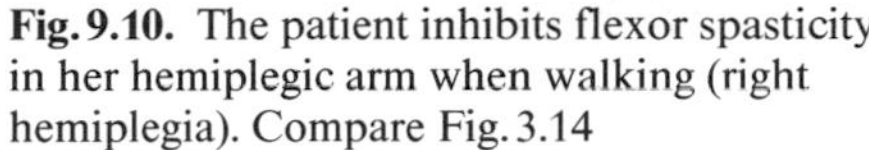

Fig. 9.10. The patient inhibits flexor spasticity in her hemiplegic arm when walking (right hemiplegia). Compare Fig. 3.14

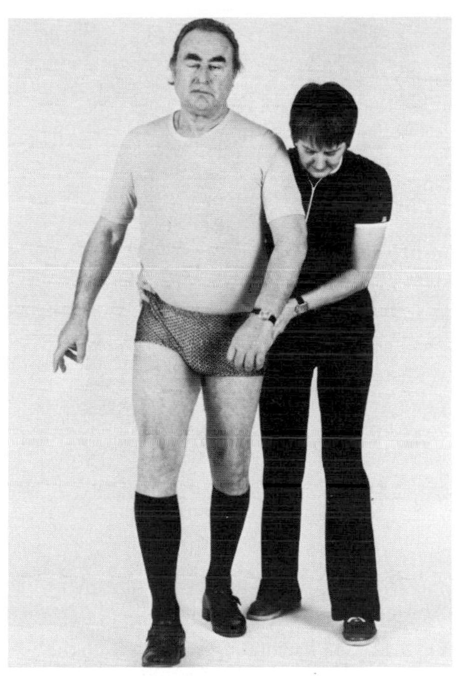

Fig. 9.11. Facilitating arm swing from the pelvis (left hemiplegia)

en postive feedback when they are correctly performed. The therapist sets the rhythm with her hands and her voice, and increases the tempo when she feels that the patient is ready to do so. As the patient's ability increases, she gradually reduces the amount of support, both manual and verbal.

Because the therapist needs both her hands on the patient's pelvis to facilitate walking in this way, she is unable to inhibit any associated reactions in the hemiplegic arm. The patient can hold his own arm behind his back with the sound hand, keeping the hemiplegic arm in extension and outward rotation (Fig. 9.10). Some patients will choose to hold their hands in this position when walking out of doors alone as well. The patient should not be asked to clasp his hands together in front of him as the position will reinforce the flexion of the trunk and hips. Later, when the patient has learned to walk more confidently and without so much effort, the arm will pull less strongly into flexion and remain at his side. When the patient is able to walk easily at sufficient speed, the therapist can use her hands on his pelvis to facilitate the arm swing by increasing pelvic rotation (Fig. 9.11).

9.2.2.2 With Both the Patient's Arms Held Behind Him, Extended and Externally Rotated

With the patient who can control hip and knee extension adequately, the therapist can facilitate the gait pattern by holding both the patient's arms behind him with the hands and fingers in dorsal extension (Fig. 9.12 a; see also Fig. 8.14 a). Her facilita-

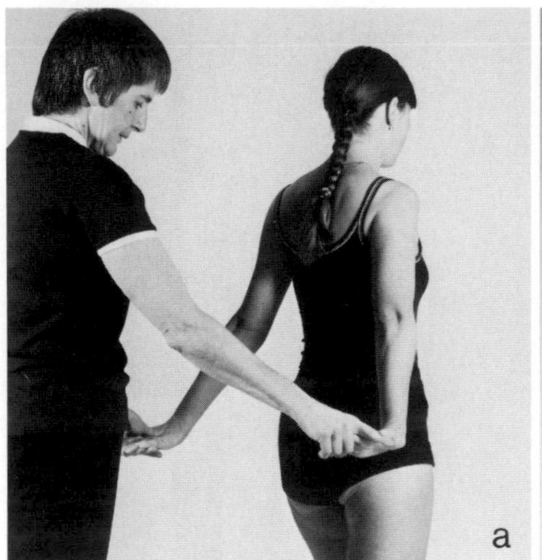

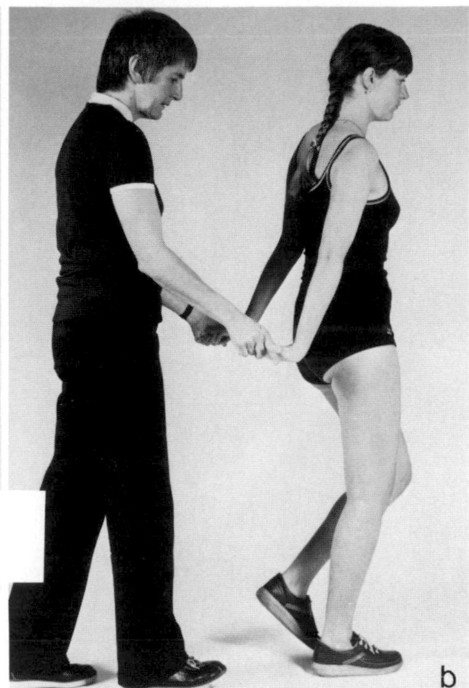

Fig. 9.12 a, b. Facilitating walking, with the patient's arms held behind her in external rotation (right hemiplegia)

tion enables the patient to extend his hips and torso more easily by counteracting the pull of the flexor spasticity in the trunk and shoulders. When the therapist holds the arms fixed in one position as the patient walks, hypertonicity is reduced. The movement of the trunk proximally against the arms inhibits the spasticity and counteracts the associated reaction in the arm (Fig. 9.12 b). Using the same grip she can facilitate rotation while walking, by moving the appropriate shoulder forwards, with the arms remaining extended and outwardly rotated.

9.2.2.3 With Rotation Assisted from the Patient's Shoulders

When the patient is able to control his hip and knee adequately himself, and the hypertonus in his arm is inhibited, the therapist can facilitate an arm swing as he walks. She places her hands lightly on the patient's shoulders, with her fingers in front and her thumbs behind. While the patient walks, she rotates alternate sides rhythmically forwards and then backwards in time with the contralateral leg, as would occur in normal walking (Fig. 9.13). It should be remembered that the arms only swing when the walking tempo is sufficient. If the patient is walking too slowly, he will actively move his arms in a stiff and artificial manner in his attempt to simulate an arm swing.

However, in certain cases the patient can be asked to swing his arms actively to overcome the tendency either to fix his sound arm against his side or to hold it stiffly in one position for increased stability. To avoid such fixation, the patient can also be asked to bounce a ball in front of him as he walks, or throw it up in the air and

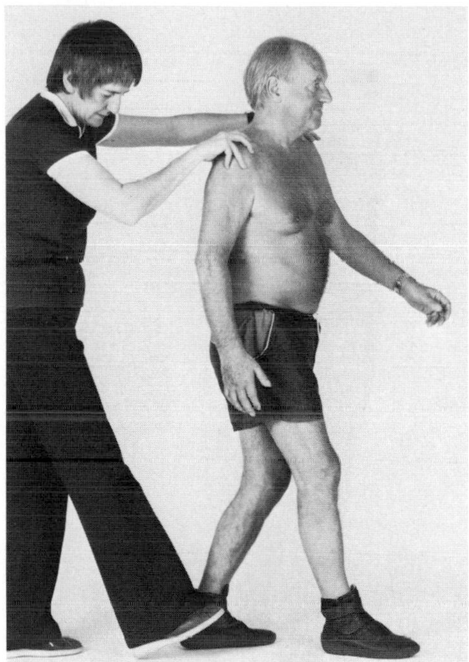

Fig. 9.13. Facilitating arm swing from the shoulders (right hemiplegia)

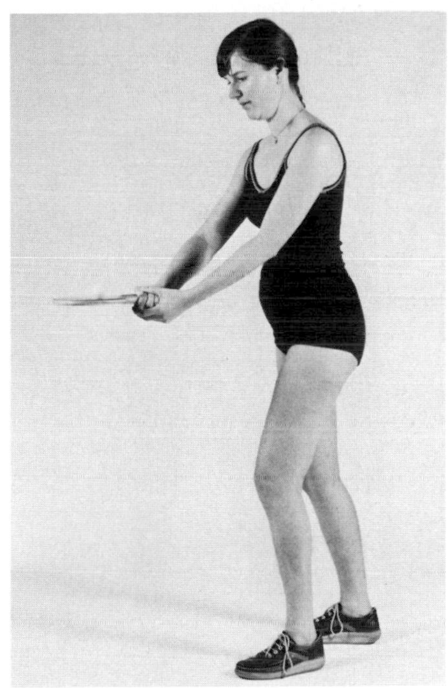

Fig. 9.14. Walking while balancing a ping-pong ball prevents associated reactions in the hemiplegic arm (right hemiplegia)

catch it again. The activity has the added effect of improving the rhythm of walking, if he bounces or throws once for each step he takes. He can also be asked to walk while balancing a ping-pong ball on a bat held with both hands (Fig. 9.14).

The patient can play a tambourine rhythmically as he walks. He taps out the rhythm of his own walking and tries to keep the beat regular. If he has active function in his hemiplegic hand he can hold the tambourine himself (Fig. 9.15), but otherwise the therapist holds it for him. By changing the position of the tambourine the therapist encourages the patient to move his head freely and not fix his eyes on the ground.

9.2.2.4 With One Arm Held Forward and Upward in External Rotation

To prevent the downward and backward pull of the hemiplegic side and shoulder, the therapist can facilitate walking by holding the patient's arm well forward in an inhibitory pattern (Fig. 9.16). His hand is held open and the elbow kept extended as he walks. The patient must be able to control his hip and knee himself because the therapist requires both her hands to support his arm in the inhibited position.

9.2.2.5 With the Hemiplegic Arm Resting on the Therapist's Shoulder

Facilitating walking with both the patient's arms resting on the therapist's shoulder is not recommended, as the position increases flexion in the trunk and hips

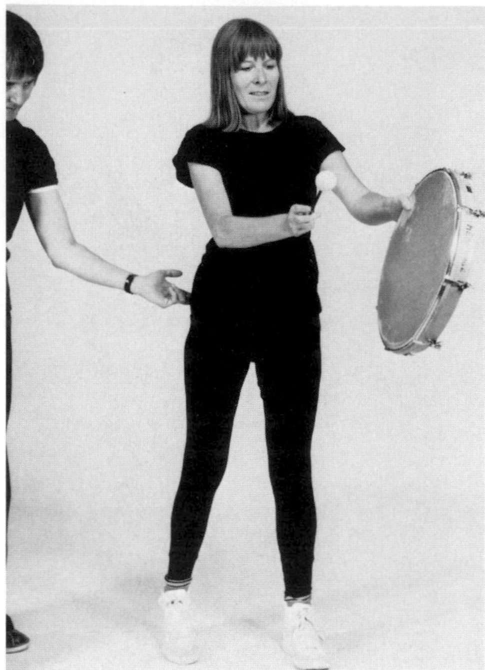

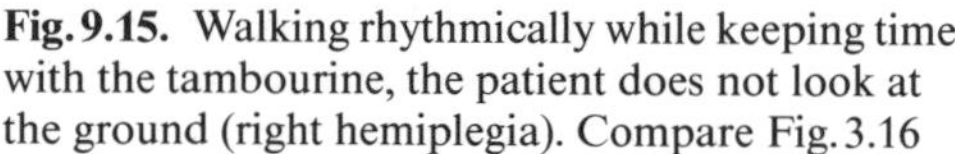

Fig. 9.15. Walking rhythmically while keeping time with the tambourine, the patient does not look at the ground (right hemiplegia). Compare Fig. 3.16

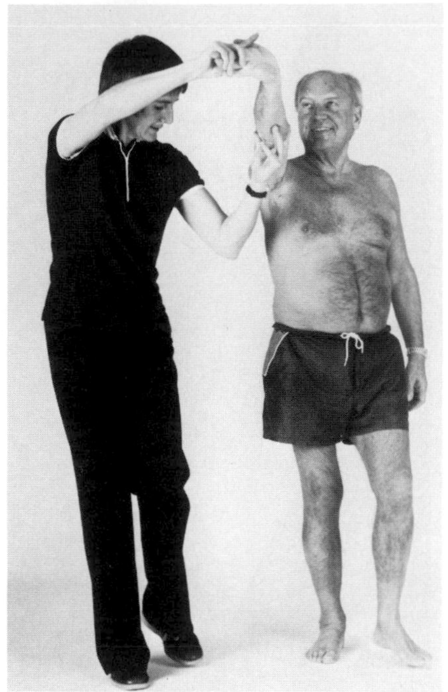

Fig. 9.16. Facilitating walking with the hemiplegic arm held forwards and upwards (right hemiplegia)

(Fig. 9.17 a). It is a normal compensatory reaction that when we lift our arms forward our hips flex to maintain equilibrium (Klein-Vogelbach 1976). The therapist therefore places only the patient's hemiplegic arm on her shoulder and splints his arm with her arm, her hand over his scapula to keep it forward. She can then use her other hand to help the patient to bring his hip forward into extension over the supporting leg (Fig. 9.17 b). This method of facilitation can be useful for achieving rotation of the pelvis over the weight-bearing leg, if the therapist asks the patient to rotate his pelvis back and forth rhythmically a few times before taking each step.

Facilitation of walking with the therapist in front of the patient has other disadvantages. Free rhythmic walking is prevented, as the therapist is walking backwards. The patient tends to lean on the therapist, so gaining extension from his arms instead of from his hips. The position can also make him dependent on someone being in front of him, and in fact he has to learn to walk with space in front of him as he must in his daily life.

9.2.2.6 With One Hand Against the Patient's Thoracic Spine and the Other Flat Against His Sternum

The patient who has difficulty in orientating his trunk correctly over his pelvis benefits from feeling the therapist's hands in front and behind him as points of reference (Fig. 9.18).

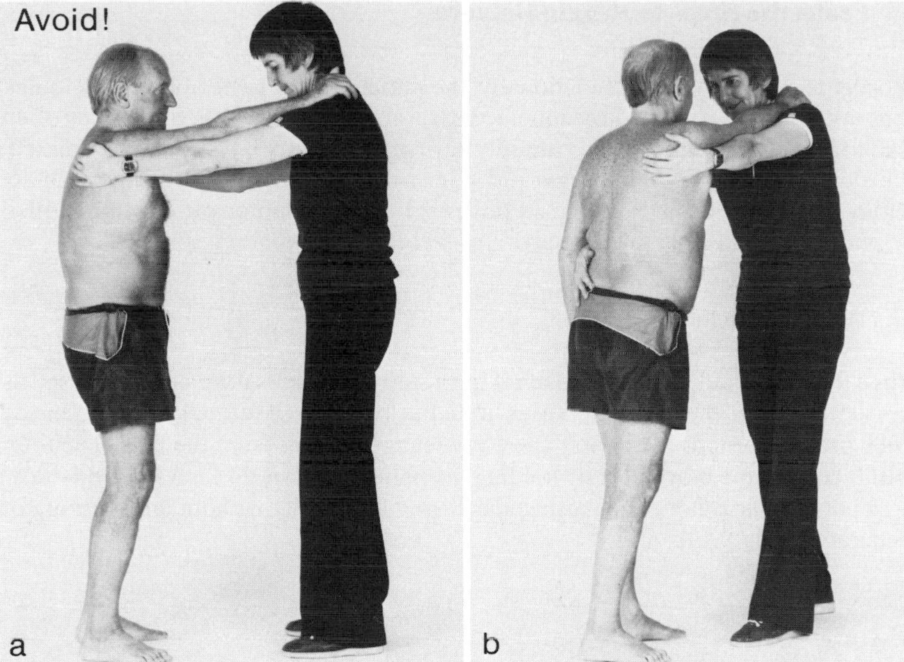

Fig. 9.17 a, b. Facilitating walking with the hemiplegic arm supported on the therapist's shoulders (right hemiplegia). **a** Supporting both arms on the therapist's shoulders increases flexion in the trunk and hips. The normal compensatory reaction is seen in the therapist's posture as well. **b** With only the hemiplegic arm supported

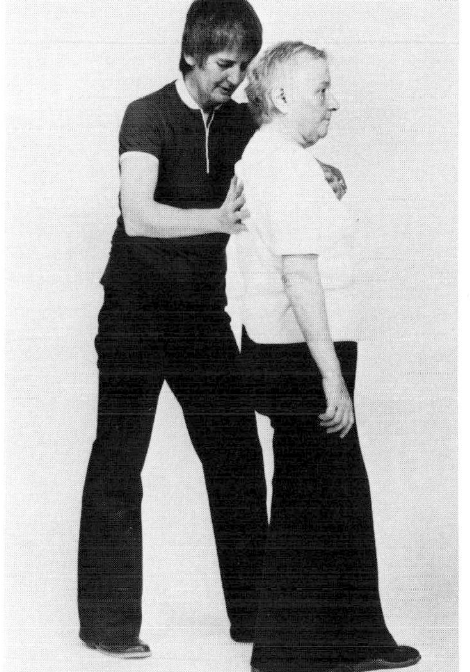

Fig. 9.18. Facilitating walking with one hand against the patient's sternum and the other against her thoracic spine (left hemiplegia)

9.3 Protective Steps to Regain Balance

In order to walk safely and functionally, the patient needs to be able to take quick steps automatically in any direction necessary, and with either leg. Such steps often need to be practised slowly and carefully at first, and the speed gradually increased. The ability to take steps backwards and sideways is also essential for functional activities. To arrange his position to sit down at table, in a motor car or on the toilet, the patient must be able to manoeuvre his feet in any direction required.

9.3.1 Walking Backwards

When the individual components of taking a step backwards have been practised as shown in Chap. 6, the patient learns to walk backwards in a normal pattern. During quick protective steps backwards the body leans forwards from the hips. The therapist facilitates the movement by holding the patient's pelvis on each side and drawing it back towards her at increasing speed, and eventually without any warning or preparation (Fig. 9.19).

9.3.2 Walking Sideways

Practising walking sideways will not only enable the patient to take protective steps, but will also improve the stance and swing phases of walking. The patient crosses

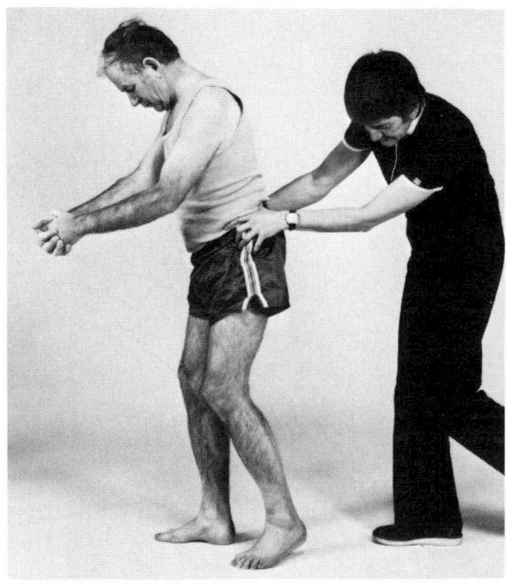

Fig. 9.19. Protective steps backwards (left hemiplegia)

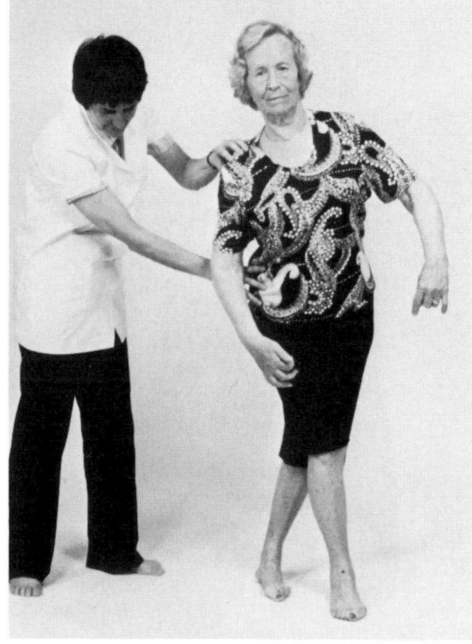

Fig. 9.20. Protective steps sideways (right ▷ hemiplegia)

one leg in front of the other as he takes each step, and the speed is increased gradually (Fig. 9.20).

9.3.3 Steps to Follow

To be fully confident and safe, the patient must be able to take quick automatic steps in any direction. The therapist facilitates such "steps to follow" with her hands placed lightly on the patient's shoulders. As he walks, she steers him unexpectedly in all directions and he follows without any resistance (Fig. 9.21). The patient should also learn to take automatic steps when the therapist indicates the direction by moving his hemiplegic arm and gives no verbal command (Fig. 9.22).

It is important to remember that, when we turn around normally, our head turns first so that we can see where we are going. Many patients do not turn their head automatically in the direction of the movement, but hold it in one fixed position instead. They only face in the new direction when the trunk has turned, bringing the head with it. The correct rotation may have to be practised by turning the head consciously at first. Practising rolling, which requires the same rotation, helps to retrain the movement. Activities such as bouncing a ball or beating a tambourine while turning round will also help to overcome the difficulty.

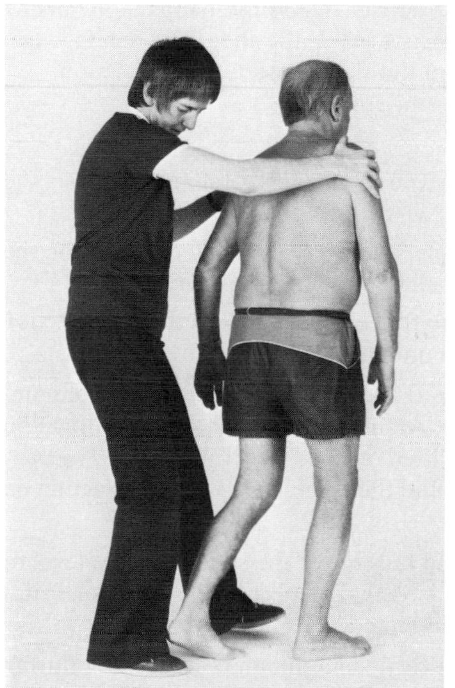
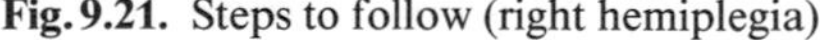

Fig. 9.21. Steps to follow (right hemiplegia)

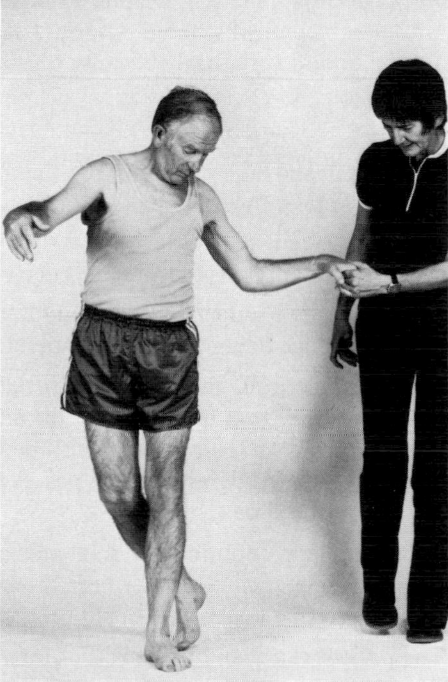

Fig. 9.22. Automatic steps (left hemiplegia)

9.4 Supporting the Hemiplegic Foot

For a correct walking pattern the patient needs a certain amount of active dorsiflexion of the ankle and toes. He also needs to be able to inhibit the over-activity of tibialis which pulls the foot strongly into supination during dorsiflexion. The swing phase, with its flexor components, is influenced by the total mass flexor synergy of the whole leg, including supination, for many patients.

With careful treatment, where the various components of walking are individually practised, the difficulty can usually be overcome. Before the patient has sufficient control himself, the foot must be held in the correct position, as he will otherwise be afraid to walk freely and will, in fact, be in danger of injuring his ankle (Fig. 9.23 a). If active dorsal flexion is inadequate, the patient will tend to flex his whole leg too strongly in order for his toes to clear the ground. The swing phase becomes distorted, and the natural rhythm of walking is lost. The decision to order a permanent calliper should not be made too early, because most patients will learn to manage without one.

9.4.1 Using a Bandage

Walking, however, need not be delayed until the patient can actively control his foot. A crêpe bandage bound firmly over the shoe will hold the foot in dorsiflexion and prevent supination, despite extensor spasticity. When the bandage is outside the shoe the patient still has a normal experience inside the shoe. The bandage can also be bound very firmly because the sole of the shoe protects the circulation.

Applying the bandage:

The patient sits on a chair and the therapist kneels in front of him and inhibits the spasticity in the foot.

With the patient's knee flexed to a right angle, and his heel firmly on the floor, the therapist supports his toes on her knee to maintain the dorsiflexion.

She wraps the bandage twice around his fore-foot to gain a good hold, the direction of the bandage being from medial to lateral underneath the foot.

The therapist pulls the bandage up tightly at the lateral border of the shoe and crosses over in front of and round his ankle. At the same time she presses down on the patient's knee to prevent his heel being lifted off the floor (Fig. 9.23 b). The bandage is not pulled tightly when it passes around the ankle, only where it is acting on the sole of the shoe.

The bandaging continues, and extends along the sole of the shoe from the level of the fifth metatarsal head to where the heel begins. The heel of the shoe is left uncovered, so that the danger of slipping is eliminated.

The patient can then bring his foot forward easily in a plantigrade position during the swing phase of gait (Fig. 9.23 c). When the patient is continually in danger of spraining his ankle, the bandage should be applied first thing in the morning and

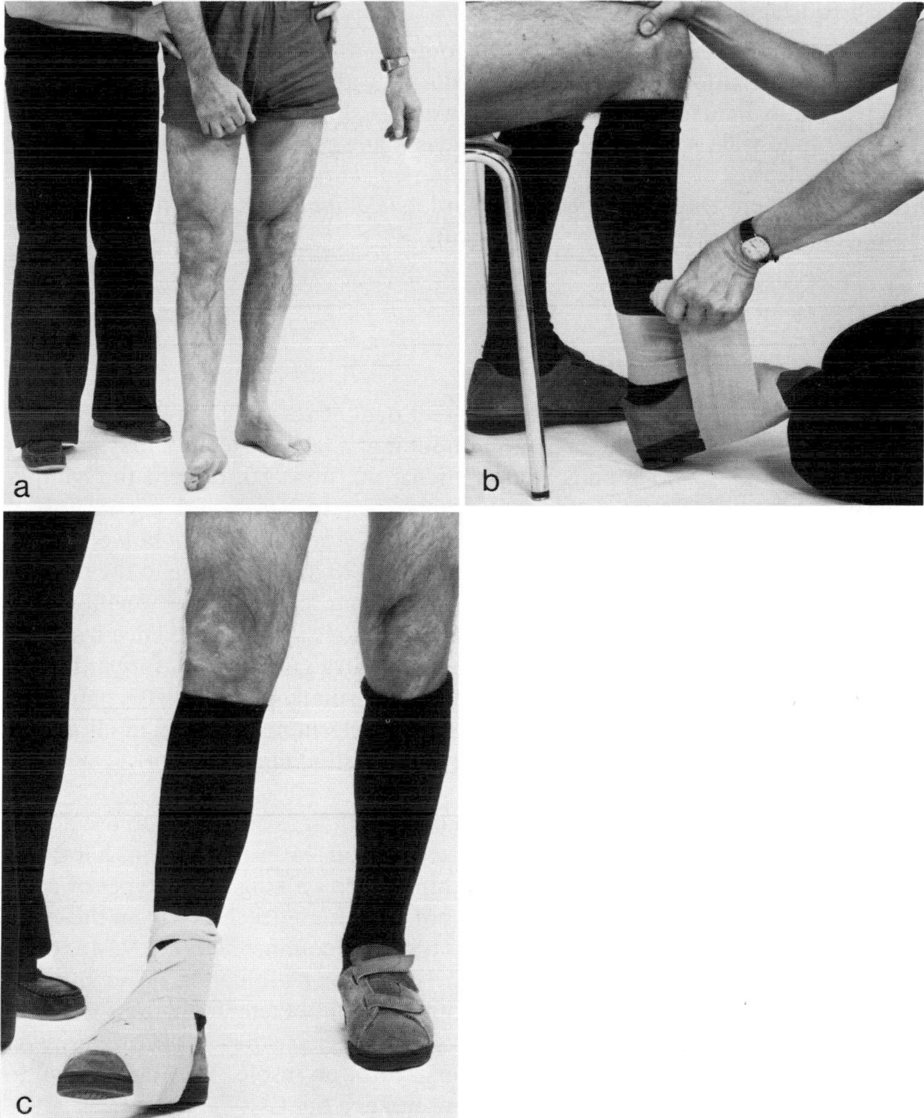

Fig. 9.23 a–c. Supporting the foot with a bandage (right hemiplegia). **a** Attempting to walk without a bandage; **b** applying the bandage – a firm pull into pronation; **c** walking, the foot safely protected and able to swing forwards easily

left on during the day. The ankle may otherwise be injured even during transfers or due to a prolonged incorrect position while he is sitting in the wheelchair. Such patients often have a localised oedema of the foot and lateral side of the ankle, caused by repeated traumas. The oedema disappears rapidly when the bandage has been applied for a few days.

The indications are as follows:

Dangerous supination or inversion of the foot in sitting, standing or walking.
Inadequate active dorsiflexion of the foot during walking.
As a temporary help for patients who have worn a calliper for some time and are trying to learn to walk without it (the bandage is made progressively less supportive).
For early attempts at learning to go up and down stairs correctly (Chap. 7).
For young patients, where the decision to order a calliper is delayed in the hope that sufficient control may be achieved eventually.

9.4.2 Using a Calliper

The decision to order a calliper carries a great deal of responsibility because most patients will find it difficult to manage without it at a later stage once they have become used to the total support. Some patients do, however, discard the calliper when they have become more confident through walking freely with it. Certainly, it is most important for the patient to be able to walk short distances at home without a calliper, e.g. for walking to his bed after having a bath, or walking to the toilet at night. A calliper is seldom required if the patient has learnt to bear weight on his hemiplegic leg without using the total pattern of extension with the knee hyperextended. He is then able to release the knee before bringing the foot forwards, and only a little active dorsiflexion is required, which is usually possible in the pattern of walking. When, however, despite prolonged and determined training in all phases of walking the supination persists and no active dorsiflexion is present, a calliper is required.

It is preferable for the patient to wear a calliper than to be obliged to use a stick if it is a case of one or the other. The former choice still leaves the patient's hand free for functional tasks, such as carrying something while walking. Many types of calliper have been described and are available, but the design developed from the original English inside iron and outside T-strap type is recommended (Fig. 9.24a, b). It has the advantage of reducing spasticity by preventing supination through direct pressure over the neck of the talus. Other forms of calliper tend to increase hypertonus in the muscles of plantar flexion and inversion because they all act primarily on the sole of the foot, either through the shoe itself or an insole. They usually fail to control marked supination unless the patient wears a boot.

The recommended calliper, which has become known through repeated usage as the "Valens" calliper, is cosmetically pleasing, particularly for patients wearing trousers, when only a fraction of the metal strut is visible.

The ankle joint of the calliper has a useful mechanism whereby tightening or loosening a small screw varies the amount of assistance given to dorsal flexion of the foot. The amount can be varied from total support to no assistance, which is important because many patients only require help to prevent the foot from supinating. Constant support of dorsiflexion at the ankle will reduce the demand for active muscle contraction.

The calliper is easy to put on with one hand and can be removed from the shoe and fitted to the patient's other shoes as well (Fig. 9.24c). Because the calliper is re-

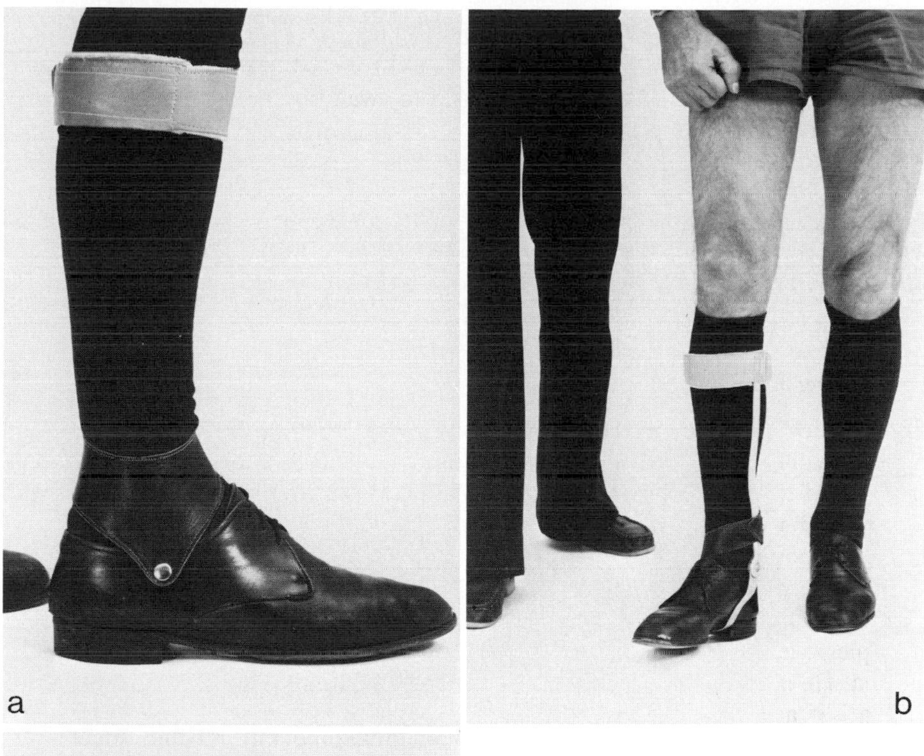

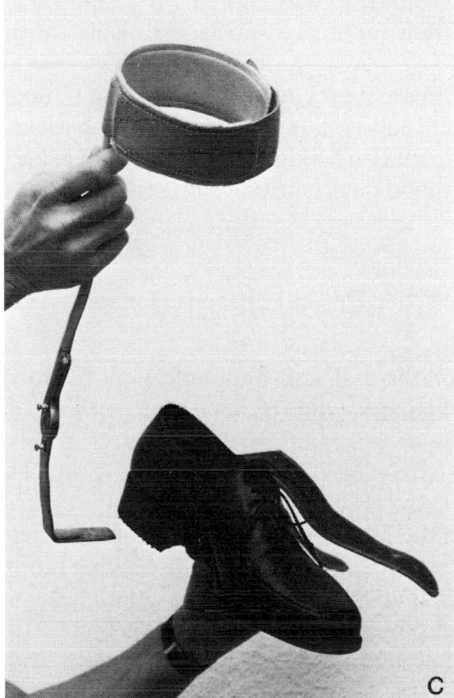

Fig. 9.24 a–c. Recommended calliper. **a** The strap prevents supination by pressure over the neck of the talus (right hemiplegia). **b** The swing phase is made easier by a variable amount of assistance to dorsiflexion (right hemiplegia). **c** The calliper can be removed from the shoe (left hemiplegia)

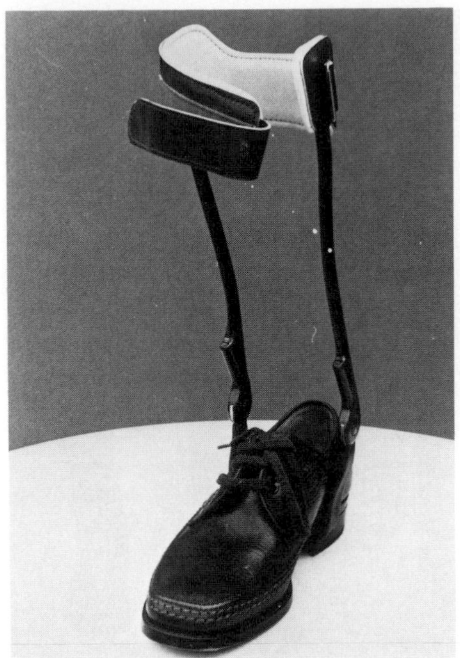

Fig. 9.25. The calliper used successfully in Hoensbroeck, Holland

movable, gait training can be continued without the calliper but with the patient wearing his normal shoes. A calliper with two upright irons with similar adjustable ankle joints will also support the foot satisfactorily if fitted to a sturdy shoe with a firm leather sole (Fig. 9.25) (Hoensbroeck 1983).

When considering different types of calliper or bracing, it is interesting to note that, during a study carried out by Ofir and Sell (1980), "the number of patients progressing in their functional ambulatory capability did not seem to change, and did not seem to be related to the kind of orthotic device or brace prescribed".

9.5 Going Up and Down Stairs

Practising the stairs has a beneficial effect on the gait, and walking cannot be truly functional if the patient is not able to manage stairs. Once he leaves the confines of his own home he is constantly confronted by steps, when entering theatres, toilets and older public buildings, and even when crossing the road. In many instances there may be no handrail (Fig. 9.26).

If stairs are included at an early stage in the rehabilitation the patient will have little difficulty in learning the activity, and will achieve independent walking more quickly. From the first attempt onwards, the patient is taught to go up and down stairs in a normal way, i.e. one foot after the other on alternate steps. At first sufficient support is given by the therapist, so that the movement occurs smoothly and rhythmically and the patient is not afraid (Chap. 7).

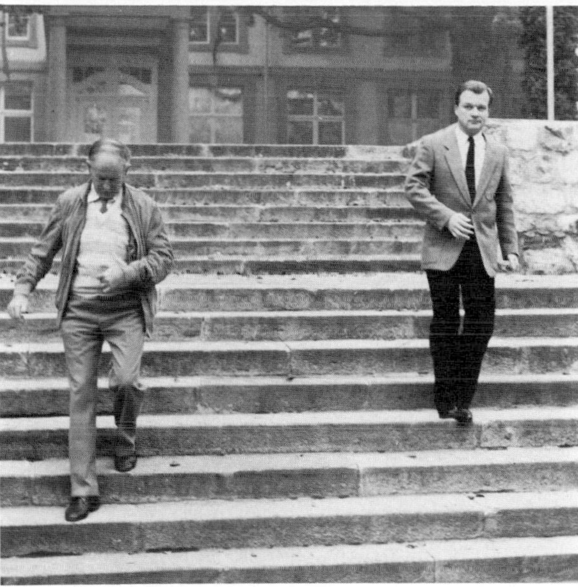

Fig. 9.26. Two patients leaving an old public building, managing the steps with no handrail available (left hemiplegia and right hemiplegia)

9.6 Using a Stick

It should not be assumed that giving the patient a stick for support will enable him to walk safely. The hemiplegic patient falls towards his hemiplegic side and backwards, when the stick would be of little help to save him. It is useful for the therapist to apply the somewhat paradoxical rule, "a patient should only be given a stick when he can walk without one". The rule implies that the patient can manage to walk in his sheltered home environment without a stick, and can therefore carry something from room to room. It implies also that he has some means of maintaining his balance, should he fall toward the hemiplegic side.

Many patients, particularly older ones, like to have a stick with them when they venture out on the street. They feel that other people will then recognise that they have balance problems and be more considerate. If it is at all possible even these problems should be overcome through further practice and experience in the actual situations. However, the fact that the patient feels confident and is prepared to go out on his own is of prime importance, and taking the stick with him is far better than his sitting indoors. The presence of a stick can also be a help for relatives who are afraid that the patient will overbalance towards his sound side and are in this way encouraged to walk on his affected side. It must always be remembered that if a person has a stick in one hand he will lean towards that side, and that the other arm tends to be in an adducted position as a result.

The ordinary wooden cane or walking-stick is the only type that is recommended, if a stick is to be used at all. It is cosmetically more acceptable, can in fact

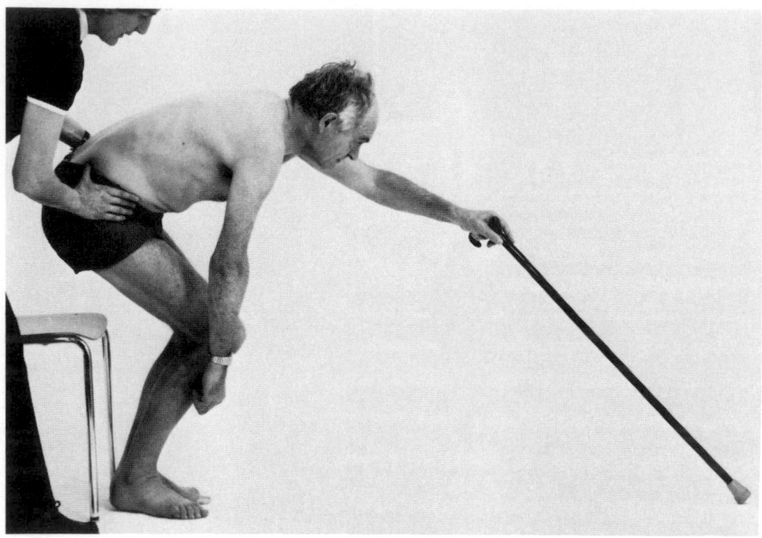

Fig. 9.27. Despite the stick the patient stands up in normal pattern

be elegant, and does not immediately draw attention to the person as an invalid. The adjustable metal walking-stick is only used to select the correct height for the individual patient. Sometimes, using a cane that is somewhat longer than the recommended height of trochanter level prevents the patient from leaning on it too heavily.

Quadripods or tripods should never be used, as they are cumbersome to manoeuvre and only offer increased support if the weight is transferred directly over them, that is, away from the hemiplegic side. The metallic appearance is definitely associated with hospitals and disability, and changes the attitude of other people towards the patient. The Canadian elbow crutch also offers no extra security for the hemiplegic patient, and again only encourages more transfer of weight towards the sound side.

Any form of manual support causes the centre of gravity to be more over the sound side and emphasises the retraction of the affected side. In some cases, the patient will almost be walking diagonally sideways and the side of the body which is constantly behind him will tend to be more and more neglected.

If the patient uses a walking-stick, he should still try to maintain certain normal patterns of movement. For example, when standing up from sitting the patient should push the cane as far in front of him as possible, with the hemiplegic arm remaining forward in extension. In this way, his head is brought forward well over his feet, using the normal pattern of coming to the upright position (Fig. 9.27). The same principle applies when he sits down again. With the feet parallel, the patient slides the stick well forwards before lowering himself on to the chair. A patient who stands up by pushing on a support immediately takes all the weight over to that side, and will assume a starting position for walking that is already asymmetrical. Often the hemiplegic foot, without any weight being taken through it, will lift off the floor.

9.7 Considerations

Walking is a natural and enjoyable activity for human beings and enhances the quality of our lives. Patients who walk functionally will achieve greater independence and maintain their mobility and level of achievement far better. Using the erect position improves circulation, muscle extensibility and activity, as well as other vital bodily functions. Those patients who do not achieve completely independent walking will still benefit from the activity in the upright position. Even if the patient can only walk with the help of another person, many aspects of daily life will be easier and more enjoyable. Being able to walk at all provides access to those places where a wheelchair would be impossible, and allows the patient a greater freedom of choice.

10 Some Activities of Daily Living

Rehabilitation aims at the highest possible level of independence in daily life for the patient with hemiplegia. For the adult patient, being independent is the first vital step to being able to return to his former life-style. Independence means no longer being an invalid, dependent on help from others for all everyday activities. Being independent enables the patient to choose where, when and with whom he would like to be at any given time, and even the choice to be on his own. The fact that he knows he can manage is important for the patient, but a little help can often go a long way and should not be rigidly withheld.

10.1 Therapeutic Considerations

1. How the patient carries out the routine activities in his daily life will affect not only the quality of his overall movement but also the maintenance of the standard he ultimately achieves. The importance of the 24-hour way of life has already been discussed (Chap. 5). It is self-defeating if, after a concentrated treatment with full inhibition of spasticity, the patient then struggles to dress himself incorrectly and marked associated reactions occur.
   All activities of daily living should be performed in such a way that associated reactions are avoided. The movements should be as economic and normal as possible, and the correct postures encouraged. Careful and repeated training, with sufficient guidance, will often be needed before the sequences are automatically carried out correctly and beneficially. They must become a part of the patient's repertoire through repeated experience, so that he reproduces them in any situation when they are required, and not only in the presence of the therapist.
2. Because the activities take place regularly, they can be a valuable recurring therapy, and form an integral part of any home programme for the patient. For the same reason, if they are performed incorrectly the detrimental effects are considerable.
3. The patient will learn more easily in familiar everyday situations, and the retrieval of previously stored functions is facilitated during actual events (Chap. 1). In daily life activities the patient can learn to plan, move and perceive. Activities such as washing and dressing help to overcome the neglect of the hemiplegic side.
4. Balance reactions are considerably improved by standing and walking during those activities which would normally be carried out in the upright position.

Every patient will have different wishes and expectations for his life. A few activities which are common to most people have been chosen, and the same principles can then be applied to individual requirements such as working conditions and hobbies. It is never too early to start incorporating the activities in the treatment programme, as long as the therapist guides the patient adequately to avoid frustration or failure (Chap. 1).

10.2 Personal Hygiene

10.2.1 Washing

The patient sits at the wash-basin, preferably on a stool or an upright chair. When he has filled the basin and checked the water temperature, he places his hemiplegic

10.1 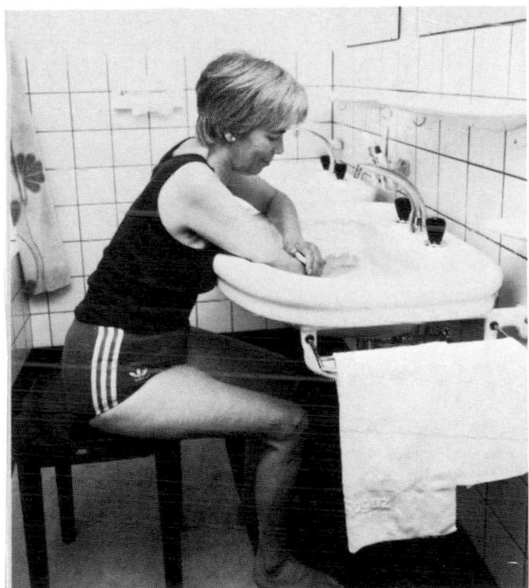

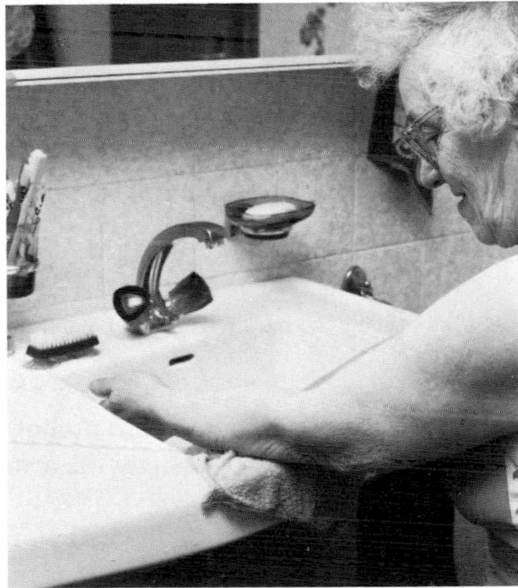 10.2

10.3 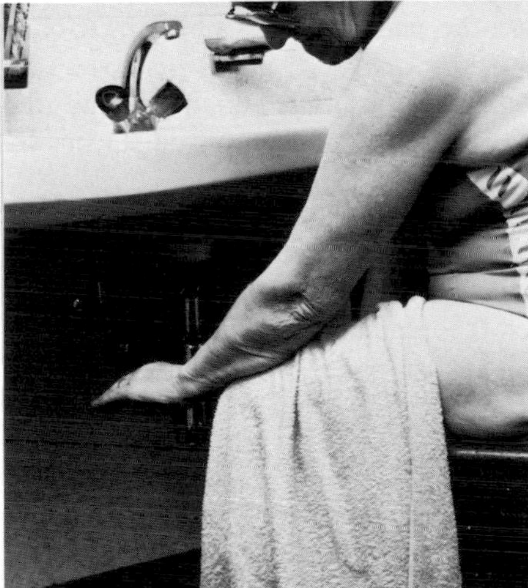

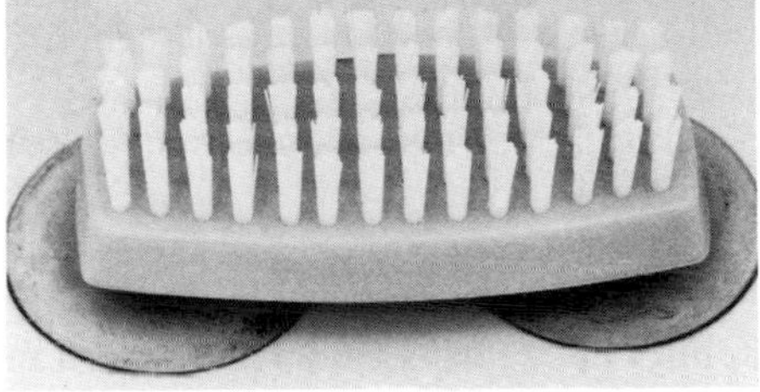 10.4

Fig. 10.1. Position at the wash-basin (right hemiplegia)

Fig. 10.2. Washing the sound arm (right hemiplegia)

Fig. 10.3. Drying the sound arm (right hemiplegia)

Fig. 10.4. Nail-brush adaptation, for cleaning nails or false teeth

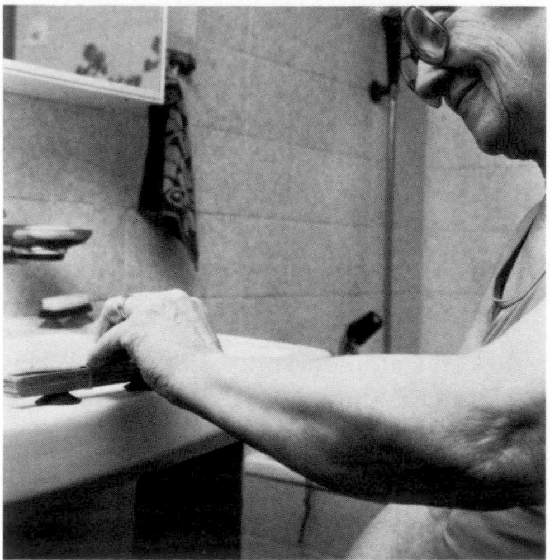

Fig. 10.5. Adapted nail-file (right hemiplegia)

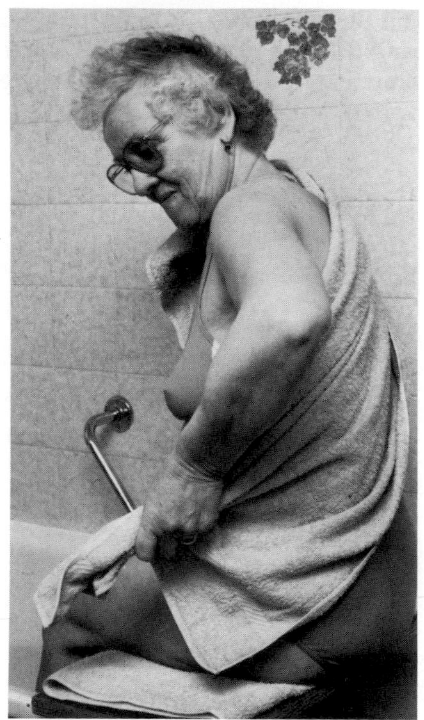

Fig. 10.6. Drying the back (right hemiplegia) ▷

arm in the basin. The downward pull of the side is inhibited, and a symmetrical upright posture achieved. Washing the arm and the axilla is also easier in this position (Fig. 10.1).

To wash the sound arm, the patient fixes the soapy face-flannel over the edge of the basin and rubs his arm and hand over it (Fig. 10.2). To dry the sound arm, he places the towel over one of his legs and moves his arm over the towel (Fig. 10.3). A nail-brush with suction caps attached enables the patient to clean his finger-nails (Fig. 10.4).

Cutting or clipping finger-nails is possible only for very few patients. A nail-file, attached to a small strip of wood, can be held in place on a supporting surface by two suction caps and enables the patient to file his nails (Fig. 10.5).

To dry his back, the patient tosses the towel over one shoulder and then reaches behind him, grasps the other end and pulls the towel down across his back. He repeats the procedure over the other shoulder. The same procedure can be used after bathing or showering, or in fact whenever the patient needs to dry his back (Fig. 10.6).

10.2.2 Brushing Teeth

At first in sitting, the patient rests his affected arm along the edge of the basin if the space is sufficient. With only a little control, the hemiplegic hand can hold the brush while the toothpaste is applied instead of balancing it on the basin. As soon as it becomes possible, the patient stands to brush his teeth. When some activity has returned he can hold the side of the basin, but otherwise can leave his arm forward in an inhibited position.

10.2.3 Having a Bath

Not only for hygienic reasons, but also for his enjoyment, it is important to teach the patient how to get in and out of the bath safely and easily, preferably without aids.

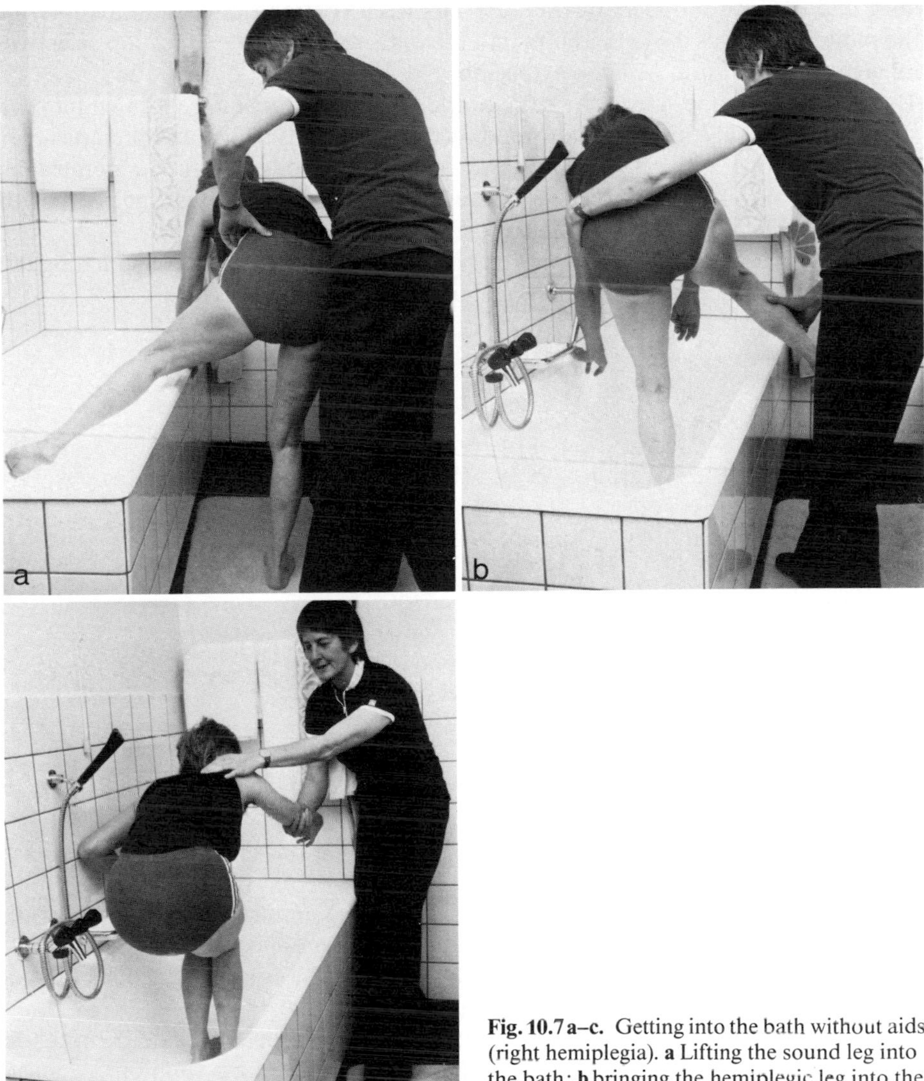

Fig. 10.7 a–c. Getting into the bath without aids (right hemiplegia). **a** Lifting the sound leg into the bath; **b** bringing the hemiplegic leg into the bath; **c** sitting down in the bath

Most patients who can walk unaided will be able to manage the following method. The patient requires help from the therapist to learn the movement sequence, which often seems difficult when attempted for the first time. The method was worked out by patients themselves and is worth practising, as it does not require a special bath or handrails.

The patient stands with his sound side to the bath, irrespective as to which end the taps and plug are situated. The water, at the correct temperature, is already in the bath. He lifts his sound leg into the bath while holding on to the side nearest to him. The therapist assists by holding both sides of his pelvis (Fig. 10.7 a).
The patient moves his sound hand to the other edge of the bath, and lifts his hemiplegic leg forward and upward into the bath. The therapist helps him to bring the knee and hip into sufficient flexion (Fig. 10.7 b). It is almost always impossible for the patient to lift his leg behind him into the bath, as the movement is too selective, i.e. active knee flexion with hip extension.
The patient holds the side of the bath, or the tap, and lowers himself down into the sitting position. The buoyancy afforded by the water assists him. The therapist, her hand placed over his scapula, leans away so that her body weight counteracts his descending movement. With her other hand she eases his arm forward to prevent an associated reaction in flexion (Fig. 10.7 c).
The patient washes himself, a bar of soap on a string around his neck facilitating the manipulation of the soap on to a flannel or his sound hand (Fig. 10.8).

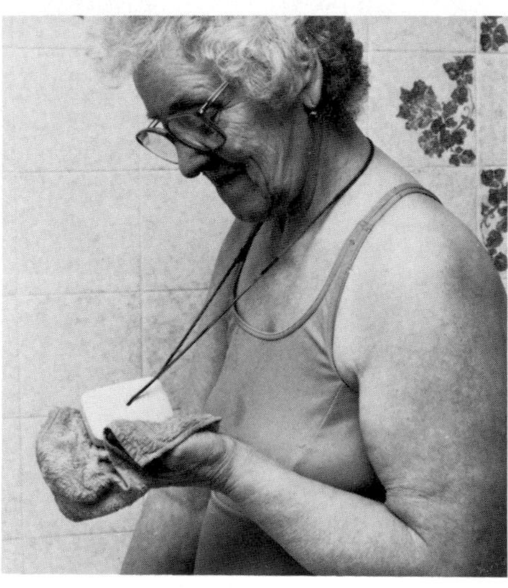

Fig. 10.8. Soap on a string (right hemiplegia)

When the washing is completed, he removes the plug and then prepares to get out of the bath by drawing his legs up into as full a flexion as possible.
The patient uses his sound hand to turn both knees to that side, the feet placed as far as possible to the opposite side of the bath.
He draws his hemiplegic arm forward across his body and as far round behind him as he can, so that the shoulder is well forward and trunk rotation achieved (Fig. 10.9 a).

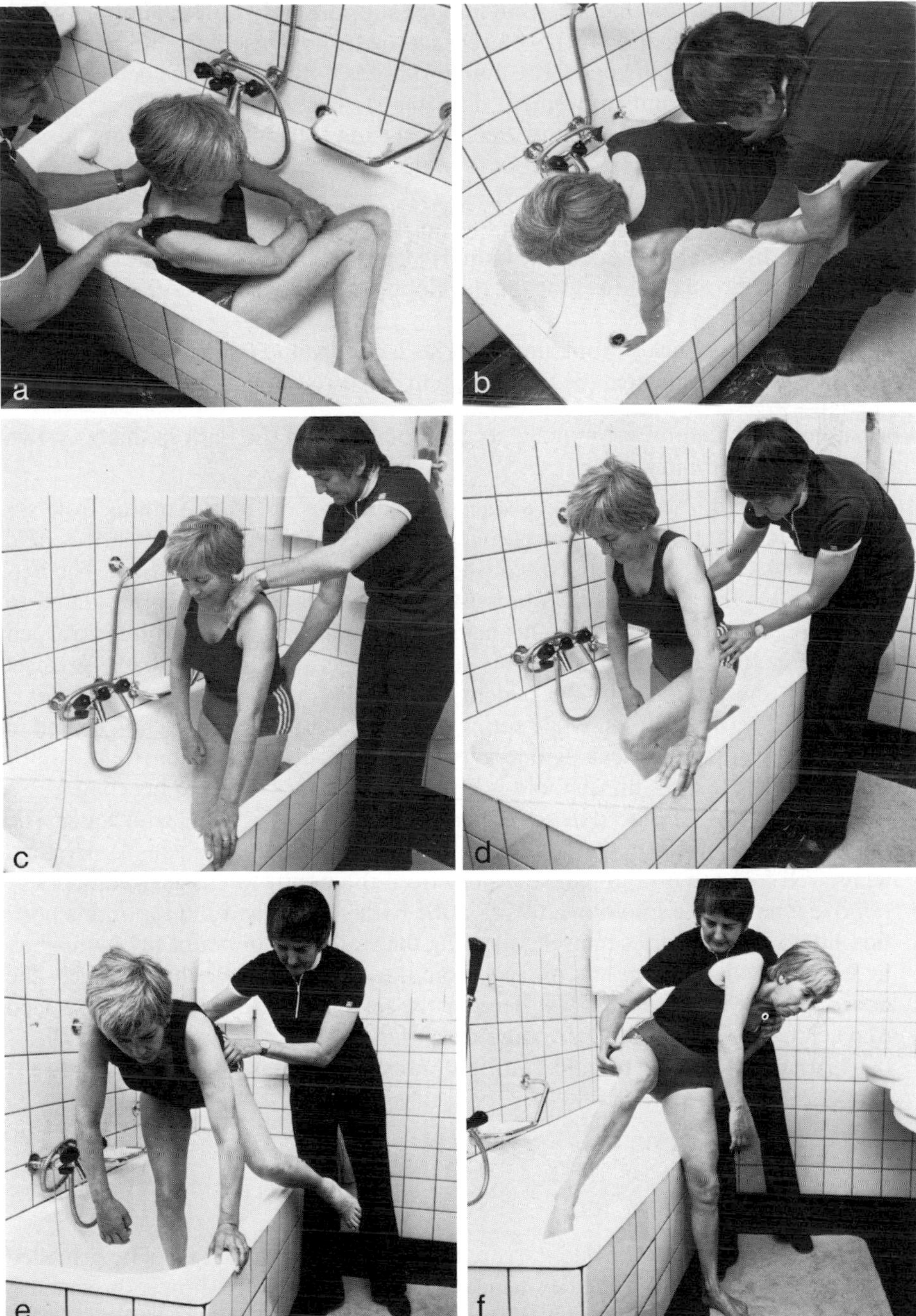

Fig. 10.9 a–f. Getting out of the bath without aids (right hemiplegia). **a** Preparing to turn around on to the knees; **b** turning on to the knees, with the therapist assisting from the pelvis; **c** coming to an upright kneel-standing position; **d** half-kneel-standing on the hemiplegic knee; **e** standing, lifting the sound leg out of the bath; **f** turning and lifting the hemiplegic leg

He then places his sound hand behind him for support, either on the bottom of the bath, or up on the end, and lifts his buttocks as he turns himself around completely to take his weight on both knees. The therapist holds both sides of his pelvis to facilitate the lifting and turning movement (Fig. 10.9 b).
He then kneels upright with his hips well forward in extension and, holding the side of the bath (Fig. 10.9 c), brings one foot forwards (preferably the sound leg) to come to a half-kneeling position (Fig. 10.9 d).
Bringing his weight forward over the foot in front, he rises to a standing position and then lifts his sound leg out of the bath. He keeps his hand on the side of the bath for support as he places the foot on the floor with outward rotation of the hip (Fig. 10.9 e).
The patient reaches back behind him, turns his hand around to grasp the bath on his sound side, and lifts his hemiplegic leg up and out through flexion (Fig. 10.9 f).

For patients who cannot yet manage to get in and out of the bath in this way, two intermediate stages can be of help.

1. For the patient who is still using a wheelchair and has difficulty coming from sitting to standing, a board is placed over the end of the bath. The board is held firmly in place by rubber knobs screwed on underneath it (Fig. 10.10 a). The patient transfers from his chair, with assistance, towards his hemiplegic side on to the board (Fig. 10.10 b) and lifts his hemiplegic leg into the bath with his clasped hands (Fig. 10.10 c). He then lifts his sound leg actively into the bath. A towel placed on the board helps the patient to slide to the middle. He then takes a shower and washes himself while sitting on the board. A shower curtain tucked in beneath his sound buttock will prevent water from running on to the floor (Fig. 10.10 d). He dries himself and is helped to transfer back into his chair.
2. A lower bath stool is placed below the board and the bath is filled with water. The patient is transferred or sits down first on to the board as in stage (1). He then leans well forward and lifts his buttocks from the board to enable the helper to remove it and guide him down to sit on the bath stool (Fig. 10.11 a). In this position he washes and dries himself, allowing the water to run out of the bath when he has finished. He then lifts his seat from the stool and the helper replaces the board on which he can sit again. Because the seat is so low, the patient may need to reach forward and hold on to the side of the bath for support instead of clasping his hands together (Fig. 10.11 b). He transfers with assistance back into his chair.

10.2.4 Having a Shower

Some patients may prefer or find it easier to take a shower. A seat must be provided so that the patient can sit while he washes himself. In a separate shower the seat can be of the folding type, attached to the wall, or a bathroom stool can be placed in the shower, in a corner for additional support (Fig. 10.12). Where the shower is over the bath, the patient must first climb into the bath as already described and have some sort of seat in or attached to the bath. The cake of soap with a string attached is once again most useful.

Fig. 10.10 a–d. Getting into the bath with assistance (right hemiplegia). **a** A board is placed over the bath; **b** transferring towards the hemiplegic side from the wheel-chair to sit on the board; **c** lifting the hemiplegic leg into the bath; **d** showering while sitting on the board with the shower curtain tucked under one buttock

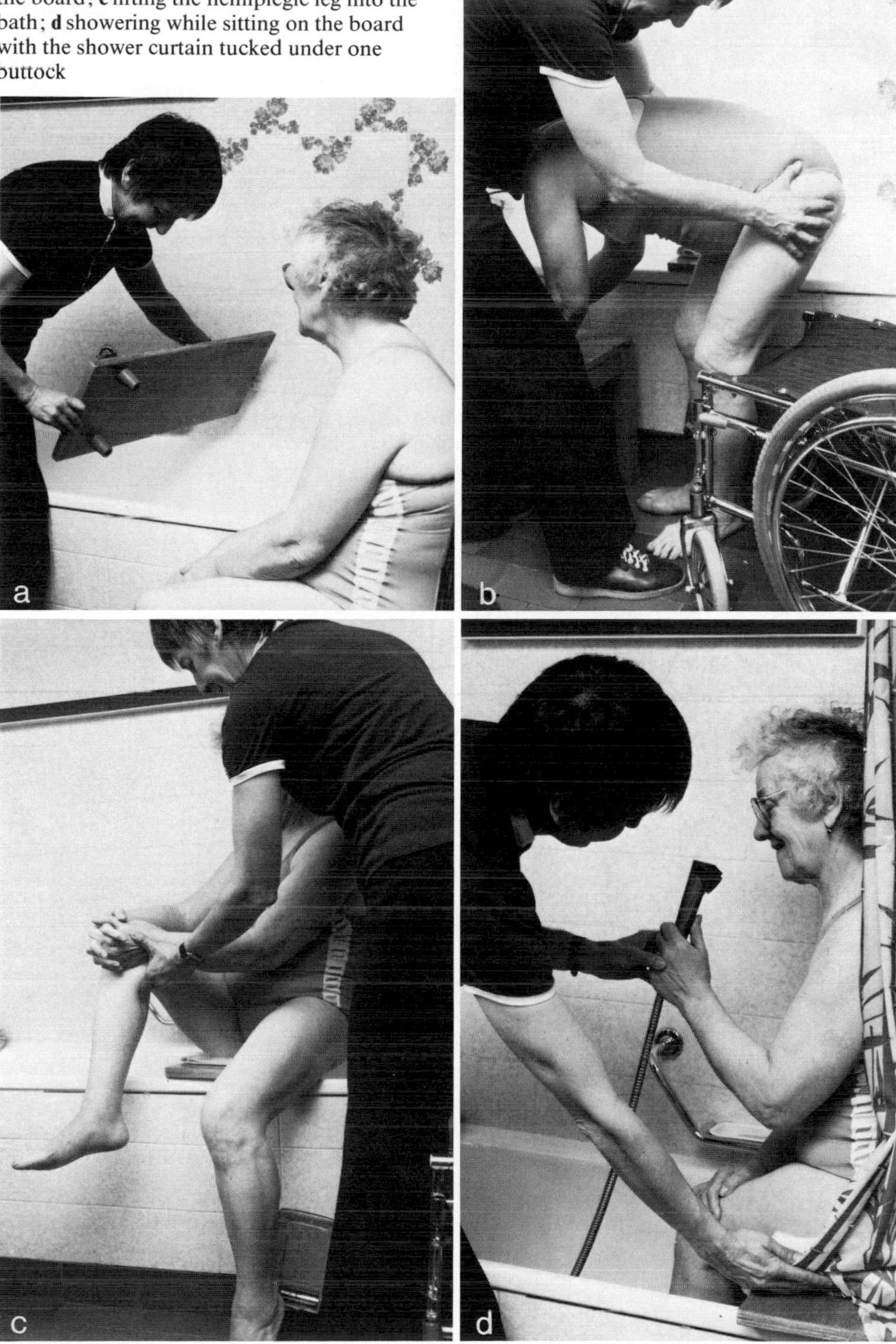

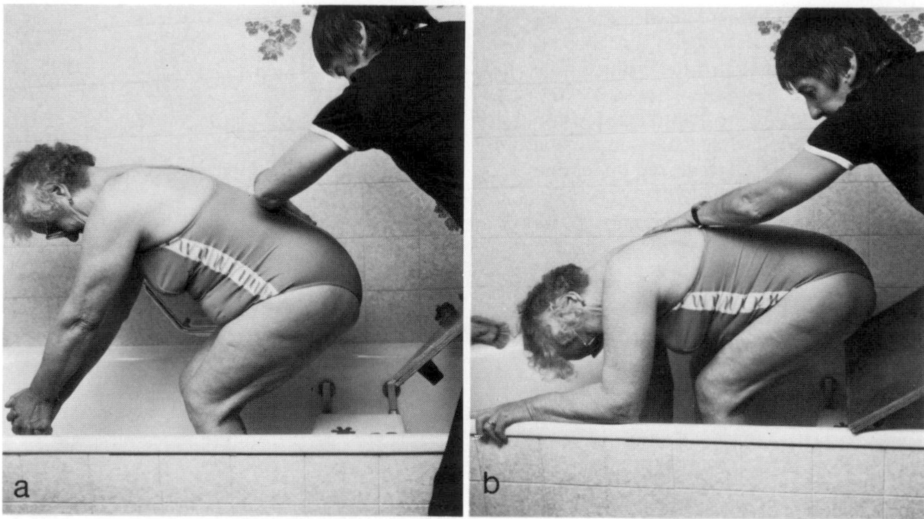

Fig. 10.11 a, b. Bathing while sitting on a low bath stool (right hemiplegia). **a** The helper removes the board and the patient sits down on a bath stool. **b** After bathing the patient lifts her buttocks so that the helper can replace the board

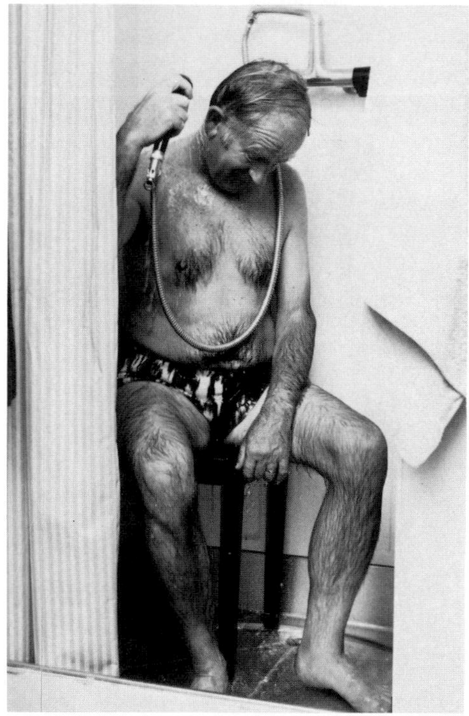

Fig. 10.12. Taking a shower (left hemiplegia)

10.3 Dressing

It must not be forgotten that getting dressed also necessitates deciding what to put on and fetching the clothes from the wardrobe (Fig. 10.13). The patient should sit on an upright chair with his feet flat on the floor, and not on the edge of his bed. The mattress is unsteady and would entail his struggling to maintain his balance, and the height of the bed itself is often unsuitable. Patients should eventually be able to put on the clothes of their choice, but loose simple clothing enables them to learn the sequence and arrangement more easily and rapidly at first (Leviton-Rheingold et al. 1980).

When the clothes are arranged in front of the patient, i.e. within his field of vision and in the correct order, the task becomes far simpler for him, being then on the recognition level (Fig. 10.14). Later, the clothes are placed ready at his hemiplegic side so that he turns towards that side as he reaches for each garment.

When the patient first starts learning how to dress himself, he need not put on all the clothes himself. This would take far too long. Instead, the therapist or nurse goes through the routine with him and he helps, with guidance, to put on one or two articles of clothing. What is important is that from the start each person who assists him should always follow the same routine. He can then learn the sequence for getting dressed.

There are many different methods of putting on clothing with one hand, but here the decision rests with the individual therapist. What is important is that the patient should succeed, without undue effort and without associated reactions appearing. The following method is recommended for the majority of patients. A simple rule is to start each sequence by first dressing the hemiplegic limb.

With the clothes placed on a chair at his hemiplegic side, the patient first puts on his underwear. He puts on his underpants in the same way as he does his trousers. For ladies, the brassière can be a problem, and one way is to insert an elastic strip at the

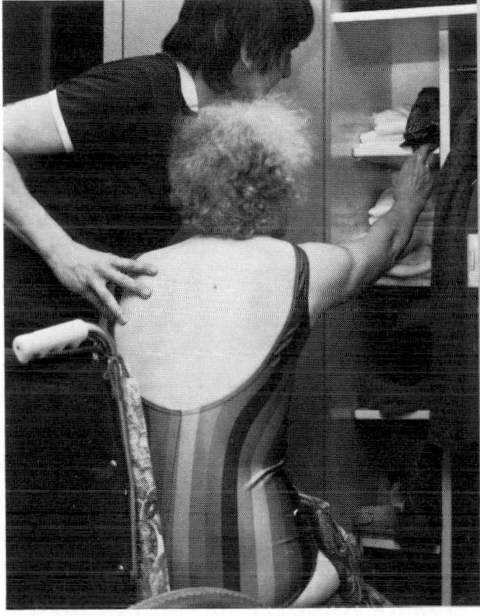

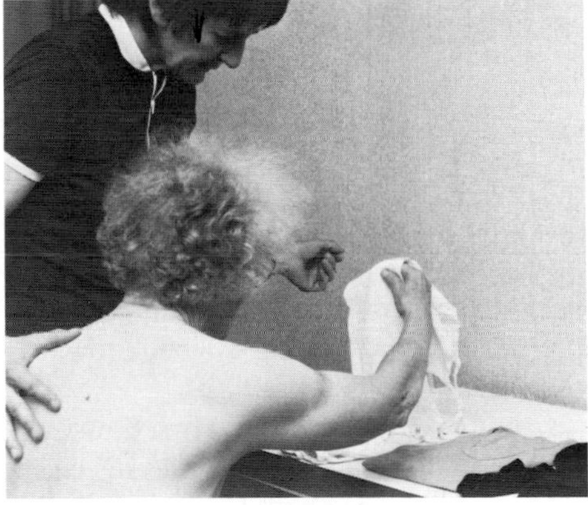

Fig. 10.14. The clothes arranged in the correct order in front of the patient (left hemiplegia)

◁ **Fig. 10.13.** Fetching clothes from the wardrobe (left hemiplegia)

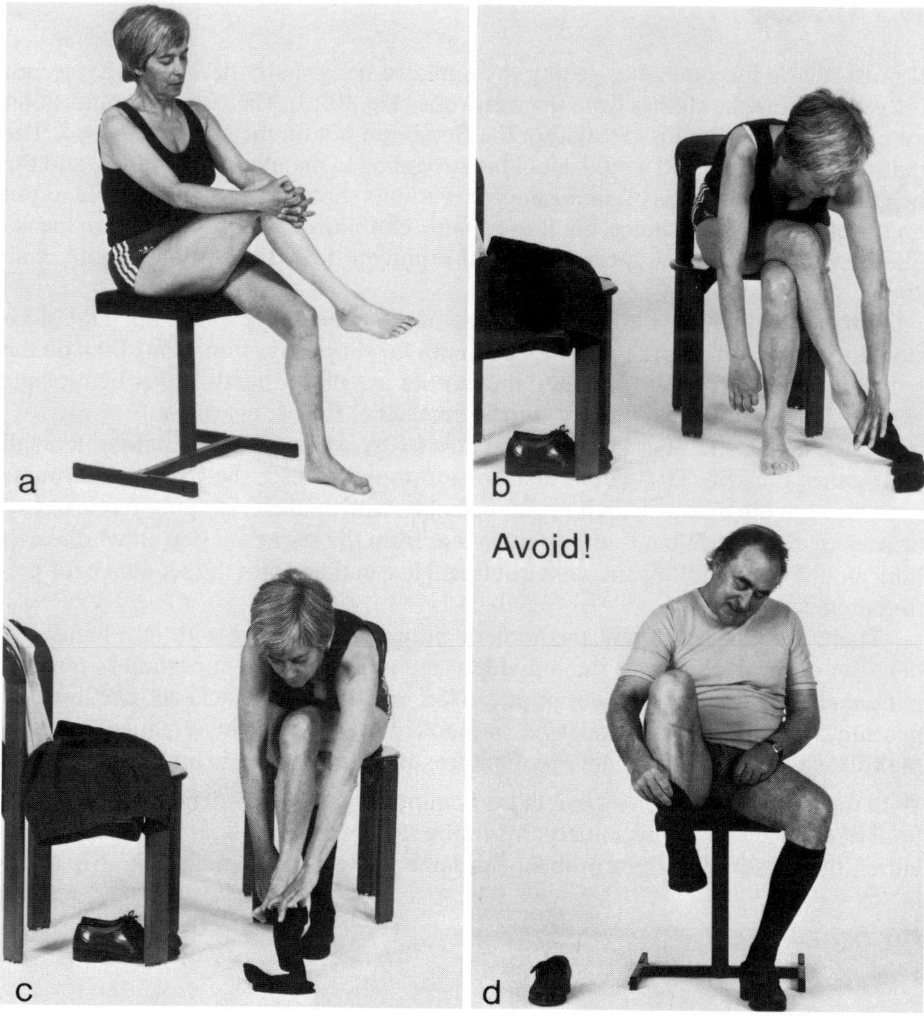

Fig. 10.15 a–d. Putting on socks (right hemiplegia). **a** Crossing the hemiplegic leg over the other leg. **b** Putting the sock on the hemiplegic foot. The arm remains forwards. **c** Putting the sock on the sound foot with the leg crossed over. **d** Associated reactions occur if the sound leg is not crossed over (left hemiplegia)

back, leave it fastened and then put it on like a pullover. Some patients can fasten the brassière by turning the back towards the front and fastening it before putting their arms through the straps.

To put on socks, the patient first crosses his hemiplegic leg over the other leg. If he is unable to do so actively, he uses his clasped hands to lift it (Fig. 10.15 a). He should never grasp his leg with his sound hand and struggle to pull it into position, as this will cause the hemiplegic side to retract strongly in an unwanted spastic pattern. He then opens the sock, using his thumb and first fingers, and leans well forward to pull it over his foot. Before doing so, he brings his hemiplegic arm forward with the shoulder protracted and the elbow extended (Fig. 10.15 b). He should put on the

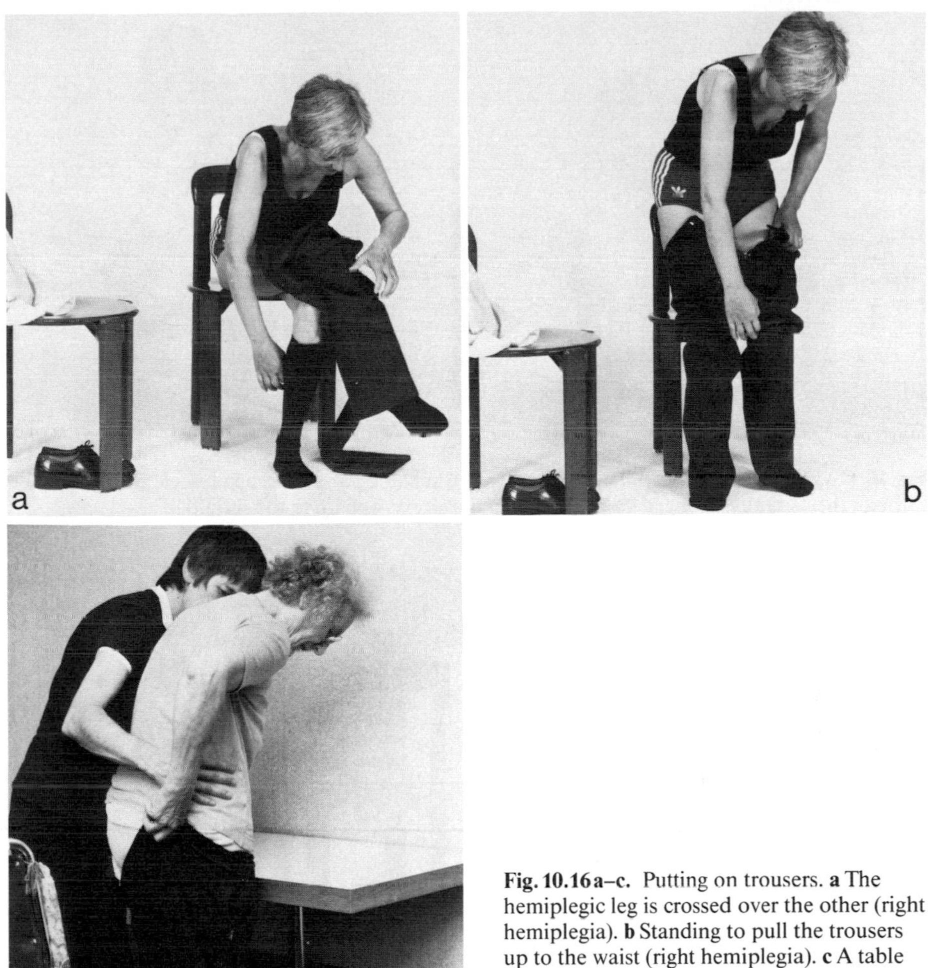

Fig. 10.16 a–c. Putting on trousers. **a** The hemiplegic leg is crossed over the other (right hemiplegia). **b** Standing to pull the trousers up to the waist (right hemiplegia). **c** A table provides security and orientation if the patient has poor balance (left hemiplegia)

other sock in exactly the same way, so that his weight is then over the hemiplegic side and associated reactions in the arm and leg are prevented (Fig. 10.15 c, d).

To put on his trousers, the patient first crosses his affected leg over the other one and pulls the trouser-leg up as far as possible (Fig. 10.16 a). When he has placed the affected foot back flat on the floor, he steps into the other trouser-leg. The hemiplegic arm remains well forward all the time.

Taking weight on both feet, he lifts his buttocks off the chair and pulls the trousers up to his waist (Fig. 10.16 b) before fastening them, either while standing or after sitting down again. His hand needs to be guided at first to ensure that the hemiplegic side is not neglected, leaving the trousers pulled down on that side. If the patient has difficulty in maintaining his balance while standing, a table in front of him is a great help. It provides security and also orientation (Fig. 10.16 c).

To put on a shirt, cardigan or jacket, the patient arranges the garment across his knees in such a way that the sleeve hangs free between his knees, creating an easy

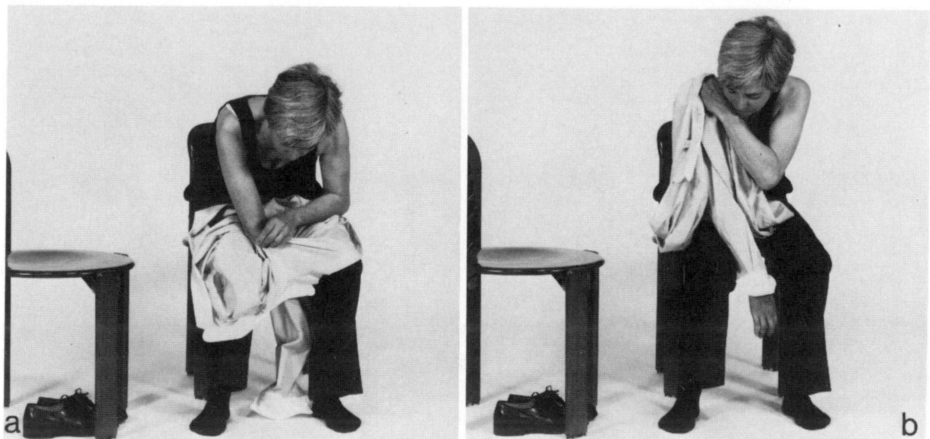

Fig. 10.17 a, b. Putting on a shirt or blouse (right hemiplegia). **a** The hemiplegic arm is pushed through the carefully arranged sleeve. **b** Pulling the sleeve well up to the shoulder

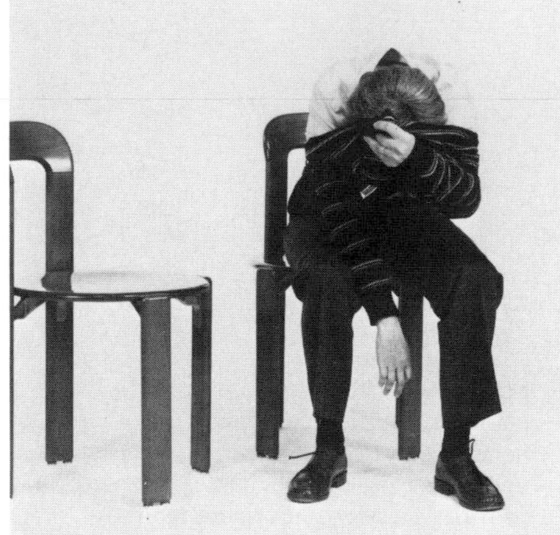

Fig. 10.18. Putting on a pullover (right hemiplegia)

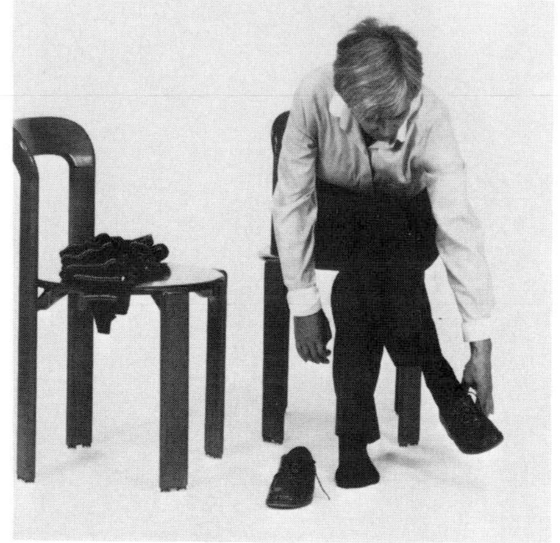

Fig. 10.19. Putting the shoe on the hemiplegic foot (right hemiplegia)

passage through which he pushes his hemiplegic hand (Fig. 10.17 a). He then pulls the sleeve well up the arm, to the shoulder (Fig. 10.17 b). The elbow remains extended due to the protraction of the scapula. The patient then reaches round to grasp the jacket and pulls it towards the other side until he can place his sound arm in the sleeve. Some patients with good standing balance find it easier to put on a shirt while standing.

The problem of fastening the button at the cuff of the sound arm is solved by sewing it on with an elastic thread. He leaves the button fastened but is able to push his arm through the end of the sleeve.

To put on a pullover or T-shirt, the patient arranges the garment across his knees with the collar furthest away from him and the label at the neck uppermost. The

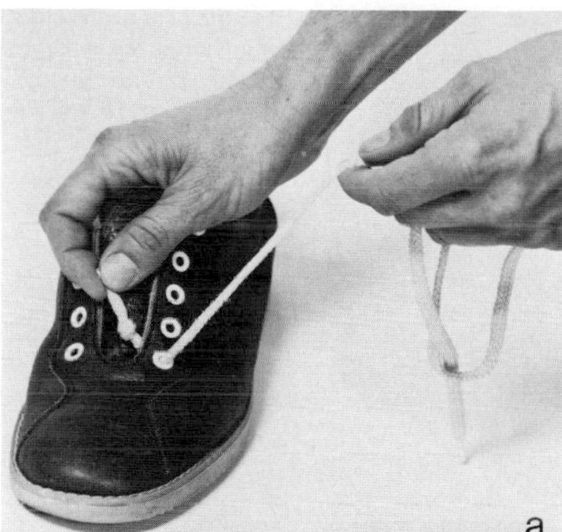

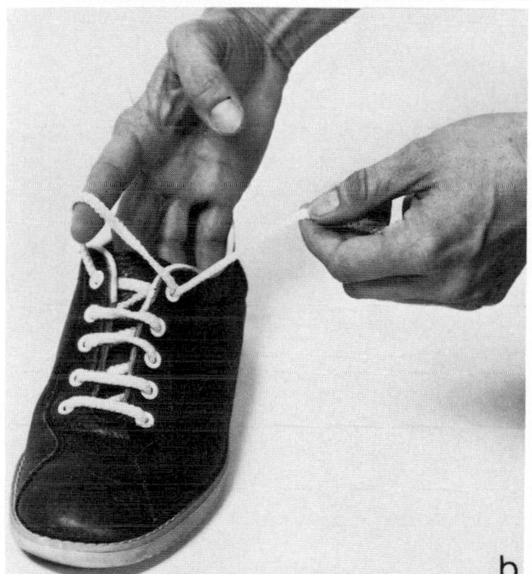

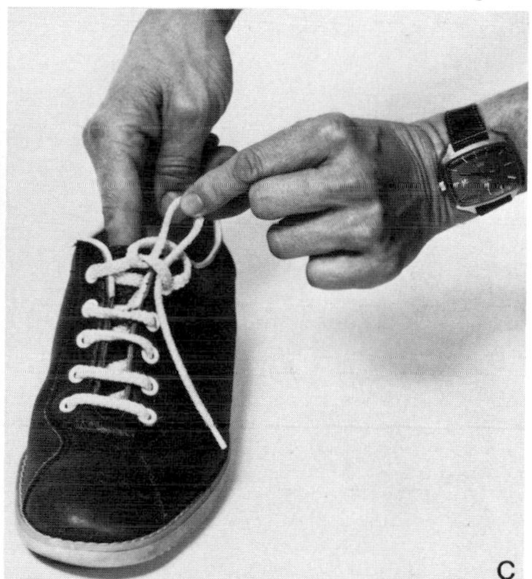

Fig. 10.20 a–c. Shoe-lace for fastening with one hand. **a** Lacing begins with a knot on the lateral side of the shoe. **b** The lace is kept firm if it is placed through the top hole twice. **c** Tying the lace

sleeve for the affected arm is once again hanging between his knees. Having placed his arm through the sleeve with the sound hand, he draws it right up to his shoulder before slipping the sound hand through the other sleeve. Grasping the back of the pullover he then places it over his head, leaning well forward so that his arm remains extended (Fig. 10.18).

The patient puts on his shoes as he does his socks (Fig. 10.19), but can fasten them when the feet are flat on the floor. If the patient is wearing lace-up shoes the lace should be threaded in such a way that he can fasten it using one hand if need be (Fig. 10.20 a–c). Moccasin-type shoes can look smart and avoid the necessity for coping with shoe-laces, and nevertheless give good support (Fig. 10.21 a). Some patients find a half-boot with a zip fastener easy to put on and welcome the added support at the ankle. Some shoes or half-boots are available with Velcro fasteners, or the patient can have Velcro straps fitted on his own shoes (Fig. 10.21 b).

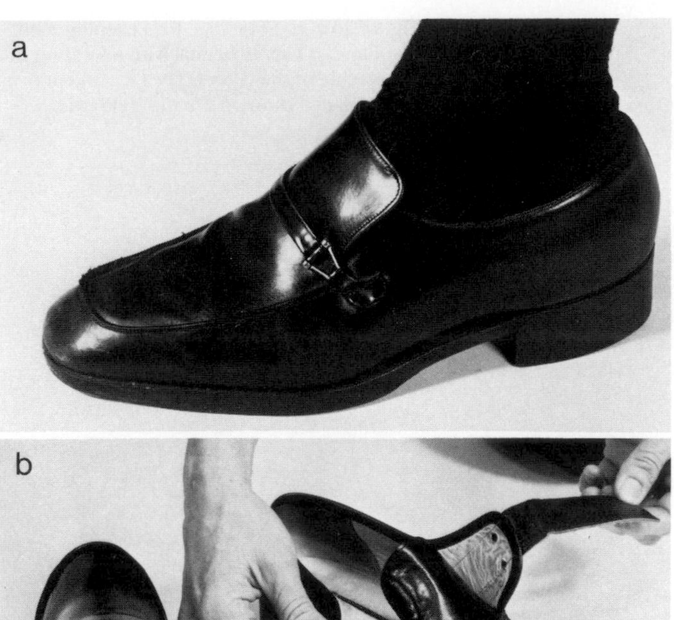

Fig. 10.21 a, b. Avoiding shoe-laces. **a** A moccasin-type shoe giving firm support; **b** Velcro straps fitted to the patient's shoes

An outdoor coat is best put on when the patient is standing, and he puts it on as he does a cardigan. If the hemiplegic arm is very spastic he may need to arrange the coat on a table, so that he can place the hand in the sleeve with the help of his sound hand.

10.4 Undressing

Undressing is simpler than dressing because the patient recognises each step which has to be taken (recognition level; Affolter 1981). The movements are carried out in the same sequence and pattern as for dressing, i.e. crossing the legs, keeping the hemiplegic arm forward in extension etc. However, the patient must now undress the sound limbs first, to enable him to free the garment from the hemiplegic side. In normal life putting our clothes away or in some order, after undressing, is a part of the routine, and should be included in the sequence for the patient.

10.5 Eating

The problems experienced by patients when eating are fully discussed in Chap. 13. It is important, in addition, that the patient be taught how to sit down and move his chair near enough to the dining-room table. He walks to the table and moves the chair sufficiently away to enable him to sit down. When seated he grasps the front of the chair between his thighs, leans forwards enough to be able to raise his seat and draws the chair nearer to the table (Fig. 10.22). The patient places his hemiplegic arm forward on the table, adjacent to his place setting. The correct position of the arm will help him to maintain an upright symmetrical posture while eating (Fig. 10.23). When some active movement returns to the hemiplegic arm the patient can use his affected hand to bring food to his mouth (such food as we normally eat with our hands). Manipulating a fork or spoon requires far finer movement and

10.22
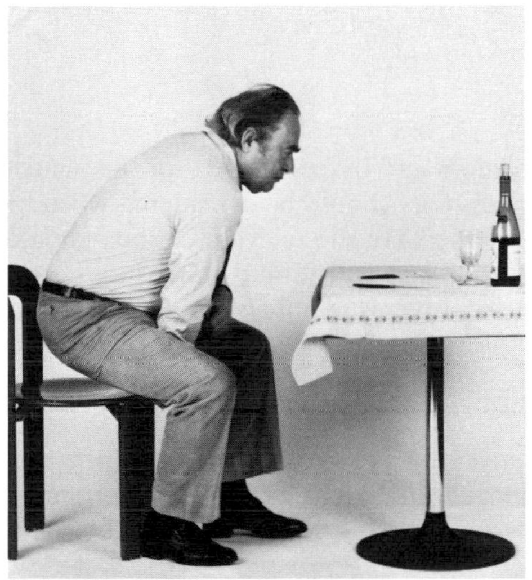

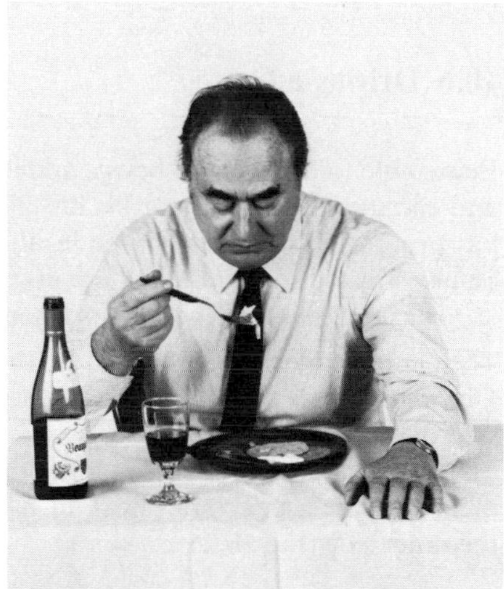
10.23

10.24
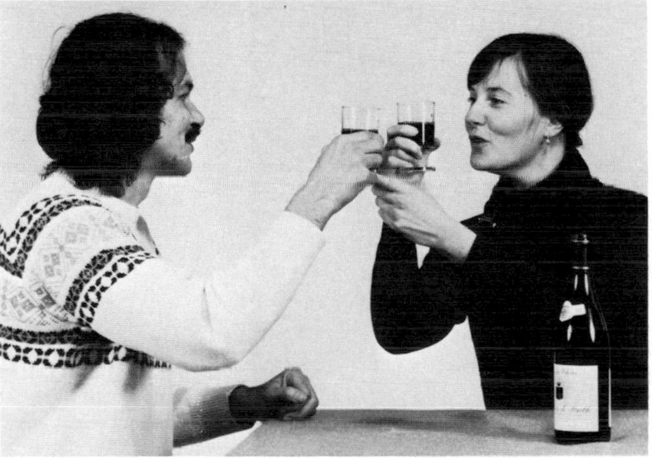

Fig. 10.22. Bringing the chair near enough to the table (left hemiplegia)

Fig. 10.23. Upright symmetrical posture for eating (left hemiplegia)

Fig. 10.24. Drinking from a glass with the hemiplegic hand (right hemiplegia)

control. Fruit, toast and biscuits are some of the easiest things for the patient to manage at first. Drinking from a glass requires only a little active movement, and the patient can even assist the activity by using his sound hand to steady the other one (Fig. 10.24). As soon as it is feasible, the patient should be encouraged to use both hands for eating with a knife and fork, even though he may have become adept at managing with the sound hand alone.

Teamwork

During the period when the patient is learning how to perform the activities of daily living in a correct and therapeutic way, it is important that all who assist him follow the same procedure. It is confusing when different members of the team give conflicting assistance or advice. For example, even if the patient is being helped while dressing hurriedly to be on time for an appointment, the same sequence of movement should be followed by the person helping him.

10.6 Driving a Car

Being able to drive again brings added freedom and independence for the patient and enhances the quality of his life. The possibility should be considered when he has progressed sufficiently. The legal requirements of the relevant country should be investigated so that the patient may drive safely, legally and competently.

The conversion of the car for a hemiplegic driver is relatively simple.

The car must have an automatic gearbox.

Driving is much easier with power steering, and a knob should be attached to the steering-wheel.

The accelerator and brake must be operated with the unaffected leg, which may mean that the accelerator pedal must be moved or have an additional extension to the other side (Fig. 10.25).

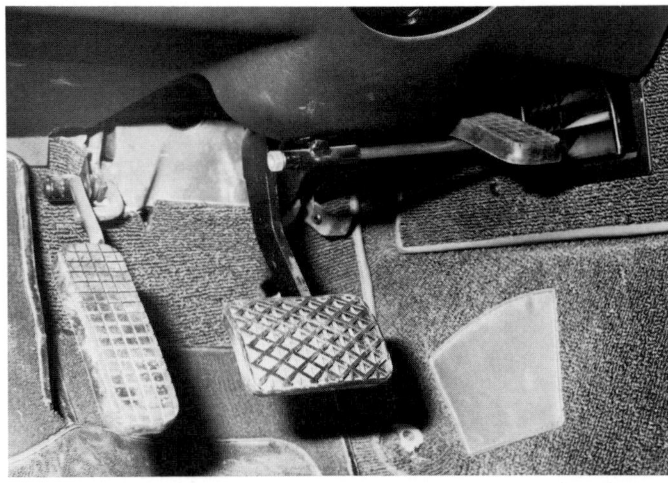

Fig. 10.25. Car adaptation. The accelerator pedal and brake can be operated with the sound foot (right hemiplegia)

Headlights and windscreen wipers must be operable without the sound hand having to move from the steering-wheel.
An arm-rest to support the hemiplegic arm helps to maintain a symmetrical posture while the patient is driving.

10.7 Considerations

Naturally, the patient's ability to stand up, walk and negotiate stairs freely and easily will add considerably to both his independence and enjoyment. Good balance is essential for carrying out all activities in his everyday life. Care must be taken that certain repeated postures do not lead to a further loss of symmetry. For example, most patients carry a sling bag to enable them to manage more easily with only one functioning hand. If the bag is carried over the sound shoulder, the patient holds that shoulder in a constant elevation to prevent the strap from slipping. The elevation of the unaffected shoulder emphasises the shortening of the affected side. When the bag is worn differently the posture is immediately improved. Such observations, and finding alternative solutions, can play an important role in maintaining the patient's level of achievement, both cosmetic and functional.

11 Mat Activities

Activities on a mat on the floor play an important role in the treatment of the hemiplegic patient. On the mat he learns to move his body again, feeling it in contact with the firm surface as he changes from one position to another. Patients with disturbed sensation have difficulty when exercising in free space, where they are completely dependent upon their own feedback systems to inform them if a movement is correct or not. The mat provides an absolute resistance, and the patient can orientate himself by changing the resistance felt against different parts of his body. The patient can move freely in a situation where he is not afraid of falling. Patients who are afraid to walk or move in the open can be helped to overcome their fear by working on the mat and learning to stand up from the floor.

A patient is not completely independent unless he can get up from the floor. Many patients have fallen when alone and have had to lie sometimes for hours, even though unhurt, until someone has found them. Activities on the mat also provide opportunities where distal spasticity can be remarkably reduced by moving the body proximally against the limbs. Patients of all ages enjoy the experience

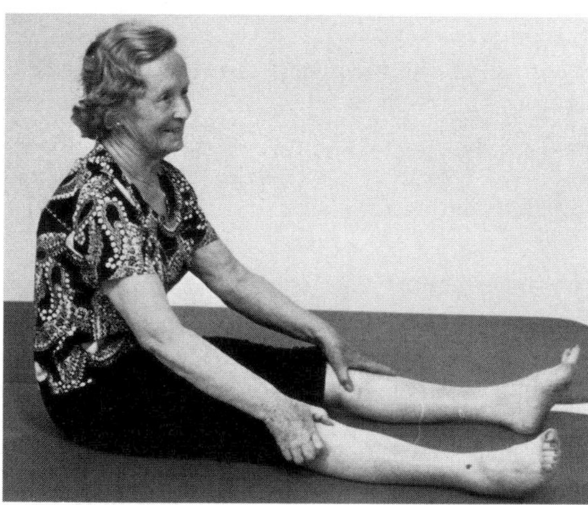

Fig. 11.1. An 80-year-old patient enjoys her mat programme (right hemiplegia)

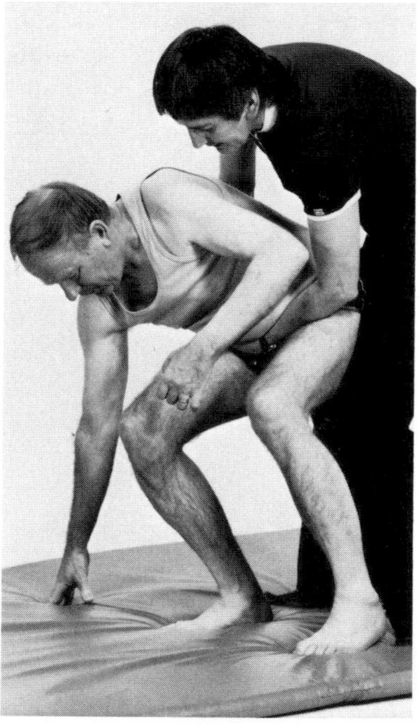

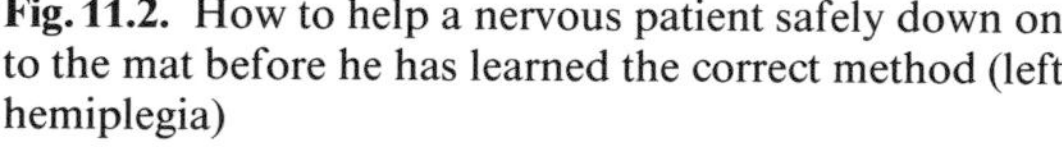

Fig. 11.2. How to help a nervous patient safely down on to the mat before he has learned the correct method (left hemiplegia)

(Fig. 11.1) and benefit from it as long as they are appropriately supported and the facilitation is adequate, particularly when they are first attempting the various activities. Gradual progression is essential.

11.1 Going down on to the Mat

The aim is for the patient to learn to kneel down on the mat, through half-kneeling on the hemiplegic leg, and then to sit down to one side. From side-sitting he can either lie down or sit with his legs in front of him. If he feels unsure at first, or if the therapist is not certain that he will be able to support himself in kneeling, the patient can be asked to go down on to the floor in any way he chooses with the necessary amount of help. The easiest way is usually with the therapist standing behind him and supporting him firmly as he puts his sound hand down on the mat, slowly bends his knees and sits down (Fig. 11.2). How he gets down on to the mat is not important at this stage, as long as it is achieved quickly, safely and smoothly. Once he is on the mat the individual components of the movement sequence can be practised.

The correct sequence is facilitated as follows:

The patient walks to the centre of the mat and takes a step forwards with his sound foot in preparation for kneeling down on the hemiplegic knee. The therapist, who has been assisting the patient with her hands on his hips, places her hands over the top of his shoulders and stands close behind him (Fig. 11.3 a). As he kneels down the therapist supports his hip firmly with her knee to prevent it from collapsing into flexion, as it will tend to do (Fig. 11.3 b). Her hands in front of his shoulders help him to extend his trunk and correct the position of the supporting hip. Once he has corrected his position in half-kneel-standing, he lifts the sound foot in front before moving it back to kneel on both knees (Fig. 11.3 c). With one hand the therapist corrects the position of the hemiplegic foot, which has often pulled into supination causing painful pressure on the big toe (Fig. 11.3 d). Her other hand remains in front of the patient's chest to ensure that he does not fall forwards.

11.2 Moving to Side-Sitting

The patient sits down on one side, first supporting himself with his sound hand. When he has learnt the movement and has sufficient trunk control, he moves from one side to the other without using his hand to help him. When the patient is moving to sit down to the right, the therapist stands behind him and places her left hand over the front of his left iliac crest. Her right hand helps him to bring his right shoulder forwards and elongate the side, while her left hand presses downwards and sideways to guide his right buttock on to the floor (Fig. 11.4 a). She moves her feet so that she can support his trunk with the inside of her right leg. Her leg assists the rotation of the trunk and prevents him from falling sideways and backwards, as he

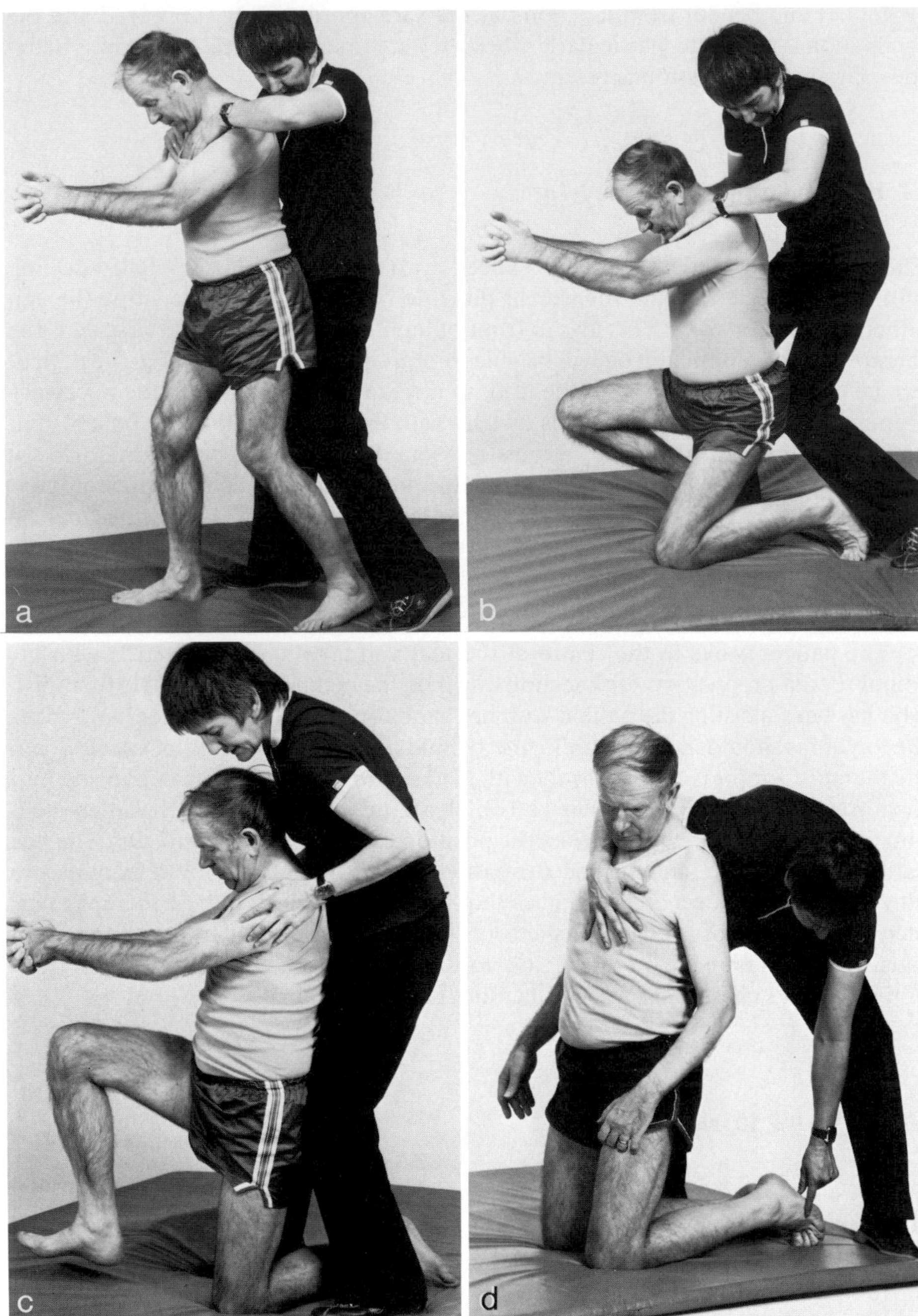

Fig. 11.3 a–d. Facilitating the recommended method of going down on to the mat (left hemiplegia). **a** The therapist stands close behind the patient and helps him to slide down over her knee on to his hemiplegic knee. **b** The hip tends to collapse or pull into flexion. **c** The therapist supports his hip in extension with her knee. The patient can then lift his sound leg. **d** He brings the sound leg back to kneel on both knees and the therapist frees his toes from pressure

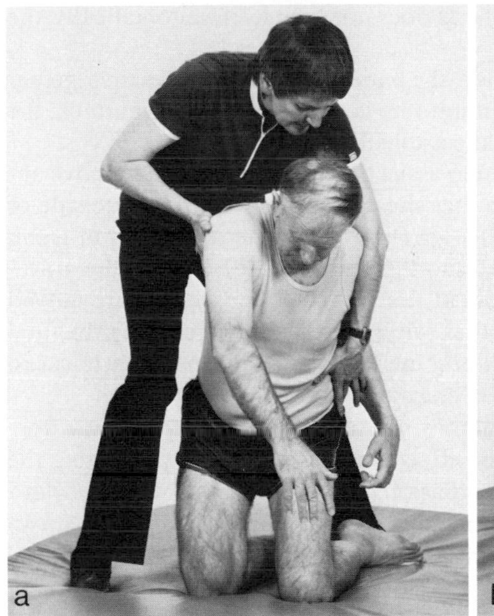

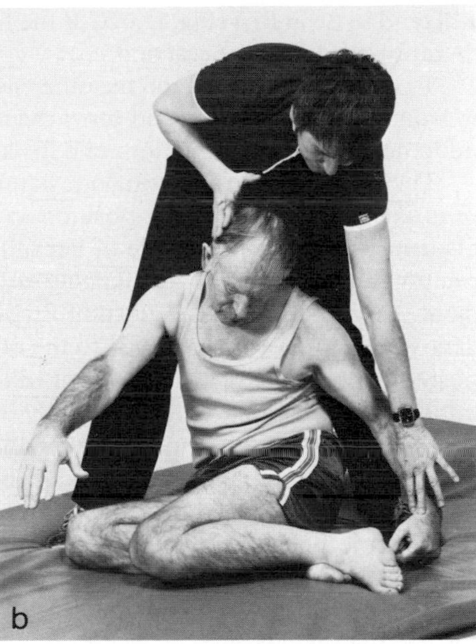

Fig. 11.4 a, b. Going down to side-sitting on the sound side (left hemiplegia). **a** The therapist facilitates trunk rotation. She has moved her feet so that she can support his trunk with the inside of her right leg. **b** Correcting the side-sitting position. The patient does not use his sound hand for support

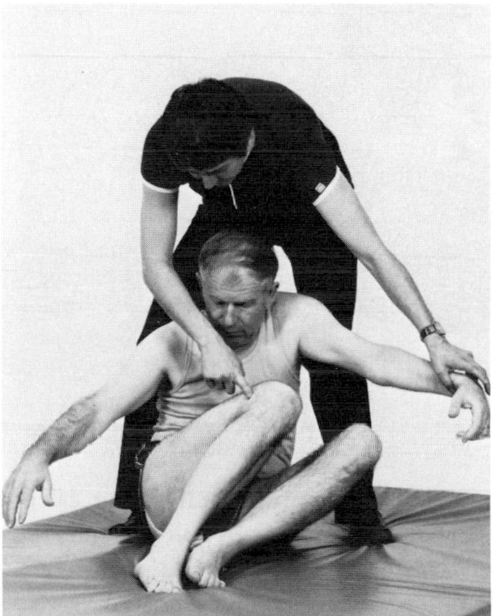

Fig. 11.5. Moving to sit on the other side (left hemiplegia)

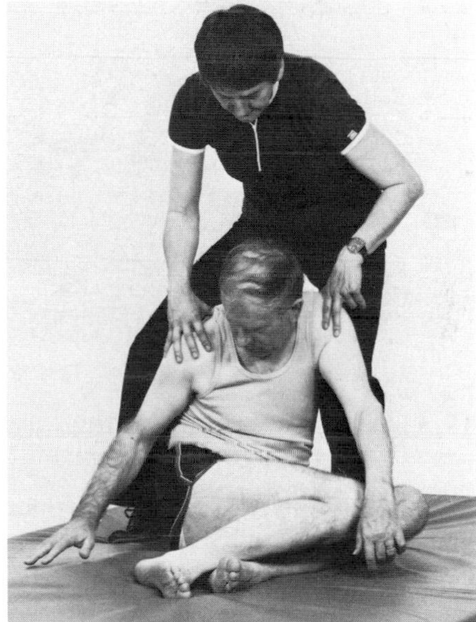

Fig. 11.6. Side-sitting on the hemiplegic side. The therapist has moved her feet so that she can support the patient's trunk with the inside of her left leg (left hemiplegia)

will tend to do at first (Fig. 11.4b). If the head does not right itself automatically, the therapist can assist the reaction.

To move so that he sits on the other side, the patient brings his knees up together in front of him (Fig. 11.5) and turns them until he is sitting on the left buttock, the underneath leg flat on the floor and his knees together.

The therapist helps by using one hand to assist the hemiplegic knee to move appropriately, and changes her position so that she can support the opposite side of his trunk with the medial side of her other leg (Fig. 11.6). Due to the loss of trunk rotation and appropriate lengthening and shortening of the side flexors, the movement may be difficult and uncomfortable at first. The patient's knees are moved gently and slowly from one side to the other, without necessarily reaching the final position immediately; the movement will become easier as trunk spasticity releases, until the patient can eventually sit fully on one side or the other.

Side-sitting on the hemiplegic side inhibits the spasticity in the trunk side flexors, and frees the scapula as a result. The effect can be increased by elevating the patient's arm fully in outward rotation, and asking him to move his weight toward the hemiplegic side and then away from it. In the same position the therapist can place the patient's hand at his side, with the elbow extended, to practise supporting his weight through his arm and extending his elbow actively (Fig. 11.7).

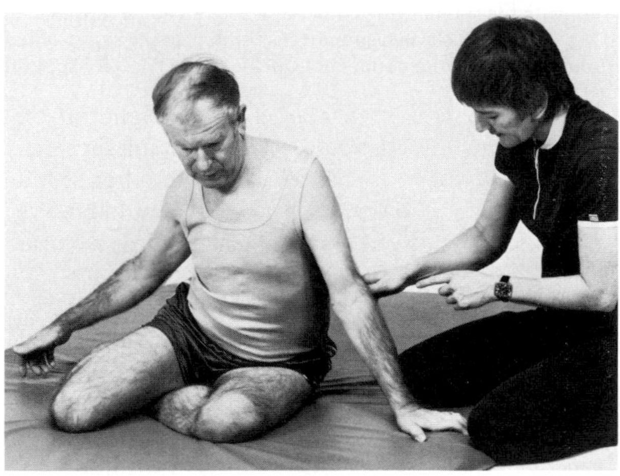

Fig. 11.7. Side-sitting, arm support sideways with the hemiplegic arm (left hemiplegia)

11.3 Activities in Long-Sitting

From side-sitting, the patient straightens his legs out in front of him and places his hands forwards on his legs. Keeping his knees as straight as possible, he slides his hands gently along his legs towards his feet. The therapist kneels in front of the patient and guides his hemiplegic arm so that the movement is performed without effort. When she feels that the whole arm is no longer pulling back from the scapula, she asks him to leave his hands resting on his legs (Fig. 11.8a). If necessary, she holds his foot in dorsiflexion. When the patient places his hemiplegic hand on the opposite leg, protraction of the scapula is achieved. He is assisted by the sensation

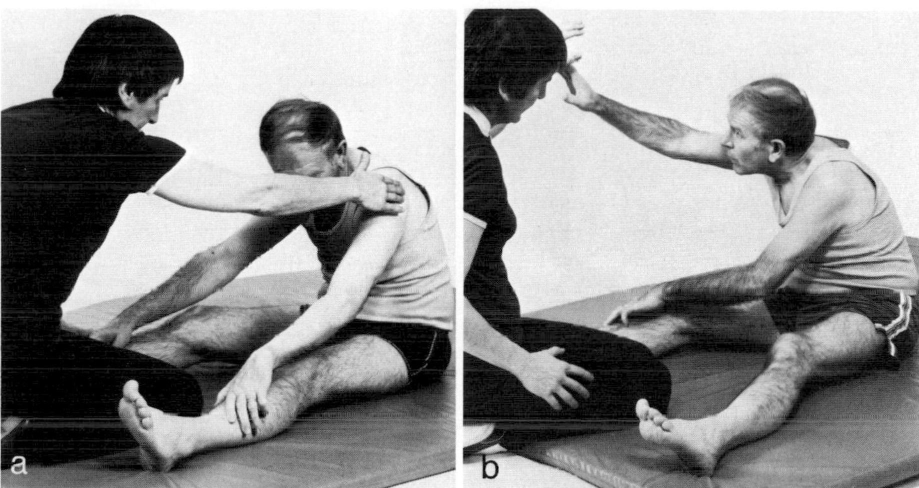

Fig. 11.8. a, b. Long-sitting, inhibiting flexor spasticity in the whole arm (left hemiplegia). **a** Leaving his hands lying on his legs. **b** The hemiplegic hand stays on the sound leg while the patient moves the sound arm actively

in the sound leg as he learns to inhibit the retraction, and in fact the whole pattern of flexor spasticity in the arm and hand. While moving his sound hand actively, he tries to let his hemiplegic hand remain in place (Fig. 11.8 b).

With his hands placed on the mat behind him, he supports his weight through his outwardly rotated, extended arms. With the therapist helping to maintain extension at the elbow, the patient transfers his weight from one side to the other, so that the scapula moves freely over the chest wall. The balls of his hands should both remain flat on the floor. Flexor spasticity is inhibited and at the same time extensor activity is stimulated.

The patient can also inhibit the spasticity around the scapula by rounding his thoracic spine, while his hands remain in the same position, both scapulae being fully protracted as a result (Fig. 11.9 a). He then extends his spine as fully as possible, inhibiting the hypertonus in the arm and shoulder as he moves his trunk against his fixed arms (Fig. 11.9 b).

The same activities can also be performed in standing and sitting positions with the hands supported on the plinth as described in Chap. 8. The patient places his hands flat on the floor between his legs in front of him and the therapist inhibits the retraction and depression of the scapula (Fig. 11.10). When she feels that the hypertonus is inhibited she asks him to leave his elbow in extension. He then allows the elbows to flex slightly before extending them actively.

With the therapist maintaining full inhibition of the arm to keep it forward in extension, the patient slowly lies down over his sound side with adequate trunk rotation. The hemiplegic shoulder remains well forward, and he tries to prevent it from pulling back as he moves (Fig. 11.11). The patient comes back up to long-sitting again, over the sound side. He brings his hemiplegic shoulder forward and the therapist keeps his arm in extension. From the supine lying position, the activities involving rolling would follow well in a movement sequence.

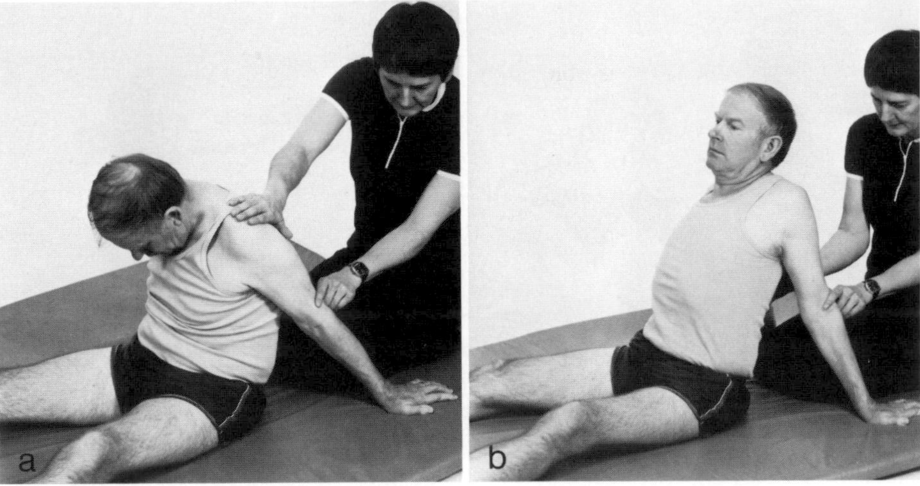

Fig. 11.9 a, b. With the extended arms supported behind him in external rotation, the patient inhibits spasticity by moving his trunk **a** into flexion; **b** into extension (left hemiplegia)

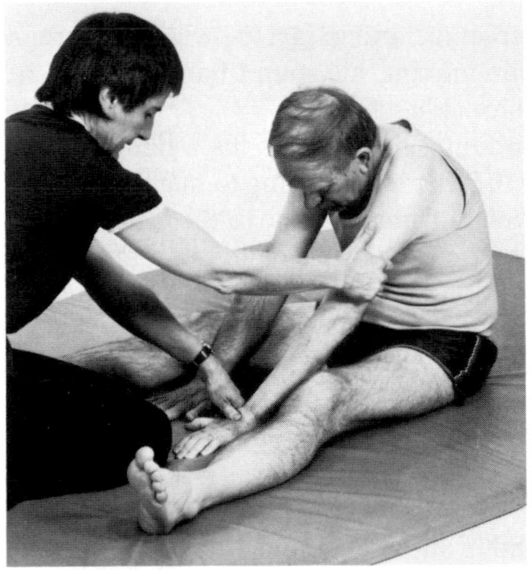

Fig. 11.10. Inhibiting retraction and depression of the scapula (left hemiplegia)

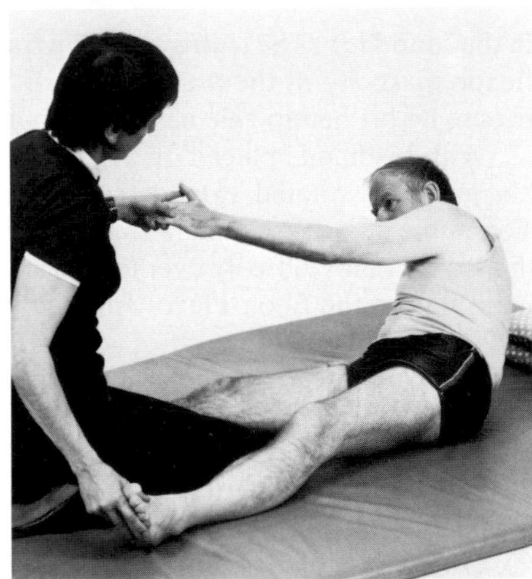

Fig. 11.11. Lying down and sitting up with trunk rotation emphasised (left hemiplegia)

11.4 Rolling

Rolling over on to the side is an easy movement for the patient and can be so facilitated that it is light and rhythmic. To either side or into the prone position the therapist must ensure that the normal pattern of movement is used. Often the untrained patient will use his sound leg to push off from the floor behind or bring it too soon on to the floor in front of him to slow the movement down. He may hold his head in too much extension or use his sound hand to support himself in front as he rolls forwards, or behind him before rolling back. The therapist adjusts her facilitation accordingly until the patient is able to roll unaided in a normal way right over into prone.

Because rolling is so beneficial it can be used in the treatment at all stages, with the appropriate amount of assistance and increasing exactness. If two plinths are placed together for additional width, rolling can be practised even before the patient is able to go down on the mat. It can be used to inhibit the spasticity before active arm movements are attempted.

11.4.1 Rolling to the Hemiplegic Side

Turning towards the affected side is the easiest movement for the patient, and he can learn to do so in the normal pattern of movement from the beginning, even when he is in bed (see Chap. 5). The vulnerable shoulder must be protected in the early stage, or if it is already painful, and the therapist cradles the patient's arm between her arm and her waist, supporting his upper arm with her hand. By doing so she keeps the scapula in protraction and the shoulder forward. With her other hand she facilitates the movement of his sound leg, which he must lift up and bring forwards over the other leg, without pushing off on the plinth or mat behind him. The patient's hemiplegic leg usually fails to rotate outwards as he rolls over it, but pulls into internal rotation, part of the spastic extension pattern. The therapist then uses her free hand placed on the patient's thigh to facilitate external rotation. She must move the hand quickly out of the way as his sound leg is brought forwards. The patient brings his sound arm forward freely. He rolls back again, the unaffected leg returning to a position of extension and abduction, lying flat on the mat.

When the movement has released the spasticity in the whole hemiplegic side, the therapist eases the arm further into abduction, until it lies flat on the mat even when the patient rolls forwards or returns to the supine position (Fig. 11.12a). Finally, he should try to leave his arm extended and abducted without the help of the therapist, and without its pulling into flexion.

For very full inhibition of the proximal spasticity, the patient rolls on to his hemiplegic side and the therapist draws his scapula into full protraction. She places her hand right over the scapula and holds its medial border forwards with her fingers (Fig. 11.12b). Holding it firmly in the corrected position, she asks the patient to roll very gently back and forth without the scapula becoming spastic. As the spasticity releases he rolls further over on to his back each time.

11.4.2 Rolling to the Unaffected Side

The therapist kneels on the patient's unaffected side to help him to bring his hemiplegic leg forward in a normal pattern. He clasps his hand together with his arms extended, to ensure that the affected arm is protected. The unaffected leg remains flat on the mat, rolling into external rotation as the other leg swings forwards.

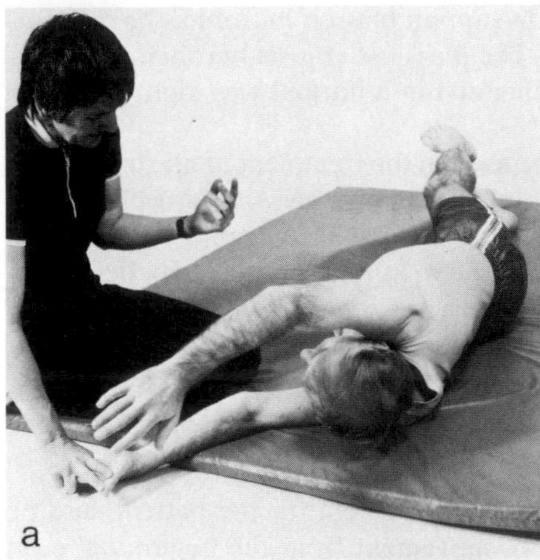

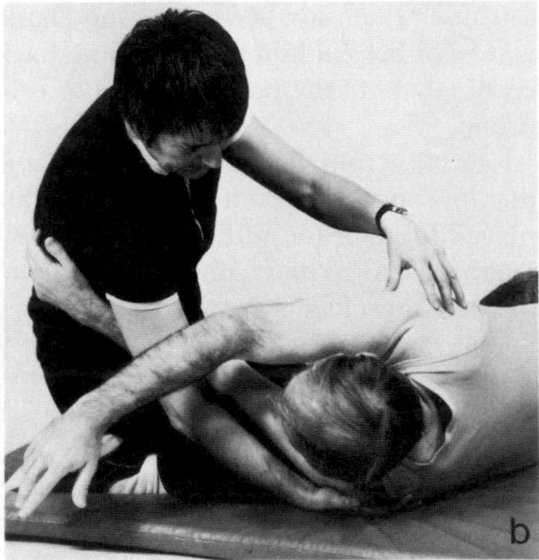

Fig. 11.12 a, b. Rolling to the hemiplegic side (left hemiplegia). **a** With the arm lying in abduction fully extended; **b** with the scapula held in full protraction

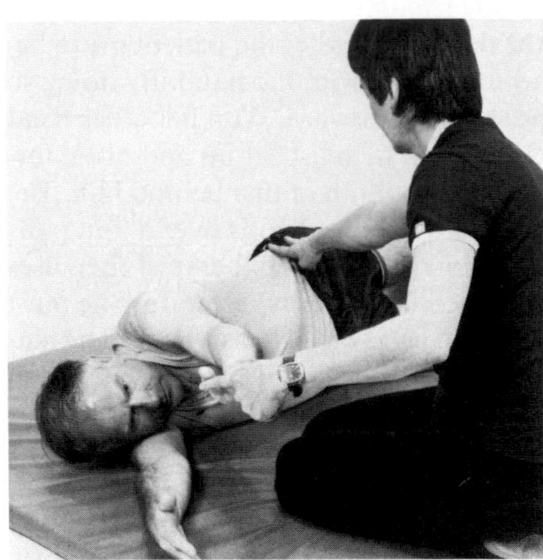

Fig. 11.13. Rolling back to a supine position from the sound side with increased trunk rotation (left hemiplegia)

When the patient is able to bring his affected leg to the front actively, the therapist holds his hemiplegic hand as he rolls back and forth with increased rotation of the trunk. With one hand she keeps his hand in dorsiflexion, while with the other she prevents his shoulder from retracting as he rolls from his side on to his back. He tries to place his affected leg far back on to the supporting surface in abduction.

When the therapist feels that the hypertonus in the arm has been reduced she holds only the patient's hand and asks him to roll back without letting his shoulder go back at the same time. With her free hand she increases the amount of trunk rotation by helping him to roll his pelvis backwards (Fig. 11.13).

11.4.3 Rolling over to a Prone Position

Rolling to prone is somehow a very positive experience for the patient, and he feels his body from a completely different aspect, against the resistance of the mat. Care

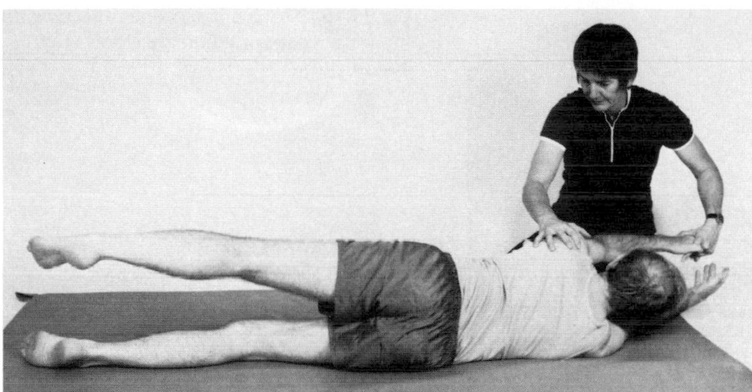

Fig. 11.14. Rolling to a prone position over the sound side (left hemiplegia)

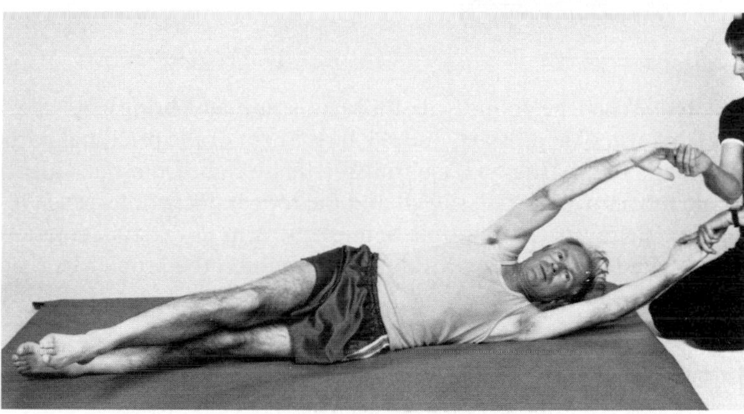

Fig. 11.15. Rolling to a prone position over the affected side (left hemiplegia)

must be taken that his shoulder is protected during the roll. As he comes into the prone position there could be an increase in flexor tone (see Chap. 3), and its influence on the arm and scapula could cause pain in the shoulder. For this reason it is safer to practise the movement with the patient rolling over his unaffected side at first, as the vulnerable shoulder can be carefully supported by the therapist.

The patient rolls over the sound side, to lie prone with his weight supported on his elbows, or with his arms extended in front of him. The therapist controls his hemiplegic arm throughout the movement, guiding it forwards into position without the shoulder retracting (Fig. 11.14).

The patient rolls over his hemiplegic side with his affected arm maintaining elevation (Fig. 11.15). He arrives in the prone position with both arms outstretched in front of him.

11.5 Prone Lying

Lying prone with the weight supported on his elbows, the patient can be helped to move in such a way that the increased tone around the scapula is reduced and selec-

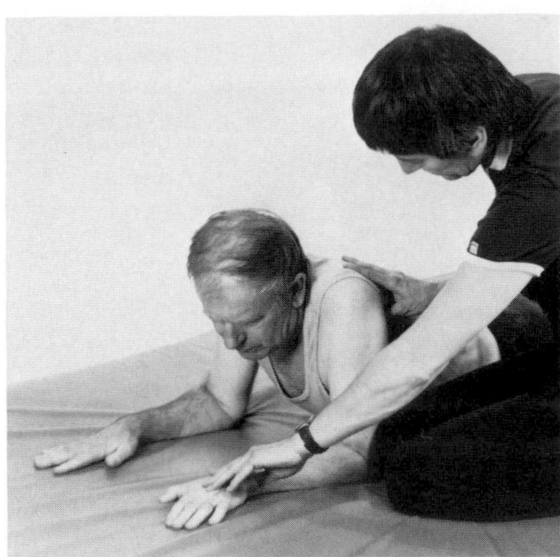

Fig. 11.16. Moving in a prone position with the weight supported on the elbows (left hemiplegia)

tive activity stimulated. When he rounds his thoracic spine and brings his chest away from the floor, his scapulae protract, and the movement of the proximal parts against the distal inhibits the spasticity. If he transfers his weight from one side to the other, the scapula moves over the chest wall and the tone in the whole arm is reduced (Fig. 11.16). The therapist can hold his hemiplegic arm in external rotation with the forearm supinated while he moves sideways, to inhibit the pronation.

11.6 Moving to Prone Kneeling

The patient moves from lying to prone kneeling by rolling over on to his sound side, flexing his knees and hips and pushing himself up with his arm to side-sitting, and then turning to support himself on his knees and sound hand.

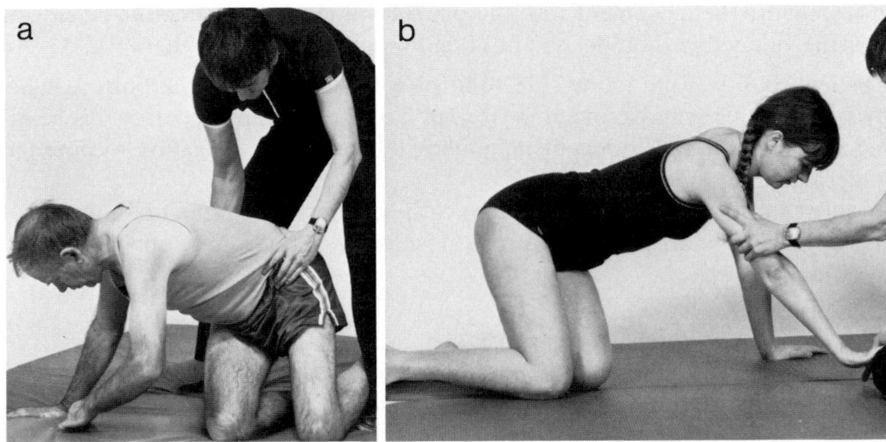

Fig. 11.17 a, b. Coming from side-sitting to prone kneeling. **a** Supported from the hips (left hemiplegia); **b** guided from the hemiplegic arm (right hemiplegia)

If the patient still has difficulty in coming to prone kneeling, the therapist stands behind him and places one hand on either side of his pelvis. She helps him to lift his buttocks from the floor and to turn round on to his knees (Fig. 11.17a). Once the patient is kneeling, the therapist moves round to the front of him and places his hemiplegic hand on the mat in the correct position. When the patient is able to move into prone kneeling on his own, the therapist kneels in front of him and guides his hemiplegic arm throughout the movement sequence (Fig. 11.17b).

Alternatively, the patient could move from kneel-standing to prone kneeling when he first goes down on to the mat. He must, however, learn the sequence of coming from lying to side-sitting to prone kneeling, so that he can stand up from the floor should he ever fall over. (Quite apart from falling over, many patients enjoy being able to sit on the grass or lie on the beach and would like to be able to stand up again easily.)

11.7 Activities in Prone Kneeling

1. With his weight distributed evenly over both hands and both knees, the patient rounds his back as fully as possible, and by so doing moves the scapulae into protraction (Fig. 11.18). The therapist helps him to maintain elbow extension with his fingers remaining fully extended. The patient then hollows his back, extending his spine, and repeats the movement. As his ability to maintain the arm in extension increases, the therapist gradually moves his hands so that the shoulder is increasingly externally rotated and the forearm supinated.
2. From prone kneeling the patient sits back on his heels leaving his hands outstretched on the mat in front of him (Fig. 11.19a). He then brings his weight forward over his arms (Fig. 11.19b). The therapist helps to maintain the correct position of his hemiplegic arm and to elongate the side of his trunk. If necessary, she uses her thigh to keep his elbow extended and stabilises his shoulder forwards

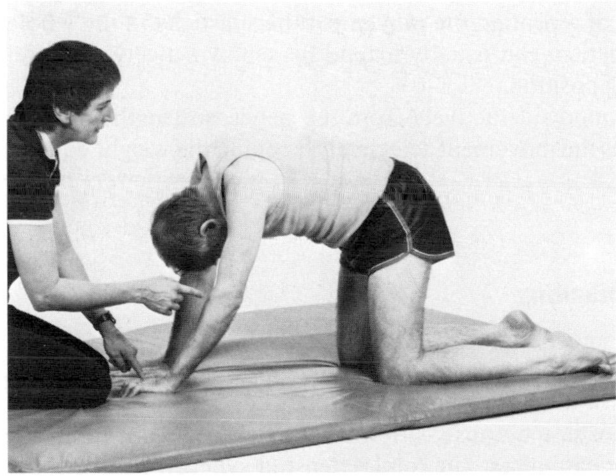

Fig. 11.18. Prone kneeling, rounding the back to inhibit retraction of the scapula (left hemiplegia)

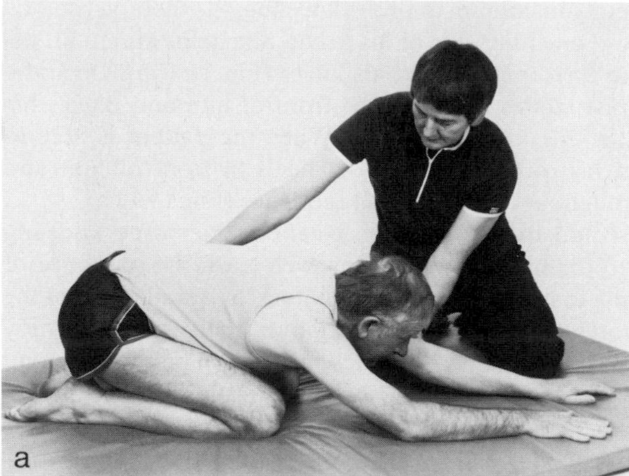

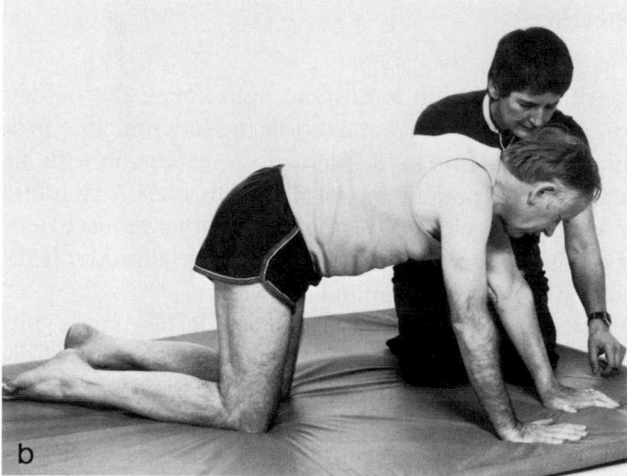

Fig. 11.19 a, b. Moving in a prone kneeling position (left hemiplegia). **a** Sitting back on the heels; **b** bringing weight forwards over the arms

with her hand. As a result of repeating the movement the spasticity in the whole side is inhibited and the patient can usually extend his elbow actively as he returns to the prone kneeling position.

3. The patient shortens his sound side actively from the pelvis, so lengthening the hemiplegic side. He repeats the movement selectively, keeping the weight equally over both knees.

11.8 Activities in Kneel-Standing

The patient moves from prone kneeling to kneel-standing, the therapist standing behind him so that she can assist the hip extension with her knees. Hip extension is difficult for patients in this position because with the knee flexed the hip control is very selective, i.e. the patient cannot use the total extension synergy, and with the

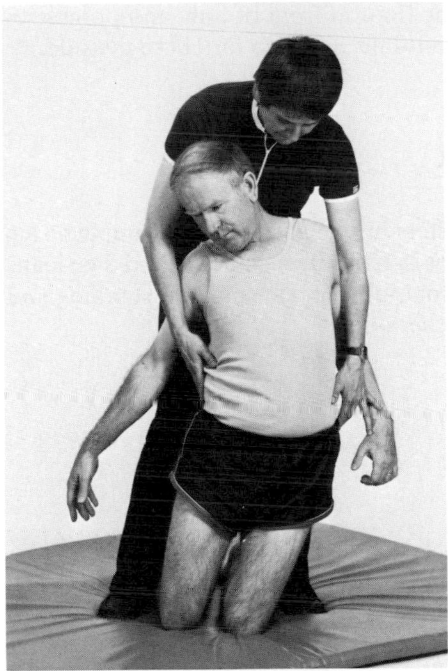

Fig. 11.20. Kneel-standing, transferring the weight over the hemiplegic leg (left hemiplegia)

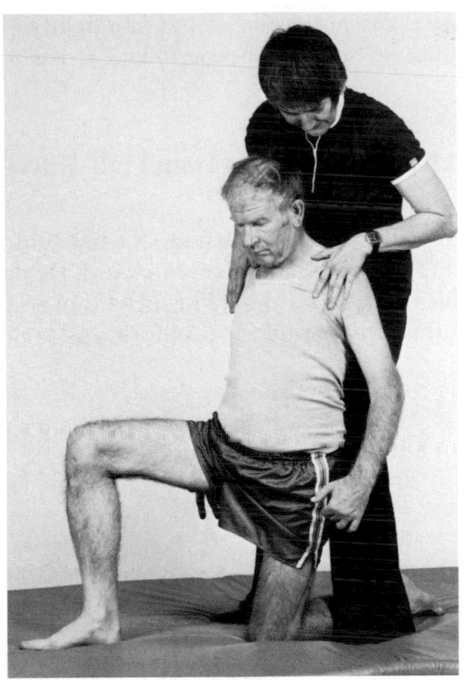

Fig. 11.21. Half-kneel-standing on the hemiplegic leg (left hemiplegia)

knee flexed there is a tendency for the whole leg to pull into flexion. It is therefore a useful position in which to work for pure hip extension. During activities in kneeling and half-kneeling the patient's arms can be left free and not clasped together, so that normal balance reactions are encouraged. The position of the hemiplegic arm is also a guide as to whether enough assistance is being given or whether the patient is having to struggle to perform the movements.

The patient moves his weight first over one leg and then the other. When he moves to the hemiplegic side the whole of that side should elongate, the hip being the most lateral point (Fig. 11.20). His hips must remain extended, and the therapist facilitates the extension with her knees. When she feels that the active control is improving, she asks the patient to keep his buttocks away from her knees, and gradually withdraws her support. With her hands she assists the lateral movement of the pelvis. With his weight well over the hemiplegic leg, the patient brings his sound foot forwards and places it lightly on the floor in front of him (Fig. 11.21).

11.9 Activities in Half-Kneel-Standing

The patient practises bringing his sound leg down again to kneel-standing and then up again to half-kneel-standing, without scraping his foot on the floor as he does so. The therapist continues to assist with hip extension and balance.

The patient taps his sound foot lightly on the floor in front of him, and progresses until he can tap it nearer to and across the mid-line, and also far out to the side.

11.10 Standing up from Half-Kneeling

To stand up from the floor, the patient transfers his weight over the hemiplegic leg and brings the sound foot forward. He pauses in half-kneel-standing and then leans his trunk forward until his head is over the foot in front. He comes to standing and brings his hemiplegic foot forwards to the other one.

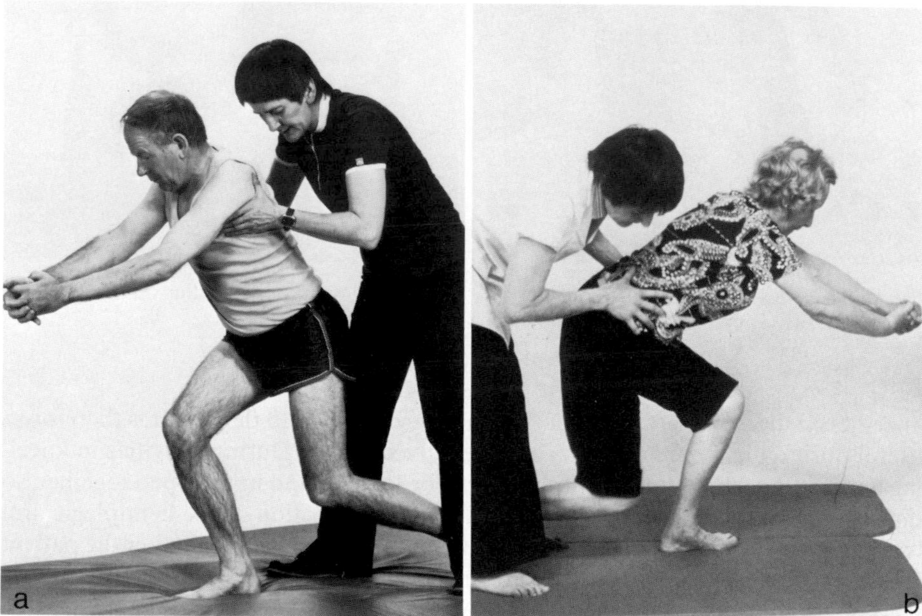

Fig. 11.22 a, b. Standing up from the floor. **a** The therapist facilitates with her hands in the patients axillae (left hemiplegia). **b** Facilitation from the pelvis (right hemiplegia)

Practising the activity with the patient's hands clasped together and the arms extended helps him to bring his weight far enough forwards. The therapist facilitates the movement by placing her hands in his axillae from behind and guiding him forward and upward (Fig. 11.22 a). She can also facilitate the movement by supporting with her hands on each side of his pelvis and helping him to come upright (Fig. 11.22 b). If the patient or therapist is anxious about standing up at first, a chair can be placed in front of him and he supports his clasped hands on it as he comes to the upright position.

11.11 Considerations

Exercising on the mat should be a pleasurable experience for the patient and care must be taken that the amount of support given in the beginning is adequate. It is easy for the therapist to make the mistake of keeping him too long in kneel-standing while practising weight transference, for example. The patient's knees begin to hurt and he will be loath to go on the mat again in the future, as he will remember the unpleasant sensation. If the patient's foot pulls strongly into flexion and causes painful pressure on his toes, a small pillow can be placed beneath his foot to relieve the pressure at first. As the movements become easier, the foot ceases to pull into flexion. It would be a pity to avoid the valuable therapeutic effect of moving on the mat simply because the first attempt was unsuccessful. Moving on the floor is, after all, the way in which we all originally learn to move in early childhood in preparation for standing and walking.

12 Shoulder Problems Associated with Hemiplegia

In many hospitals and rehabilitation centres all over the world, hemiplegic patients suffer from severe pain in the shoulder, and the problem is most distressing for both the patient and the staff. The pain has been described as affecting up to 70% of the patients (Caldwell et al. 1969).

As Roper (1982) says, "the painful shoulder is a major impairment to the entire rehabilitation programme, because the patient with an adducted medially rotated shoulder makes no attempt to use the affected arm and often fails to participate in walking training." "The patient who has pain when he moves will remain immobile. If he also has pain at rest he usually withdraws from any active rehabilitation programme" (Braun et al. 1971).

The sequelae of the pain are even more extensive:

The patient cannot concentrate on learning new skills, as he is constantly distracted by the pain.

He has difficulty in regaining independence in the activities of daily life because the pain and stiffness interfere with dressing and washing, turning over in bed etc.

Balance reactions are prevented both in sitting and standing, and the patient is afraid to move freely to carry out the tasks required of him.

His morale is drastically lowered, and like any other person with constant pain he becomes depressed. A vicious circle ensues. The patient is unable to sleep, and then cannot co-operate fully in the therapy sessions. As a result he makes little or no progress, and with the lack of success he becomes more depressed.

Pain itself can inhibit muscle activity, and it is very difficult to stimulate the return of active movement in the hemiplegic arm while pain persists.

Fortunately, shoulder pain can be avoided with proper early management and treatment, and should it occur or already exist it can be overcome. With so many adverse effects the correct treatment of the shoulder should surely have a high priority in the overall rehabilitation. Having suffered a stroke with all its devastating consequences, the patient should not have to live with pain as well.

Before treatment can be carried out successfully, it is necessary to understand both the normal shoulder mechanisms and the problems which arise in association with hemiplegia. The problems can be divided into three distinct categories, and may be observed in isolation or as a combination of two or even all three.

The subluxed shoulder.
The painful shoulder.
The shoulder-hand syndrome.

The successful treatment varies according to the problem, and care must therefore be taken to differentiate between them.

12.1 The Subluxed or Malaligned Shoulder

The subluxed shoulder is in itself not painful. It is, however, extremely vulnerable and can easily be traumatised. Malalignment of the shoulder is very common, especially where there is a total paralysis of the upper limb, and has been described as occurring in up to 73%, 66% and 60% of groups of hemiplegic patients with severe paralysis of the arm (Najenson et al. 1971; Najenson and Pikielni, 1965; Smith et al. 1982).

During investigations carried out at King's College Hospital in 1976, it was found that all hemiplegic patients with a total paralysis of the arm showed a malalignment of the shoulder when X-rayed in an upright sitting position within the first 3 weeks after onset of stroke (Fig. 12.1 a). Despite the sometimes marked luxation, all patients had full pain-free range of motion at the shoulder joint, and it was interesting to note that when the arm was fully elevated, the head of the humerus was seen on X-ray to be correctly located in the glenoid fossa (Fig. 12.1 b).

The patients did, however, experience a dragging discomfort or ache if the arm was left hanging at their side too long. The ache was immediately relieved if the arm was elevated passively or supported on a table in front of them. As these patients had no pain and were being positioned and carefully treated from the beginning of their illness, it could be hypothesised that subluxation occurs spontaneously when the patient starts sitting or standing up against gravity in the early stages following a stroke, and not as a result of traumatic or incorrect handling.

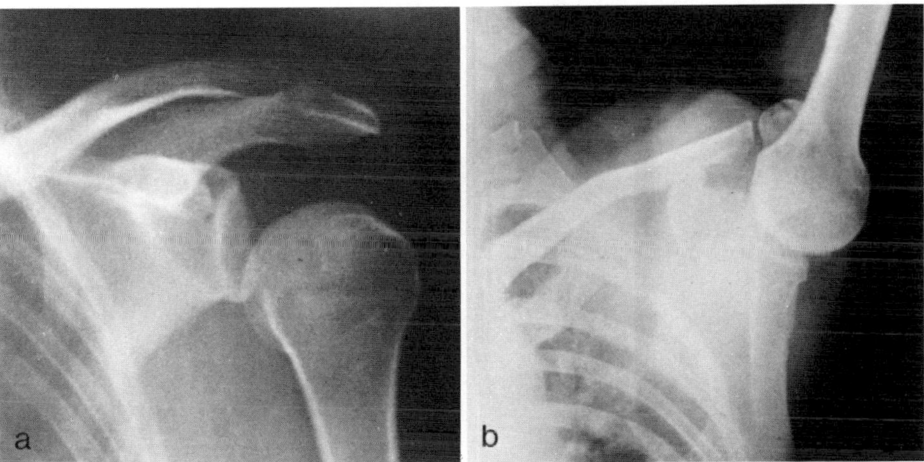

Fig. 12.1 a, b. X-rays from the patient series at King's College Hospital. **a** Subluxed shoulder; **b** position corrected when the arm is in elevation

Roper (1975) described a large series of patients with hemiplegia who where admitted to Rancho Los Amigos Hospital for surgery to relieve severe shoulder pain. None showed radiological evidence of shoulder subluxation. As these patients had had their hemiplegia for 2 years or more, it could be postulated that subluxation becomes progressively less with the passing of time, i.e. as the muscle tone returns, until it usually disappears altogether and "certainly is extremely rare when the patients are reviewed after neurological stabilisation has occurred" (Roper 1982).

12.1.1 Causative Factors in Hemiplegia

The shoulder joint needs to allow an enormous range of movement in order for fine skilled manipulations to be performed by the hand and fingers. Stability has therefore been sacrificed in favour of mobility, the socket being relatively small compared to that of the hip joint. Two-thirds of the humeral head are not covered by the

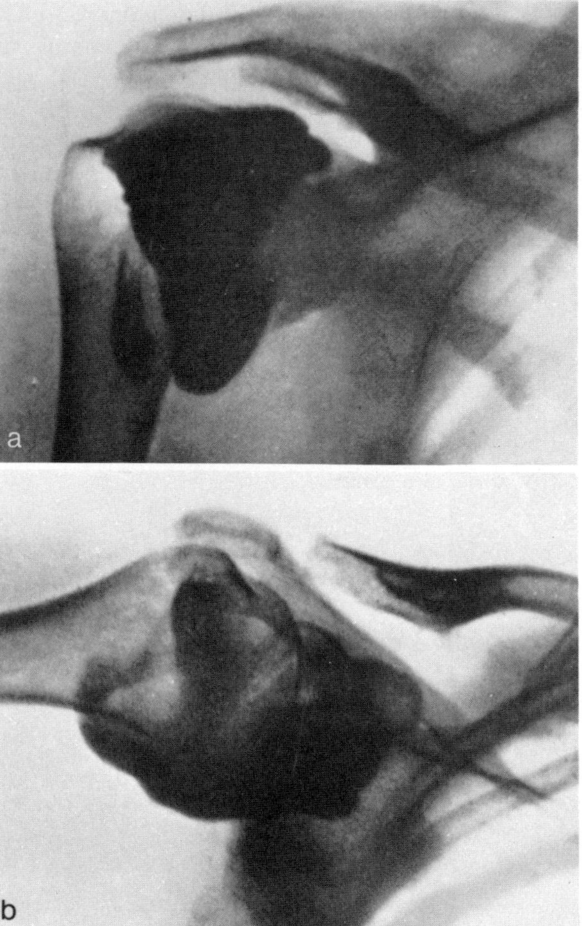

Fig. 12.2 a, b. Arthrogram: normal shoulder. **a** Arm adducted, superior portion of capsule taut; **b** arm abducted, superior portion of capsule lax

glenoid fossa. The loss of stability has been partly compensated for by a strong surrounding musculature (Zinn 1973).

Both Basmajian (1979, 1981) and Cailliet (1980) have described fully and clearly the factors preventing downward displacement or subluxation in the normal state, as well as explaining its occurrence in hemiplegic patients. In the normal correct orientation of the scapula the glenoid fossa faces upwards as well as forwards and laterally. The upward slope of the fossa plays an important role in preventing downward dislocation because the head of the humerus would need to move laterally in order to move downwards. With the arm in an adducted position, the superior part of the capsule and the coracohumeral ligament are taut and passively prevent the lateral movement of the humeral head and so its downward displacement (Fig. 12.2 a). Basmajian describes the "locking mechanism of the shoulder joint". The supraspinatus reinforces the horizontal tension of the capsule when the arm is loaded.

When the arm is lifted sideways in abduction or forwards, the superior capsule becomes lax (Fig. 12.2 b), eliminating the support, and the joint stability must be provided by muscular contraction. The locking mechanism cannot operate when there is abduction of the humerus. The integrity of the joint then depends almost exclusively on the rotator cuff muscles "which should be called the guardians of the shoulder" (Basmajian 1981).

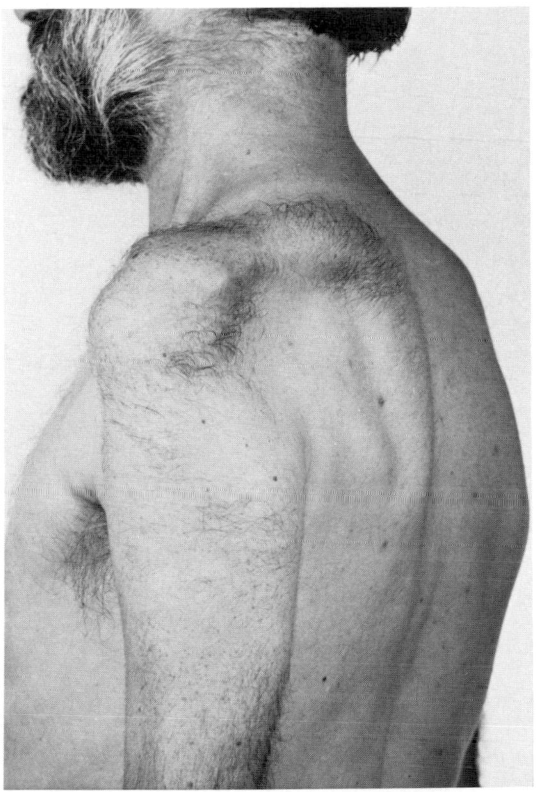

Fig. 12.3. Patient with brachial plexus lesion of 9 years' duration

The muscles most important in preventing subluxation of the glenohumeral joint are those whose fibres run horizontally, in particular the supraspinatus, the posterior fibres of the deltoid and the infraspinatus. A patient who has a paralysis of the shoulder muscles following a brachial plexus lesion does not necessarily demonstrate subluxation. The passive locking mechanism of the shoulder joint is intact if the glenoid fossa remains in its normal orientation and the capsule is taut. The patient is able to maintain the correct position of the scapula actively (Fig. 12.3).

In hemiplegia, patients who have a subluxation of the shoulder have lost not only the passive locking mechanism when the arm is hanging at the side, but also the support from reflex or voluntary activity in the relevant muscles. A combination of the following signs is evident:

1. The shoulder girdle droops with loss of tone or activity in the elevators of the scapula, particularly in their combined action with the serratus anterior to elevate the glenoid fossa with scapular rotation forwards. The fossa therefore slopes downwards (Fig. 12.4a).
2. Viewed from behind, the scapula is seen to lie closer to the vertebrae, but particularly the inferior angle is adducted, and lower than that of the scapula on the other side (Fig. 12.4b).
3. The vertebral border of the scapula is pulled away from the ribs, and significantly there is a resistance to passive correction of the winging (Fig. 12.5). It must be assumed, therefore, that despite the apparent flaccid appearance of the upper limb, tone has increased in certain muscle groups. Even if the increase in tone is rela-

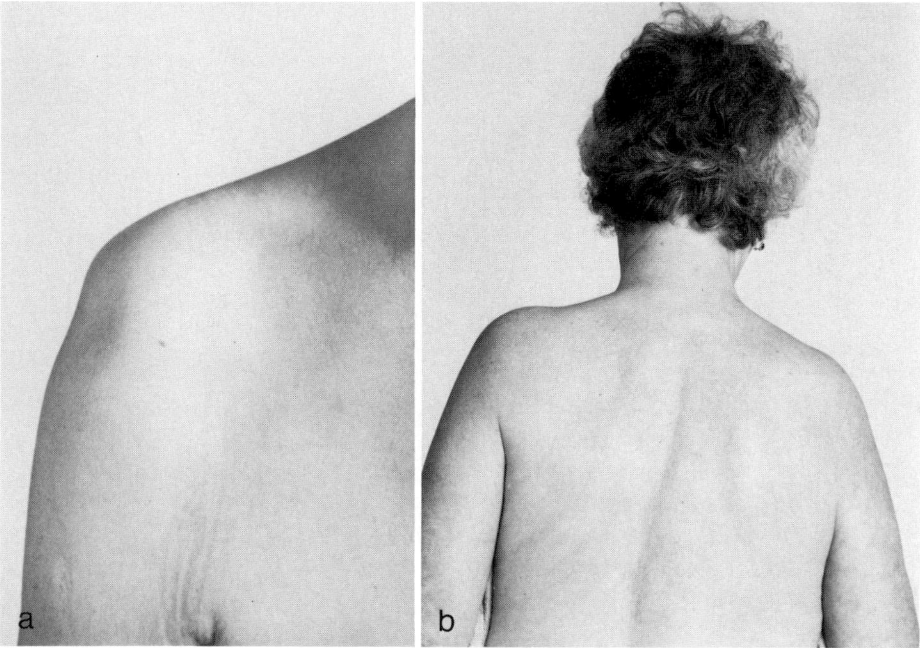

Fig. 12.4 a, b. The shoulder girdle droops on the hemiplegic side (right hemiplegia). **a** Anterior view showing typical subluxation; **b** posterior view showing position of scapula

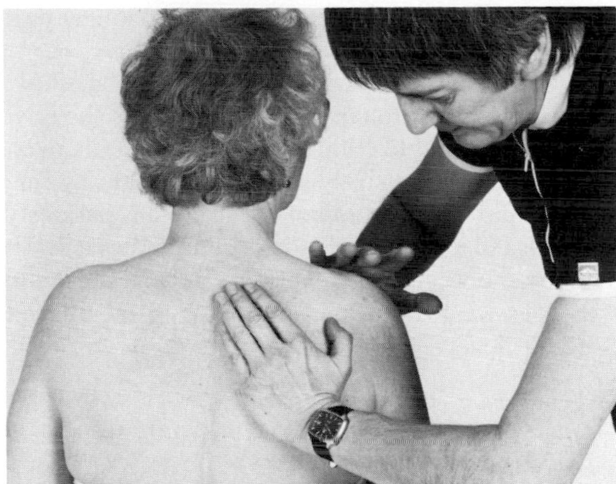

Fig. 12.5. Resistance to passive correction of the winged scapula (right hemiplegia)

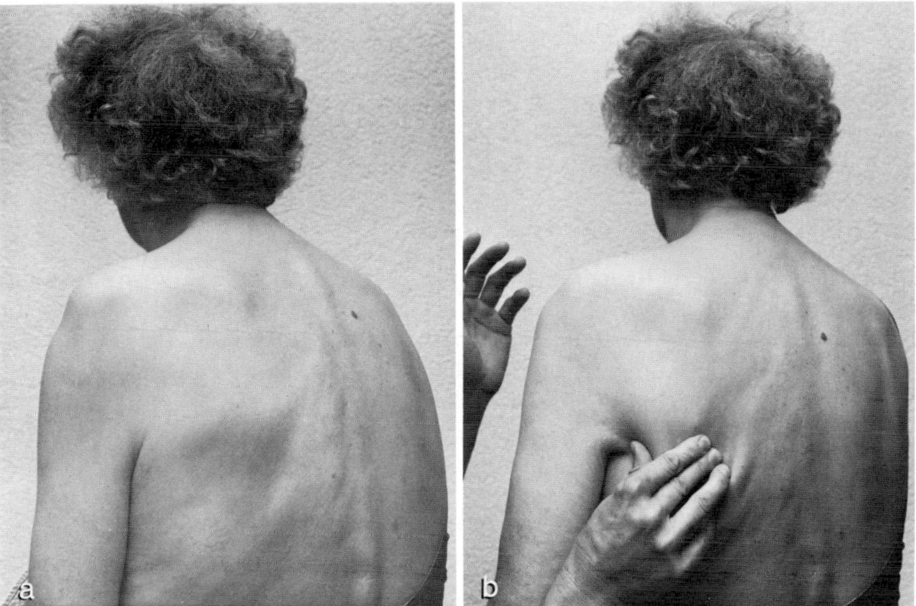

Fig. 12.6 a, b. The effect of the position of the scapula (left hemiplegia). **a** Rotated downwards with its inferior angle adducted – marked subluxation evident. **b** With the inferior angle pulled away from the vertebrae – subluxation corrected

tively slight, its effect is marked because of the hypotonus in the antagonists. The unopposed increase in tone in the pectoralis minor could be responsible for pulling the vertebral border of the scapula away from the ribs, causing the resistance to correction, and also for adding to the change in angulation of the glenoid fossa with downward rotation of the scapula. Because the scapula rotates downwards and adducts or retracts, the humerus finds itself in a position of relative abduc-

tion as the arm remains against the side of the body. The capsule is no longer taut and the head of the humerus is free to slide down the fossa.
4. The supraspinatus, infraspinatus and posterior portion of the deltoid all show marked atrophy and do not spring into activity to take over the action of the now lax capsule. Subluxation is therefore inevitable (Fig. 12.6a). The effect is even more noticeable if the patient's arm is raised passively in abduction, causing further relaxation of the capsular restraint. If the position of the scapula is passively corrected by the examiner, who holds the inferior angle firmly and draws it sufficiently away from the vertebrae, the shoulder is no longer luxated. Because the arm is once more adducted, the passive locking mechanism is re-established (Fig. 12.6b).

12.1.2 Treatment

The aim of treatment is threefold:

1. To restore the natural locking mechanism of the shoulder by correcting the position of the scapula and thus the glenoid fossa.
2. To stimulate activity or tone in the stabilising muscles around the shoulder.
3. To maintain full pain-free range of passive movement without traumatising the joint and the structures which surround it.

12.1.2.1 Correcting the Posture of the Scapula

After inhibition of any hypertonus which is rotating the scapula downwards and posteriorly, the patient is taught to elevate his shoulder anteriorly, in the direction of his nose (see Fig. 8.13). "Restoration of scapular posture to normal results in the restoration of a passive (but effective) function of the shoulder (glenohumeral) joint – the locking mechanism of the shoulder joint" (Basmajian 1979, 1981).

The therapist releases the spasticity by using those activities which move the trunk proximally against the scapula distally, e.g. rolling over the hemiplegic side, weight-bearing through the arm and transferring weight sideways, moving the scapula manually in the desired direction. When moving the scapula into full elevation with protraction, the therapist needs to move both shoulders forwards at the same time. The patient otherwise rotates his sound shoulder backwards and the protraction of the affected side is only apparent and not complete.

Positioning is important, both day and night. The patient should sit with his arm supported forward on a table when he is not moving around. He is encouraged to elevate the arm frequently during the day, using his sound hand to assist full elevation.

A sling should not be used, as it does not reduce the subluxation (Fig. 12.7) and can have deleterious results. In a careful study involving an albeit small group of new hemiplegic patients, Hurd et al. (1974) found no appreciable difference between the patients treated with a sling or without, using the parameters of shoulder range of motion, shoulder pain and subluxation. Friedland (1975) agrees that "there is no need to support a pain-free shoulder in order to prevent or correct subluxation since the sling does not prevent, improve, cure or reduce such a deformity".

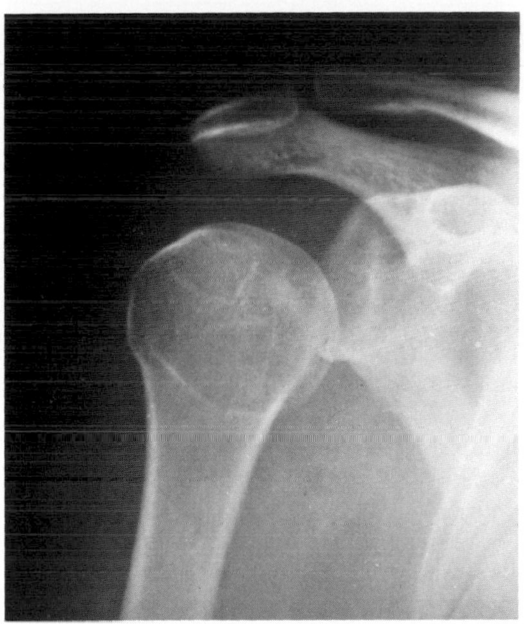

Fig. 12.7. X-ray taken with patient wearing a sling shows no reduction of subluxation

Voss (1969) describes the consensus of a group of therapists who condemned slings for interfering with body image, immobilising the arm, reinforcing flexor tone, impairing postural support and impeding normal gait. Semans (1965) describes clearly the deleterious effects that "tying the arm against the body in a sling" may have.

1. Fosters anosognosia or functional dissociation from total body movement.
2. Accentuates and encourages the spastic (flexor) pattern of the arm.
3. Prevents postural or supportive use of the arm as in turning over, rising from a chair or steadying an object for the other hand.
4. Prevents compensatory arm swing or guidance from the involved side during gait instruction.
5. Deprives patient of discriminative exteroceptive and proprioceptive input, resulting in hyperaesthesia from unbalanced spinothalamic input.
6. Increases the tendency to venous and lymphatic stasis resulting from immobility.

Many alternative means of supporting the shoulder have been developed and advocated, but each has its disadvantage. Most tend to compromise an already endangered circulation, either by compression in the axilla or by the use of a cuff-type support to take the weight of the arm. A support developed in Holland avoids compression but, like the sling, deprives the arm of input through participation and attention. Observation of hundreds of patients during the last 10 years, for whom no form of support was used, indicates convincingly that careful active treatment and correct handling and positioning achieve the best results.

12.1.2.2 Stimulating Activity or Tone in the Stabilising Muscles Around the Shoulder

All the activities described in Chap. 8 for stimulating the return of function in the arm can be used to activate the muscles which stabilise the shoulder joint. Particularly useful are those where weight is taken through the affected arm, and activity is stimulated reflexly through compression of the joints (Fig. 12.8). The therapist must use her hands to ensure the correct alignment of the scapula with elongation of the hemiplegic side.

In addition, activity in the relevant muscles can be more directly encouraged by carefully graded stimulation.

The therapist supports the patient's arm forwards, and with her other hand she taps the humerus head briskly and firmly upwards (Fig. 12.9 a). Tone and activity are increased in the deltoid and supraspinatus muscles by eliciting a stretch reflex from below.

With the arm held forwards, the therapist gives quick, repetitive compression through the ball of the hand, and the patient is asked to keep his hand forward and not to let the shoulder go back (Fig. 12.9 b).

The therapist strokes her hand firmly over the infraspinatus, deltoid and triceps muscles, moving quickly in the direction from proximal to distal (Fig. 12.9 c).

Brisk stroking with ice may stimulate activity in the relevant muscles when applied before an active movement is attempted.

12.1.2.3 Maintaining Full Pain-Free Range of Passive Movement

The maintenance of full pain-free range of movement without traumatising the joint and the structures which surround it can be achieved by carrying out accurately the activities described in Chaps. 5 and 8. The activities involve not only passive movement of the scapula and arm, but also how the patient is assisted when he moves in bed or transfers into a chair, and his position when lying or sitting.

As Smith et al. (1982) so rightly point out, "correct handling of the patient in the early stages of a stroke is crucial in preventing the consequences of malalignment of the shoulder".

At no time should pain in or around the shoulder joint be produced during an activity. Pain indicates that some structure is being compromised and the therapist must alter her support at once. Correcting the position of the scapula is invariably the solution.

12.1.3 Conclusion

It should be remembered that subluxation of the shoulder is commonly seen in the stroke patient. Subluxation is not painful as long as the scapula is mobile (B. Bobath 1978). The flaccid or hypotonic hanging arm will sublux, but this is not a factor to which any undue concern ought to be given (Johnstone 1978), and the subluxation is harmless as long as passive range of motion is not painful (Mossman 1976). The subluxed shoulder is in itself not painful (Davies 1980) (Fig. 12.10 a, b). It is, however, most important that the unprotected subluxed shoulder or malaligned shoulder should not develop into a painful shoulder with limitation of passive or active range of movement.

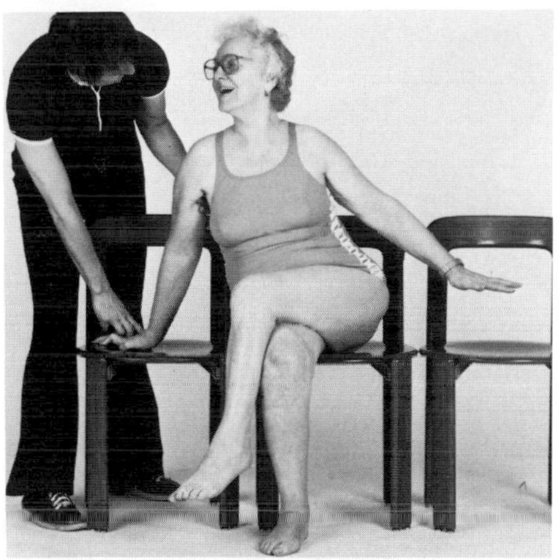

Fig. 12.8. Weight-bearing through the hemiplegic arm (right hemiplegia)

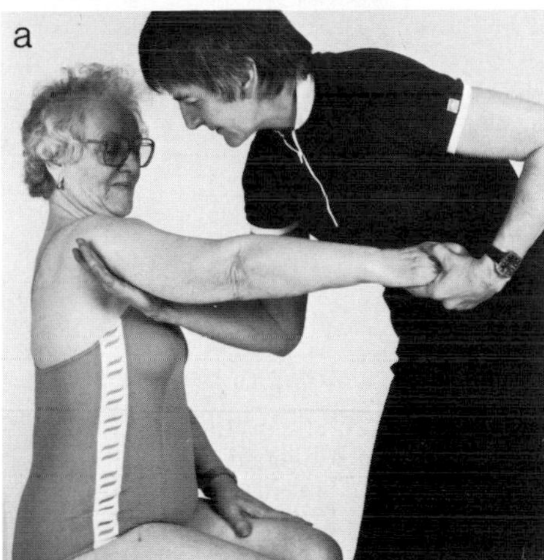

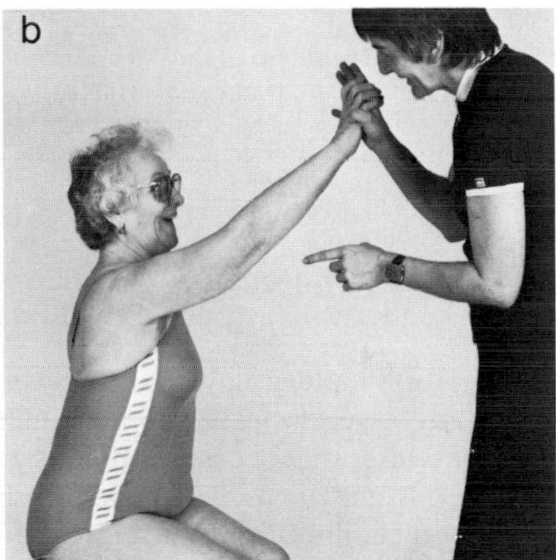

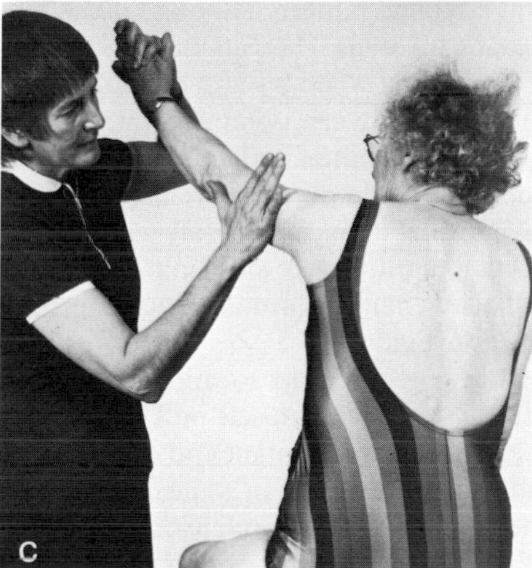

Fig. 12.9 a–c. Stimulating activity in the muscles which stabilise the shoulder.
a Tapping the head of the humerus upwards.
b Repetitive compression through the ball of the hand. The patient has no voluntary activity in her arm (right hemiplegia).
c Quick stroking from proximal to distal (left hemiplegia)

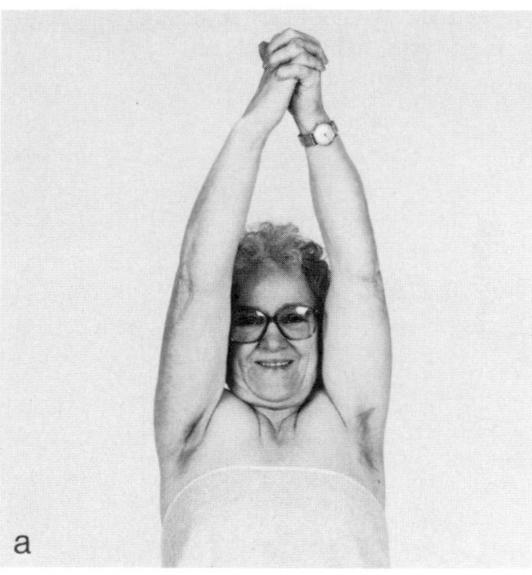

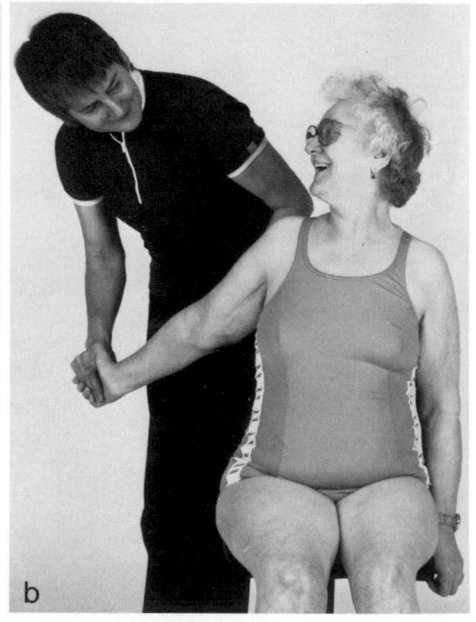

Fig. 12.10 a, b. The subluxed shoulder is in itself not painful (right hemiplegia). **a** Full self-assisted elevation is pain-free. **b** No pain is elicited even in an extreme position

12.2 The Painful Shoulder

The painful shoulder may occur fairly early following a stroke or can develop at a much later stage, even after several months. The upper limb may appear to be somewhat flaccid or show considerable spasticity. Subluxation may or may not be present, but as most hemiplegic patients show evidence of subluxation in the early stages of their illness it would logically follow that many with pain in addition will also demonstrate such a malalignment.

Pain at the shoulder usually develops in a typical pattern, although it can also occur suddenly as a result of a specific traumatic incident. The patient starts to complain of a sharp pain at the end of range of movement, when his arm is being moved passively during therapy or during an examination. He can point accurately to the painful localised area. If the causative factors are not eliminated, the pain increases over a period, or rapidly, and the patient describes pain on all movement, particularly elevation of the arm and abduction. He may experience pain only with the arm in certain positions or even when lying in bed at night. Severe sudden pain may occur, not only at full range of movement, but also when the arm is being lowered to the side again, or at certain stages during the movements.

The patient finds it increasingly difficult to give the exact location of the pain and indicates the deltoid area by rubbing his hand over the muscle bulk. If the therapeutic approach is not altered the patient has pain day and night and cannot tolerate his arm being moved at all. He complains of diffuse pain, in some cases involving the whole arm and the hand as well. The pain must be very intense indeed, for it can reduce proud strong men to a state of helpless weeping, begging the therapist not to move the arm or aggressively refusing to allow the arm to be touched at all. Some may try to avoid therapy altogether.

The pain must not be accepted as a part of the illness. It was not present at onset, so clearly something must have happened to cause it.

12.2.1 Causative Factors

"The shoulder is essentially a composite of seven joints, all moving synchronously and incumbent upon each other to ensure complete pain-free movement" (Cailliet 1980). Any interruption of this co-ordinated interaction could cause pain or restriction of movements. In order to understand the disturbed mechanism which causes pain in the shoulder following hemiplegia, certain aspects of the normal shoulder mechanism require special consideration.

The scapulohumeral rhythm described by Codman (1934) and Cailliet (1980) enables the arm to be lifted smoothly into full elevation (Fig. 12.11). When the arm is at the side of the body when standing normally, the scapula and humerus can be said to be in the position of 0°. As the arm is abducted a ratio of 2:1 exists between scapula rotation and glenohumeral movement. This would mean that when the arm is abducted to 90°, 60° of the movement take place at the glenohumeral joint and 30° are due to scapula rotation. Full elevation of the arm to 180° is performed with 120° of glenohumeral movement and 60° due to scapula rotation. The movement occurs in a smooth rhythmic pattern which the normal muscle tone allows unimpeded. The scapula rotates to change the alignment of the glenoid fossa, and without the rotation, the arm cannot fully abduct or elevate overhead.

External rotation of the humerus is essential if the arm is to abduct fully, as it allows the greater tuberosity to pass behind the acromion process. "With the arm internally rotated the greater tuberosity impinges against the coraco-acromial arch and blocks further abduction at 60°" (Cailliet 1980). A downward gliding move-

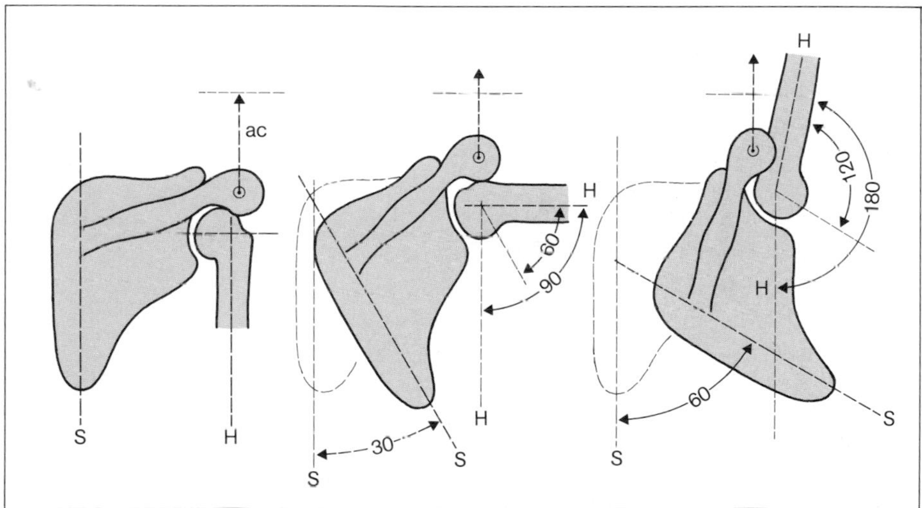

Fig. 12.11 The scapulohumeral rhythm (Codman 1934). *H* Humerus; *S* scapula

ment of the head of the humerus in the glenoid fossa must accompany the external rotation if the greater tuberosity is to pass freely under the coraco-acromial hood.

In hemiplegia, if the patient suffers from pain and loss of range of movement at the shoulder, one or all of these mechanisms has been disturbed by abnormal and unbalanced muscle tone. In the upper extremity the spastic pattern of flexion predominates. Of particular relevance to the mechanism of pain are the components of depression and retraction of the scapula and medial rotation of the humerus.

12.2.1.1 Loss of the Scapulohumeral Rhythm

When the patient's arm is lifted away from the body, there is a delay in scapula rotation. The structures located between the acromion process and the head of the hu-

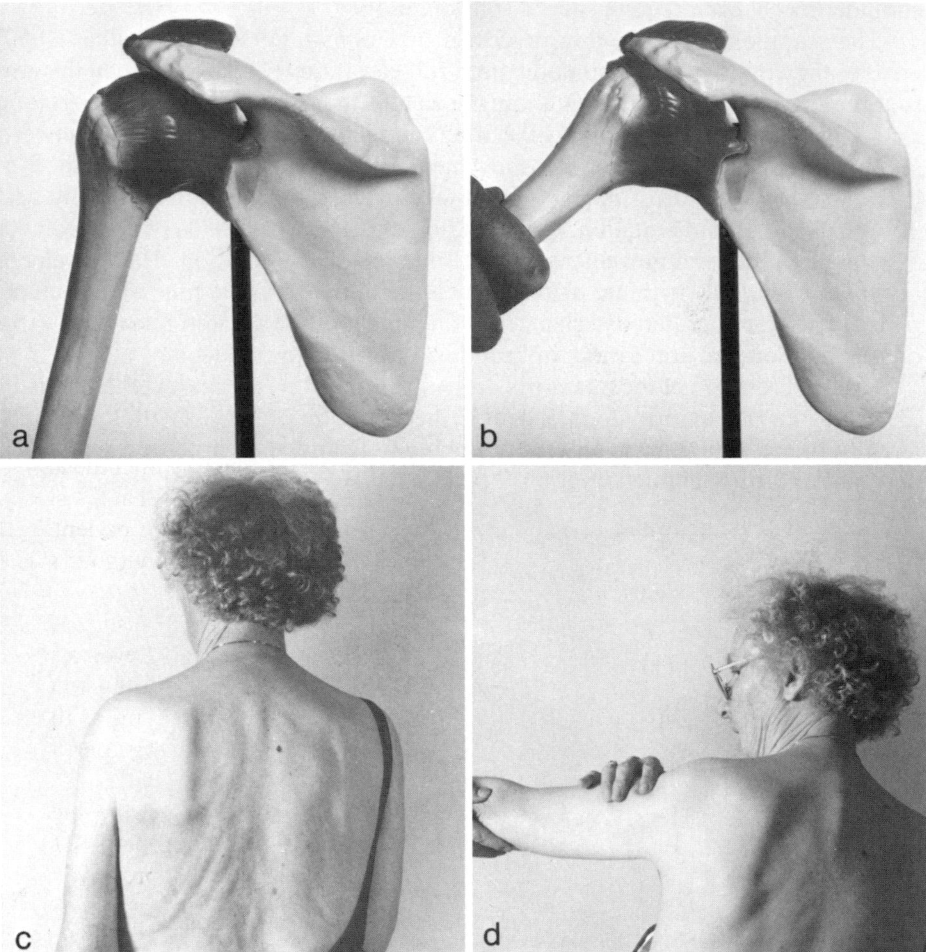

Fig. 12.12a–d. Loss of the scapulohumeral rhythm traumatises the shoulder (left hemiplegia). **a** Model of shoulder joint with humerus in a neutral position. **b** Model of shoulder joint showing mechanism of trauma when the humerus is abducted. **c** Patient with her arm at her side. **d** When the arm is lifted the scapula fails to rotate and the patient experiences pain at the shoulder

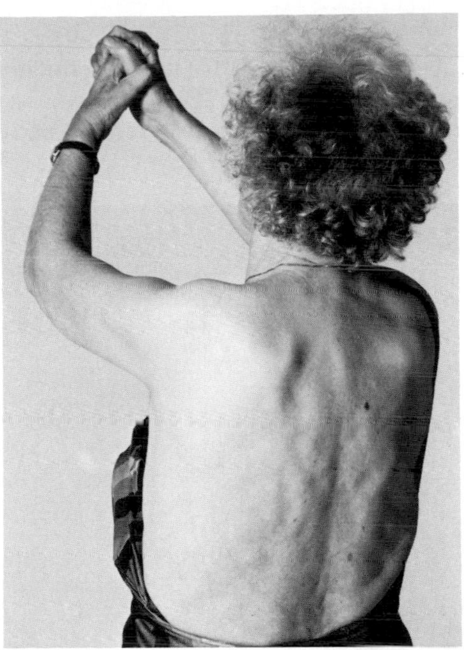

Fig. 12.13. Self-assisted arm activity performed incorrectly

merus are mechanically squeezed between the two hard bony elements. A model of the shoulder shows clearly the pinching effect when the humerus is lifted sideways and the scapula remains fixed (Fig. 12.12a, b).

Similarly, when the patient's scapula does not move sufficiently when the arm is being lifted passively, a trauma occurs and the patient experiences pain at the site of the compressed structures (Fig. 12.12c, d). The same may occur if the patient performs his self-assisted arm movement incorrectly, through flexion, without sufficient protraction and rotation of the scapula (Fig. 12.13).

The delayed scapula rotation is due to an increase in tone in the muscles which retract and depress the scapula. The arm may appear to be flaccid, but even a slight increase in tone proximally at the scapula is sufficient to delay its simultaneous rotation. Where the tone in the muscles surrounding the scapula is the same as that of the muscles in the arm itself, the rhythm remains and both move together at the same speed, providing a natural protection.

For example, if a patient is equally spastic proximally and distally, the "heavy" arm can only be moved slowly into abduction, which allows the scapula time to rotate slowly as well. Some patients with marked hypertonus will therefore have absolutely no pain or limitation of movement. In the same way, patients with marked hypotonus may also be pain-free despite having had no therapy as such. The flaccid arm can be lifted easily and the freely moving scapula accompanies it like a shadow. Any imbalance, with the tone around the scapula greater than that around the shoulder joint itself, will produce pain due to trauma if the patient is incorrectly handled.

12.2.1.2 Inadequate External Rotation of the Humerus

The patient's arm fails to rotate externally, due to the spastic pull of the powerful internal rotators of the shoulder. The greater tuberosity impinges against the coraco-acromial arch during passive movement and causes pain. The patient often experi-

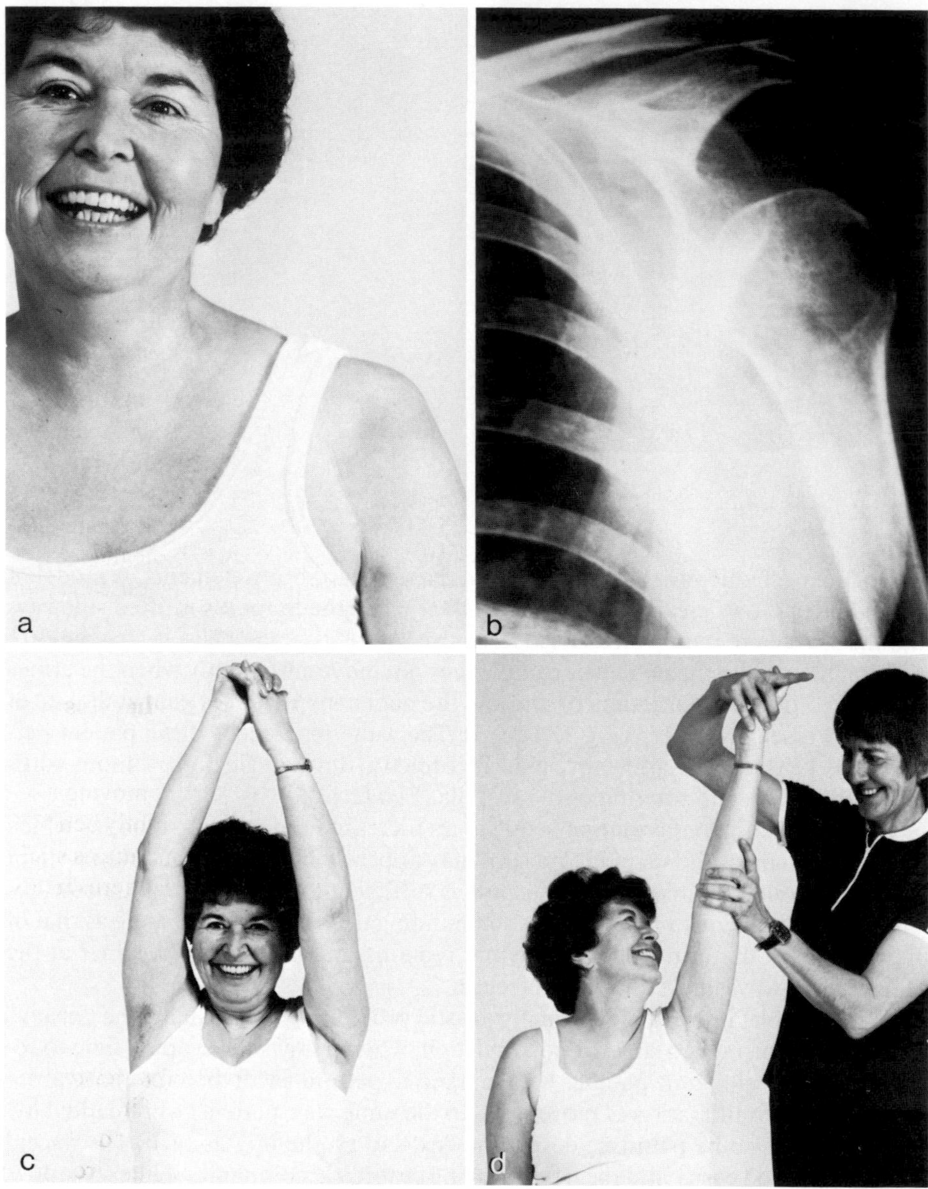

Fig. 12.14. a Patient a year after Sever's procedure (left hemiplegia). **b** X-ray taken in the same position confirms gross subluxation (Courtesy of R. Dewar). **c** Self-assisted arm elevation is pain-free. **d** Even extreme elevation with external rotation does not cause pain despite the subluxation

ences pain and tenderness if local pressure is applied to the tuberosity. A common mechanism of rupture of the rotator cuff is a "pinching of the tuberosity cuff ligament insertion zone against the acromion which occurs when the arm is forcibly abducted without concomitant external rotation to clear the tuberosity from the acromion" (Bateman 1963).

Convincing evidence of pain being caused by insufficient external rotation of the arm during elevation and not due to subluxation is presented in Fig. 12.14. The patient sought surgical intervention 1 year after the onset of her illness because of extreme pain in her hemiplegic shoulder and because the treatment described in this chapter was not available to her at the time. On examination, the surgeon noted a "very fixed internal rotation adduction shoulder contracture" (R. Dewar, personal communication).

A left Severs procedure was performed under suitable general anaesthesia, and the operation report states:

The arm was then externally rotated and the fibres of the subscapularis were identified. The fascia overlying this was bluntly retracted and the subscapularis was then divided sharply, without dividing the capsula, approximately 1.5 cm medial to its insertion on the humerus. The pectoralis major was then identified and divided approximately two inches medial to its attachment on the humerus.

The pain was relieved and full range of movement restored by releasing only two muscles whose action is internal rotation and adduction of the shoulder. A year after operation the subluxation was still clearly visible (Fig. 12.14a) and an X-ray confirmed a gross subluxation of the hemiplegic shoulder (Fig. 12.14b). Nevertheless, self-assisted arm activity was possible without discomfort, and external rotation of the shoulder was seen to be greater than that of the sound side during the movement (Fig. 12.14c). Even when the therapist moved the arm passively into full elevation with external rotation, no pain was elicited (Fig. 12.14d).

12.2.1.3 Lack of the Downward Gliding Movement of the Head of the Humerus in the Glenoid Fossa

Less commonly, pain is experienced although the scapula is seen to be moving adequately. On palpation, the head of the humerus can be felt to be held tightly beneath the acromion process. Any attempts to abduct the arm will then cause pain, as spasticity prevents the necessary downward movement of the head of the humerus in the fossa.

12.2.2 Activities Which Frequently Cause Painful Trauma

1. *Passive range of movement without the scapula being brought into the necessary position and the humerus into external rotation.* The therapist or nurse lifts the arm from its distal end, causing soft tissue compression (Fig. 12.15a) instead of controlling the scapula (Fig. 12.15b). Once pain has been elicited a vicious circle follows. Pain and fear increase flexor tone in man, and so the patient who has experienced pain during passive movement will have an increase in flexor tone even before the exercise is performed again. The increase in tone in the spastic pattern

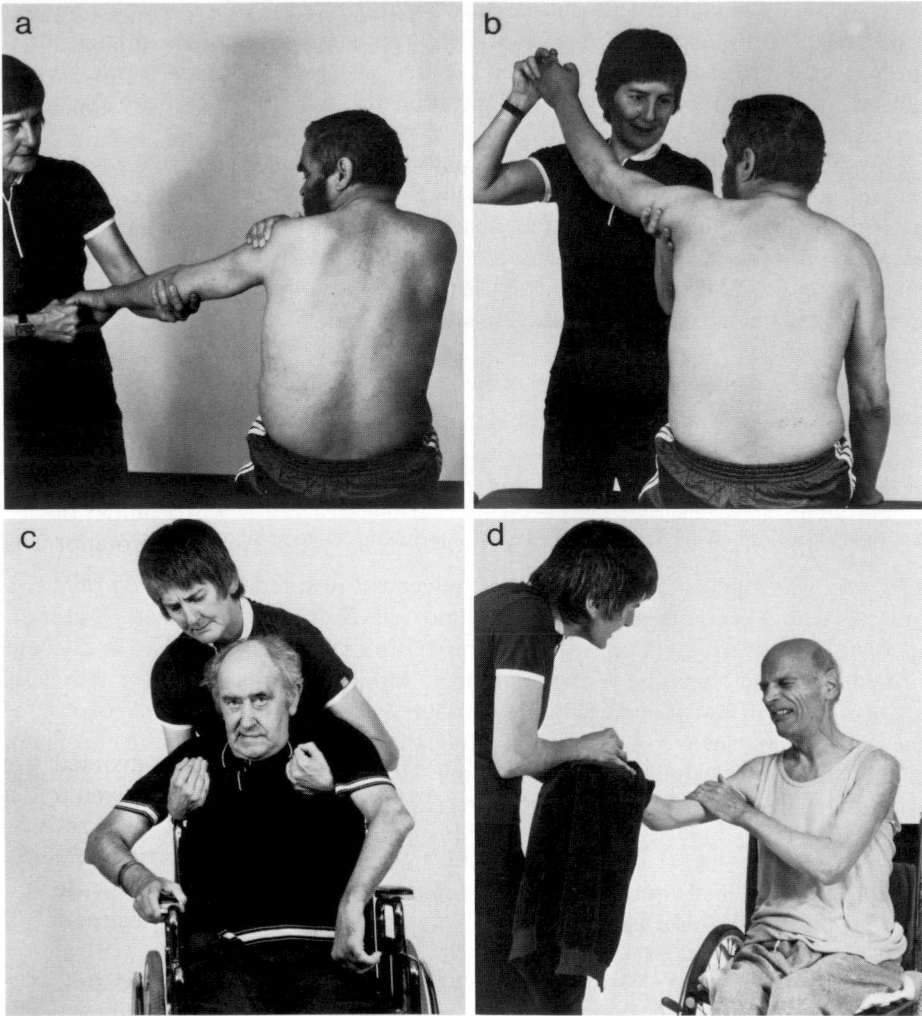

Fig. 12.15 a–d. The shoulder is easily traumatised if the therapist fails to support it adequately. **a** When lifting the arm without rotating the scapula. **b** correct support of the scapula renders the movement pain-free (left hemiplegia). **c** when lifting the patient back in the wheel-chair incorrectly (left hemiplegia). **d** when putting the patient's arm in the sleeve (right hemiplegia)

of flexion fixes the scapula in depression and the arm in internal rotation. Any attempt to force the elevation of the arm will result in increasingly severe trauma.

2. *Assisting the patient to transfer from bed to chair by pulling on his arm.* If the nurse or therapist is assisting a patient to transfer and is holding his arm, she is unable to support the heavy trunk and, as the patient moves, the weight of his body forces abduction of the shoulder. The shoulder is easily damaged. The same occurs when the patient is being helped to walk, and assistance is given either by holding his hand and arm or by his affected arm being supported across the helper's

shoulders. Any loss of balance or sudden movement immediately causes the arm to be forcibly abducted and the humerus approximates with the acromion.

3. *Lifting the patient back into the wheelchair incorrectly.* The helper attempts to correct the patient's posture after he has slipped down in the chair. She stands behind him and, placing her hands under his arms, she attempts to heave him back into the chair (Fig. 12.15 c). The unprotected hemiplegic shoulder is forced into abduction by the weight of his body. The same occurs when the nurse attempts to lift the patient out of the bath when he is not yet able to assist with the movement actively.
4. *Lifting the arm from the hand during nursing activities such as passive dressing* (Fig. 12.15 d), *washing the axilla or turning the patient in bed.*
5. *Using reciprocal pulleys.* It has often been mistakenly assumed that if the patient was encouraged to pull his hemiplegic arm up into abduction *and* elevation, using his sound hand, he would maintain full range of motion of the shoulder. On the contrary, he traumatises his own shoulder by attempting to force the inwardly rotated arm upwards. Najenson et al. (1971) and Irwin-Carruthers and Runnals (1980) describe the resulting injury to the structures around the shoulder during pulley exercises. "Shoulder pulleys do not provide adequate scapular rotation and humeral external rotation and should not be used as a means of passive elevation of the affected arm" (Griffin and Reddin 1981).

12.2.3 Prevention and Treatment

When the predisposing causes of the painful shoulder are carefully avoided, the condition can be prevented altogether. Particular attention should be given to the patient's position when lying in bed or sitting in the chair, and to how he is assisted when he moves. All passive movements of the arm must be preceded by full mobilisation of the scapula, and then the scapula supported in such a way that the glenoid fossa continues to face upwards and forwards during movements of the arm distally.

Any position or activity which causes pain must be changed immediately and carried out in such a way that the pain is eliminated. It is far better not to move the arm at all than to move it causing pain. The patient informs the therapist immediately when any movement is hurting him, and she is guided by his feedback and can avoid damaging the sensitive structures. The patient's information about the pain is the only way she knows for certain that all is well.

12.2.3.1 Overcoming Early Signs of Pain

If a patient who has hitherto been free of pain unexpectedly complains of pain in the shoulder one day, the therapist should work to achieve full range of movement without pain on the same day. She pays special attention to mobilising the scapula and using trunk rotation to inhibit the hypertonicity before moving the arm. The patient should be encouraged to continue with his self-assisted arm exercises, and the therapist checks that he is performing them carefully and correctly without eliciting pain (Fig. 12.16).

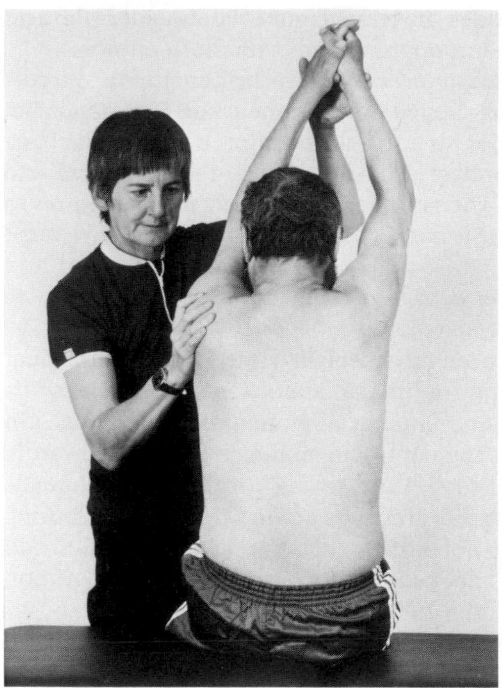

Fig. 12.16. Correcting the patient's self-assisted arm activity (left hemiplegia)

The encouragement to keep moving the arm is important, because when something is painful we all tend to hold that part still and, what is more, in flexion. For example, if someone knocks his elbow against the door-frame, he flexes his arm tightly against his body and holds the elbow with his other hand. His whole posture becomes one of flexion. If the patient has pain in his shoulder he holds it in flexion and is loath to move it. Flexor hypertonus increases and fixes the scapula even more strongly in depression and retraction, and the shoulder in internal rotation. If the vicious circle is not interrupted, passive range of movement will almost certainly be more painful on the following day. It is most important to prevent repeated trauma, and particular attention should be paid to the transfers, how the patient is helped to dress and how he is being assisted by others when walking. His positioning in bed should be checked and he should lie as much as possible in the corrected position on the hemiplegic side, with his shoulder well forward in protraction.

12.2.3.2 Management of the Severely Painful Shoulder

For a patient who has already developed a stiff, painful shoulder before the correct treatment programme was instituted, the approach is different. The patient arrives for his first treatment session and will often tell the therapist immediately that his shoulder is very painful, asking her at the same time not to move his arm. It is most important that she respects his wishes and restrains her immediate impulse to see how restricted the movement actually is. If she lifts the arm it will certainly hurt him, and the patient/therapist relationship will be off to a bad start. Inevitably, from the time the patient first complained that his shoulder was hurting him, doctors and therapists alike will have moved the arm to assess the range of movement; and each time he will have experienced pain.

The therapist should leave the arm alone and treat all other aspects of the patient's disability until she has gained his full trust and confidence. To achieve this goal the patient needs to experience success, be it in balance, walking, climbing stairs or some other activity. The time will vary from patient to patient, and may even require weeks, but it is time well spent. The stiff shoulder did not develop overnight, and another week or two will not be detrimental to the end result.

If the patient is afraid because he anticipates pain, the pain will be produced earlier when the arm is moved. Fear increases flexor tone in all people; we tend to crouch down when we are afraid. The patient likewise will have increased tone in the already hypertonic flexor groups, including those which depress and retract the scapula and rotate the humerus internally. The therapist should tell the patient that she will not pull on his arm, and reassure him with conviction that the pain will be completely overcome by their work together.

12.2.3.2.1 Positioning in Bed. The patient with a stiff painful shoulder has usually been nursed in the supine position. The side-lying positions are essential for freeing the scapula, but will need to be introduced gradually. The patient is positioned on the hemiplegic side, with perhaps only a quarter of a turn possible at first. He is asked to lie in that position for 15 minutes or until he experiences pain, and is then helped to turn again. The time is extended over the next few days, and it is surprising how quickly the full side-lying position can be achieved. The same applies to lying on the sound side.

12.2.3.2.2 General Activities. The patient who has a stiff and painful shoulder will also need to improve other movement sequences. For example, he will have difficulty in transferring weight over his hemiplegic side correctly. The therapist works on all the activities described in the previous chapters to improve his balance, gait and movement without effort.

12.2.3.2.3 More Specific Activities. The shoulder is moved without the arm being used as the moving lever. Particularly beneficial are those activities where the scapula and shoulder move from their proximal components, instead of the arm being lifted from the hand distally:

1. The therapist facilitates weight transference toward the hemiplegic side in sitting, emphasising the elongation of that side of the patient's trunk. She sits beside the patient, and with one hand in his axilla asks him to bring his weight towards her. As he does so, she uses her hand to elevate the shoulder girdle. The movement is repeated rhythmically, and each time the patient attempts to move further over his affected side. The elongation of the side inhibits the spasticity which is preventing the scapula from moving freely. The trunk moves against the scapula. The effect is further increased if the patient's hand is placed flat on the plinth beside him, and he takes weight through his extended arm. The therapist maintains the elbow in extension for him.
2. The therapist kneels in front of the seated patient and asks him to lean to touch his feet, letting his hands hang forward. The patient concentrates on not pushing with his feet, and may only be able to come as far as the therapist's knees at first.

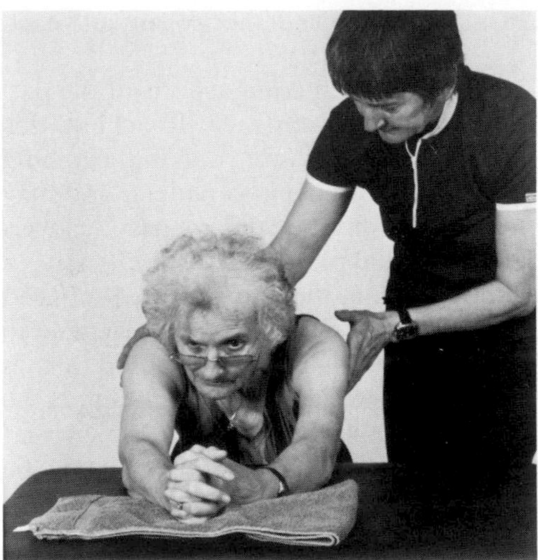

Fig. 12.17. Pushing a towel forwards with clasped hands (left hemiplegia)

She facilitates the movement by placing her hands over his scapulae, and by remaining close to him. When the patient can touch his toes, his shoulder will have moved to 90° without the hand having been lifted.

3. The patient, still seated, is helped to clasp his hands together and then to place them on a large ball in front of him. He leans forward, moving the ball away from his knees, and back again. The actual movement is taking place through flexion of the hips, but the shoulder is moving further into elevation at the same time. Because the hands are supported, no pain is elicited, and the patient can control the amount of movement, moving the ball back toward him if the shoulder starts to hurt.
4. Sitting with a table or the plinth in front of him, the patient places his clasped hands on a towel, which he pushes forward as far as he can. The friction-free surface facilitates an easy movement without effort, and once again the shoulder is being moved by the motion of the trunk (Fig. 12.17).
5. Rolling from supine over the hemiplegic side inhibits spasticity in the trunk and upper extremity. The therapist uses one of her hands to hold the hemiplegic shoulder well forward in protraction. With her other hand she helps the patient to roll gently and smoothly towards the affected side. The patient starts by rolling only part of the way, and then back again, to avoid hurting his shoulder. As he rolls back the therapist lifts his arm from the bed or plinth so that the fully abducted position is avoided to begin with. The patient continues to roll easily back and forth, while the therapist eases his arm into further elevation. When the activity ceases, the therapist holds his arm upwards in the newly achieved range, and the patient clasps his hands together and carries out self-assisted movements into further elevation.
6. While the patient lies supine with his hemiplegic leg flexed and leaning over the other leg, the therapist facilitates a gentle rocking motion of the pelvis (Fig. 12.18 a). The rhythmic rocking rotates the trunk and releases the spasticity in the whole side.

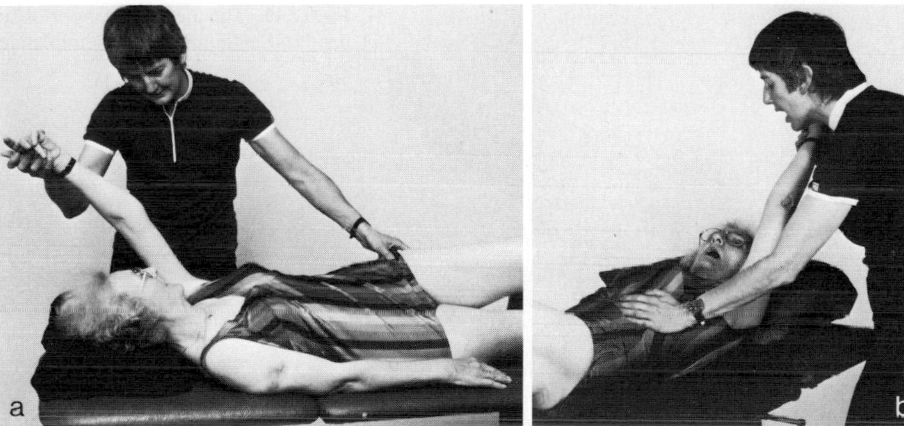

Fig. 12.18 a, b. Inhibiting hypertonus to free the scapula for movement (left hemiplegia). **a** Rhythmic rotation of the pelvis; **b** assisted expiration

The therapist holds the patient's arm in a comfortable degree of elevation with the elbow extended, and as the patient continues to rotate his pelvis she perceives a relaxation in the muscles around the shoulder. She eases the arm into further elevation, watching the patient's face carefully as she does so. Should any tension be observed in his facial expression, she immediately brings the arm a little way out of the elevated position.

The therapist's voice is very important during the activity. With a low soothing tone she reduces the amount of effort the patient is using to rotate his pelvis, and also reduces the overall hypertonicity. An amazing amount of elevation can be achieved in this way, as long as the patient is sure that the therapist will not suddenly pull his arm into a painful range of movement.

7. With the hemiplegic leg lying flexed and relaxed against the other leg, the therapist assists the patient with deep expiration. Placing one hand on his ribs, with her fingers pointing in the diagonal direction of the rib movement, she assists deep expiration by pressing downwards towards the mid-line as he breathes out. With her other hand she holds his laterally rotated arm in the maximum amount of painless elevation (Fig. 12.18b). The assisted movement of the ribs moves the thorax against the scapula and shoulder and inhibits the spasticity surrounding them. The arm can be moved easily into further elevation thereafter. Asking the patient to produce clear sustained vowel sounds as he breathes out not only adds interest but helps to improve the quality of his voice and breath control at the same time.

12.2.3.2.4 Increasing the Range of Passive Movement. When the patient has sufficient trust in the therapist and the scapula is able to be moved easily, the arm itself can gradually be encouraged into passive and, later, active elevation. It is essential that the hemiplegic side be elongated and protracted before the arm movement is attempted. The affected leg must remain flexed and leaning against the other leg, ensuring that the pelvis is forward on that side and that spasticity has been sufficiently inhibited in the whole affected side. If the leg does not remain relaxed in the

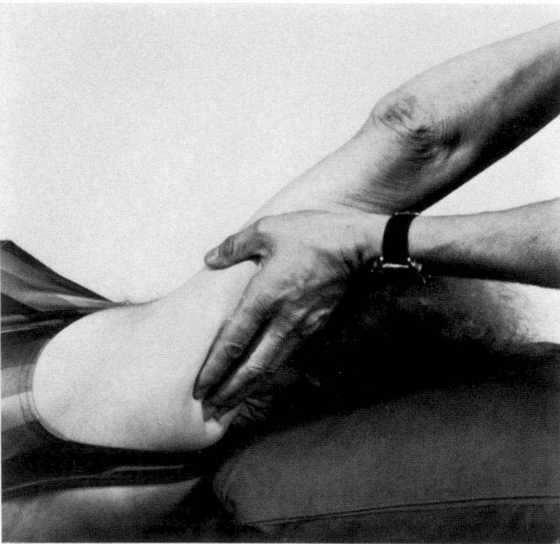

Fig. 12.19. The therapist supports the head of the humerus (left hemiplegia)

inhibitory position the therapist should on no account move the arm, as she may elicit pain in the shoulder as a result. The therapist moves the arm carefully forwards and upwards, with the shoulder externally rotated and the elbow extended. If the patient is at all apprehensive he can be asked to move his own arm as far as he can without pain, using his sound hand to do so, with his hands clasped together. In this way external rotation is assured, and the patient knows that he can stop the movement at any time. He is in charge of the procedure, so to speak.

The therapist then knows at what stage the patient first begins to feel discomfort. She takes over the patient's arm with one hand, maintaining the protraction and external rotation with slight traction. With her other hand she supports the head of the humerus in such a way that her fingers prevent it from impinging against the neighbouring bony prominence (Fig. 12.19). Her fingers also assist the downward gliding movement of the humeral head in the glenoid fossa to permit further painless elevation.

Goal-orientated movements help the patient to move without fear of pain. Because he is relaxed and concentrating on the activity, there is less spasticity in flexion and he can move his arm more freely and fully. He can, for example, push a ball or hit a balloon to a partner, using his clasped hands. Either standing or sitting he can push a ball to knock over skittles or aim at a given goal or container.

12.2.3.2.5 Self-Assisted Arm Activity. Finally, the patient must learn to move his own shoulder correctly, using his sound hand to move the hemiplegic arm into elevation. When not carefully instructed, many patients try to lift their arm through flexion, and in so doing traumatise their shoulder, or give up trying after the first few painful attempts.

If the patient lifts his arm with the scapula retracted and the elbow flexed, he will reproduce the mechanism of pain. Because the arm is pulling down in flexion and adduction, it is heavy and the patient needs much effort to lift it. The effort further increases the hypertonicity. With the help of the therapist he learns to push his arms well forward first to ensure protraction of the scapula. Then with the elbows extended and the palms of the hands together, he brings his arms into as much elevation as possible. At first he may only be able to lift them a few inches from the table in front of him, but quality of movement is more important than quantity if he is to achieve success. The patient is encouraged by all members of the team, by other patients and by his family to repeat the movement correctly many times throughout the day. Once he is able to move his arm successfully himself, and does so on his own, the shoulder rapidly becomes pain-free and the problem disappears.

12.2.3.2.6 Additional Treatment Possibilities. If the programme described is carefully followed, the shoulder pain can be completely eliminated within 2–3 months, and often far sooner. It is interesting to note that the soft tissue structures surrounding the shoulder joint have not actually shortened. Full range of passive movement is rapidly regained once pain has disappeared.

12.2.3.2.6.1 *Injection of a Local Anaesthetic with or Without a Cortisone Preparation.* Injecting the exquisitely painful shoulder may provide a temporary relief for the patient, but it is clear that if the underlying cause of the pain is not corrected, the relief will be short-lived. The anaesthetic effect is undesirable when administered before attempts at passive range of movement. As already mentioned, the only way in which the therapist can know whether she is causing trauma is by the patient informing her when something hurts.

12.2.3.2.6.2 *The Use of Ice.* Ice has been advocated to relieve spasticity, and should be applied with wet iced towels around the whole scapula and shoulder, if it is to be effective. The time and effort involved usually do not warrant its use, as the measures described will ensure a rapid and more lasting result.

12.2.3.2.6.3 *Passive Mobilisation.* Some of the techniques of passive mobilisation as described by Maitland (1973) can be useful in gaining relief of pain and range of movement, if used in addition to the total regime. The techniques are particularly useful for the following:

Where pain rather than stiffness is the predominant feature. Passive accessory movements, i.e. those joint movements which we are unable to perform actively and selectively, are the most beneficial in the treatment of pain. Irwin-Carruthers and Runnalls (1980) describe their experiences using a combined treatment of inhibition followed by mobilisation with carefully graded passive accessory movements to the shoulder joint.

Where pain is only experienced at the end of the full range of movement, probably because the head of the humerus fails to move downwards in the glenoid fossa.

Where pain is no longer present but final elevation appears to be mechanically blocked at the end of range. Once again the head of the humerus is probably failing to glide downwards to allow the full movement.

12.3 The "Shoulder-Hand" Syndrome

The sudden development of a swollen painful hand is a disturbing and disabling condition arising as a secondary complication following hemiplegia. According to Davis et al. (1977), it affects abount 12.5% of the patients and occurs most common-

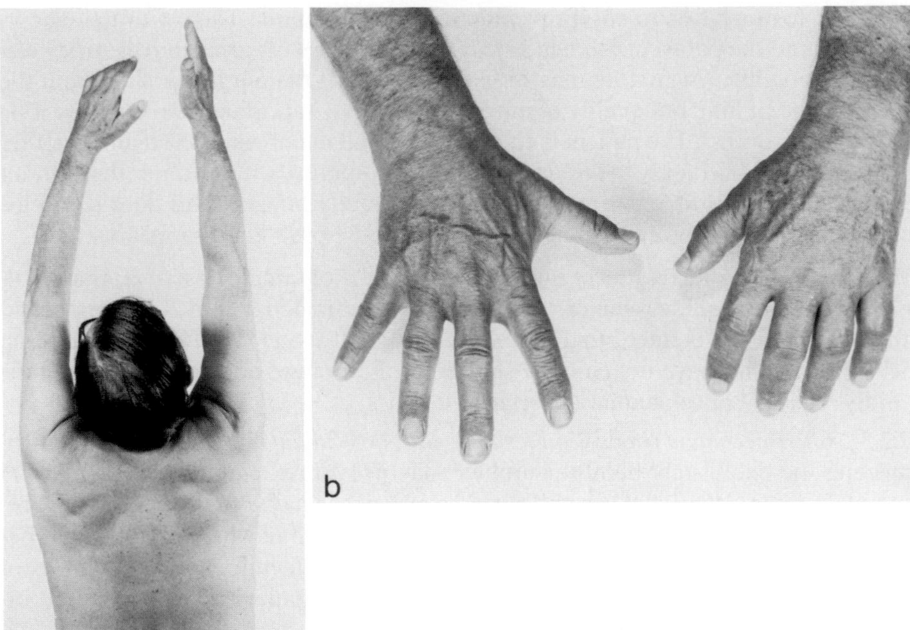

Fig. 12.20 a, b. Painless shoulder movement despite marked hand symptoms (left hemiplegia)

ly between the 1st and 3rd months following onset of stroke. The painful condition interferes with the patient's overall rehabilitation, but even more seriously, if untreated leads to a permanent fixed deformity of the hand and fingers which limits any functional use in the future. Different names have been given to the condition, and these have tended to add to the confusion as to its cause.

It is important that the causes of the condition be understood, because only then can preventative measures be adopted or successful treatment be carried out. The first step is to consider the symptoms occurring in the hand as separate from those of the painful shoulder. If, as has been described, between 60% and 80% of patients suffer from a painful shoulder, it can be assumed that the 12% who develop a swollen hand would often fall within this group. The reasons for the painful shoulder are those explained earlier in the chapter. If it is accepted that the pain in the shoulder is the result of the mechanical factors described, then it is easier to understand and treat the problems which arise from a different mechanism in the wrist, hand and fingers. It is also easier to explain the findings of Moskowitz et al. (1958) when using stellate ganglion blocks and high thoracic sympathectomy in the treatment of the syndrome. The hand symptoms were relieved but, as the authors noted, "Symptoms referable to the shoulder, including pain and limitation of motion, were not favourably affected by either the blocks or the sympathectomy." Davis et al. (1977) describe their successful treatment of 68 patients using oral steroids in addition to their rehabilitation programme, and mention that: "Two patients not included in this study had signs and symptoms only in the hand and were treated successfully using the same methods ..." If the patient's shoulder has been carefully protected and moved as described earlier in the chapter, the shoulder movement is full and painless (Fig. 12.20a), despite the pronounced hand symptoms (Fig. 12.20b).

12.3.1 Symptoms Arising in the Hand

12.3.1.1 Early Stage

The patient's hand quite suddenly becomes swollen, and a marked limitation of range of movement occurs rapidly. The oedema is predominantly apparent on the dorsum of the hand, including the metacarpophalangeal joints, and also in the fingers and thumb (Fig. 12.21). The skin loses its creases, particularly over the knuckles and the proximal and distal interphalangeal joints. The oedema is soft and puffy and usually ends just proximal to the wrist joint. The tendons of the hand cannot be seen. The colour of the hand changes, having a pink or lilac hue, particularly noticeable if the arm is left hanging down at the patient's side. The hand feels warm and sometimes moist. The nails start to undergo changes, and appear whiter or more opaque than those of the other hand.

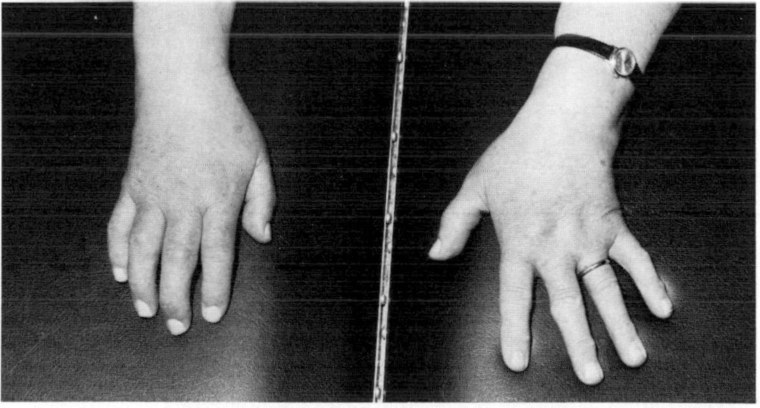

Fig. 12.21. Typical appearance of the swollen hand (right hemiplegia)

Limitation of range of movement is noted as follows:

Loss of passive supination with pain usually felt at the wrist (Fig. 12.22a).

Dorsal extension of the wrist is limited and pain is experienced on the dorsal aspect when an attempt is made to move passively into an increased range. The pain is also elicited during weight-bearing activities in therapy, when the arm is extended and the hand supported flat on the plinth.

There is marked loss of flexion of the metacarpophalangeal joints, with no bony prominences visible (Fig. 12.22b).

Abduction of the fingers is very restricted and the patient has increasing difficulty in clasping his hands together. The fingers of the sound hand appear to be too large to fit into the spaces between the fingers of the other hand.

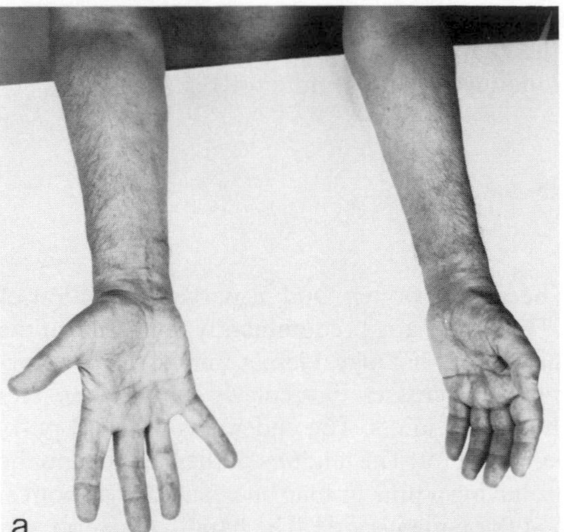

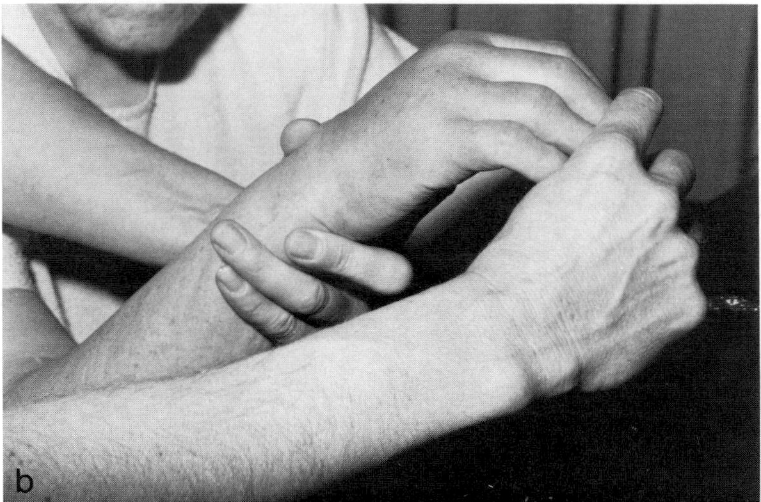

Fig. 12.22 a, b. Limitation of range of movement. **a** Loss of supination, particularly at the wrist (left hemiplegia); **b** loss of flexion of the metacarpophalangeal joints (right hemiplegia)

The proximal interphalangeal joints are stiff and enlarged. Very little flexion is possible and there is a loss of full extension as well. Pain is experienced when attempts are made to flex the joints passively.

The distal interphalangeal joints are extended, and there is little or no flexion possible. Even if these joints have stiffened in slight flexion, any attempt at passive flexion is painful and limited.

12.3.1.2 Later Stages

If the hand is not correctly treated during the early stages, the symptoms become more marked. Pain increases until the patient cannot tolerate any pressure being applied to his hand or fingers at all. Osteoporotic changes may appear on X-ray. A marked hard prominence appears centrally on the dorsal aspect of the intercarpal area and its junction with the metacarpals.

12.3.1.3 Final or Residual Stage

The untreated hand becomes fixed in a typical deformity. The oedema disappears completely, as does the pain, but the mobility is permanently lost.

The wrist is flexed with ulnar deviation, and dorsal flexion is limited. The prominence over the carpal bones is solid and more obvious without the oedema (Fig. 12.23 a).
Supination of the forearm is severely limited (Fig. 12.23 b).
No flexion of the metacarpophalangeal joints is possible, and the amount of abduction is negligible (Fig. 12.23 c). The web space between thumb and index finger is reduced and inelastic.

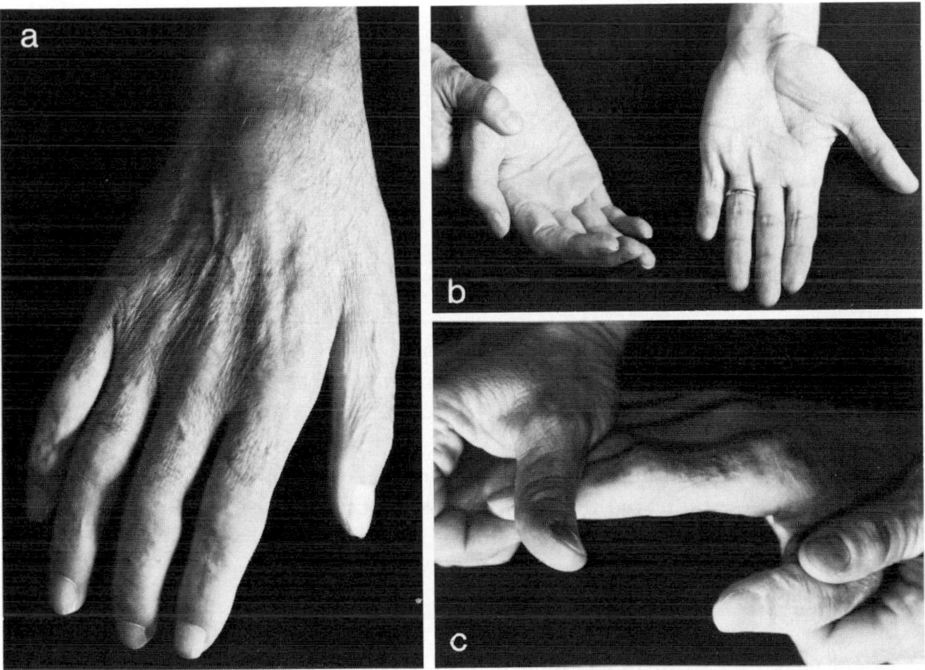

Fig. 12.23 a–c. Final or residual stage (right hemiplegia). **a** Oedema disappears; the prominence over the carpal area is solid; there is flexion of the wrist with ulnar deviation and the fingers stiffened **b** Gross limitation of supination. **c** No flexion of the metacarpophalangeal joints

The proximal and distal interphalangeal joints have fixed in a slightly flexed position, but allow little to no additional flexion.
The palm of the hand is flat and there is marked atrophy of the thenar and hypothenar muscle groups.

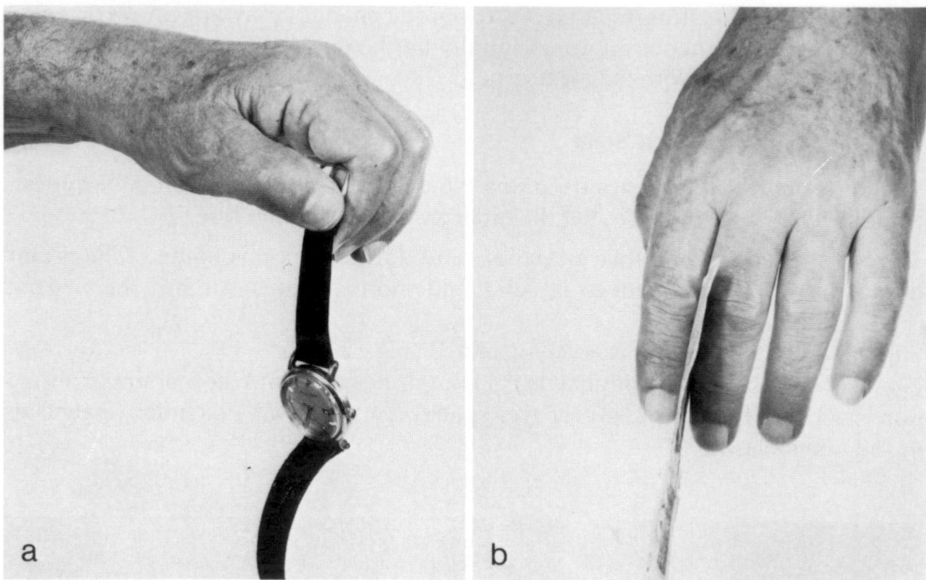

Fig. 12.24 a, b. There is often voluntary movement in the swollen hand (left hemiplegia). **a** Pinch grip; **b** selective adduction of the fingers

"The oedema, containing protein, converts into a diffuse cobweb-like scar tissue that adheres to the tendons and joint capsules and prevents further movement. The joints undergo disuse atrophy of the cartilage with thickening of the capsule" (Cailliet 1980).

During surgery on a hand in this stage at King's College Hospital, London, it was discovered that the ligaments of the interphalangeal joints had actually ossified, and laboratory examination revealed true bone formation. The swollen hand should be treated in the early stages so that the final stage can be prevented at all costs. It is particularly significant with regard to future function, because clinical observations have indicated that many patients suffering from the condition later reveal selective voluntary movement (Fig. 12.24 a, b). Davis et al. support these observations, as 70.5% of their cases had only "partial motor loss".

12.3.2 Causative Factors in Hemiplegia

Although much has been written about the shoulder-hand syndrome in hemiplegia, very little has been convincingly postulated or proved as to its cause. It would be an oversimplification to attach sole blame to the loss of motor activity or the dependent position of the arm. Many more patients would then manifest this relatively infrequent complication. After remission of the symptoms following treatment, patients may continue to have a complete loss of motor activity and a dependent arm position but show no recurrence of their original symptoms.

Something specific must occur which triggers off the syndrome, and it is then only perpetuated by the inactivity and the dependent position of the arm. The sudden onset of symptoms experienced by many patients who previously had no pain or limitation of movement supports this supposition. A logical hypothesis is that a mechanical happening causes a primary oedema or an oedema secondary to trauma, and the inadequate muscle pump fails to resolve it. The vicious cycle of oedema, pain, loss of range of movement and sympathetic nervous system involvement follows. Various causes of oedema in the hand could precipitate the shoulder-hand syndrome.

12.3.2.1 Prolonged Plantar Flexion of the Wrist Under Pressure

The patient lies in bed or sits in his wheelchair for long periods with his arm at his side and the wrist, unnoticed, in a position of forced plantar flexion (Fig. 12.25 a, b). The plantar flexion is extreme because the antagonist muscles are hypotonic and because there is more than just the passive weight of the arm pressing on the wrist from above. Hypertonicity in the muscles which retract and depress the shoulder girdle and those which adduct and inwardly rotate the arm add significantly to the pressure on the unprotected wrist. The effect is more pronounced when the patient is sitting in his wheelchair, as his whole body weight typically leans towards the affected side.

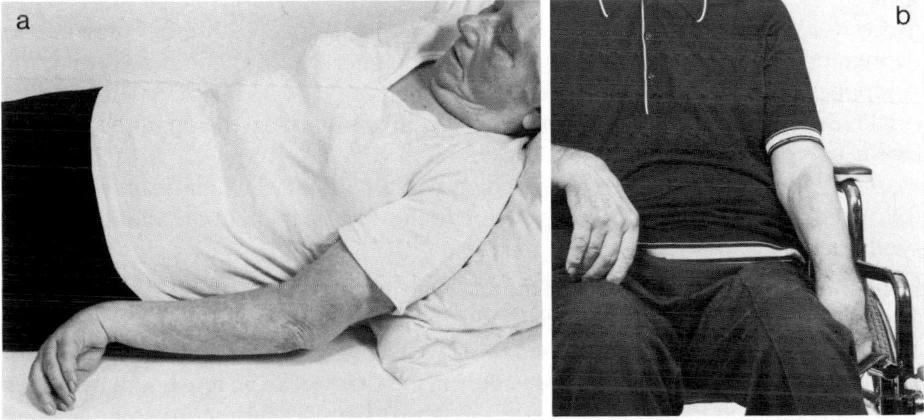

Fig. 12.25 a, b. Commonly observed positions of forced flexion of the wrist (left hemiplegia). **a** In bed; **b** in the wheel chair

Venous drainage of the hand is severely compromised by forced plantar flexion of the wrist. The X-rays of a normal hand and wrist illustrate how one of the large veins is actually blocked altogether in the flexed position when a downward force is exerted by the arm. For the experiment, a contrast medium was injected into the vein distally on the dorsum of the hand. With the wrist in a neutral position the contrast medium was seen to flow freely (Fig. 12.26 a). The subject then flexed her wrist, with the

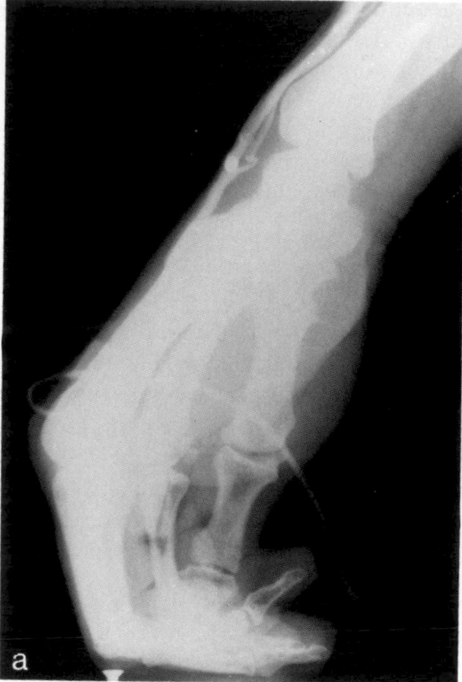

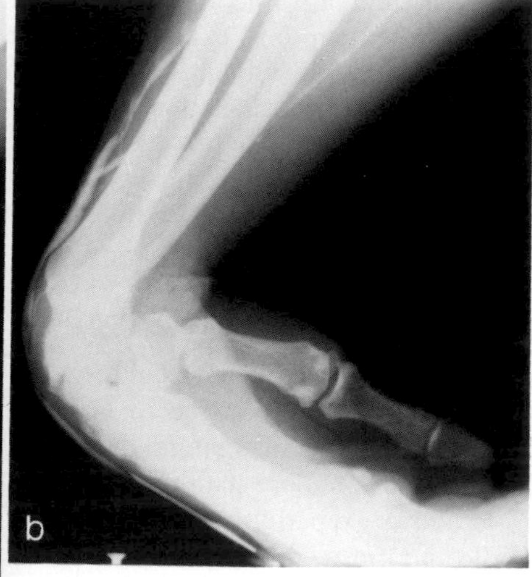

Fig. 12.26 a, b. X-rays of normal subject's wrist with contrast medium injected into a dorsal vein. **a** Wrist in neutral position – medium flows freely. **b** Wrist in forced flexion – flow interrupted

metacarpal heads pressing down on the table. She exerted additional pressure by depressing her shoulder and tensing the adductors of the arm, imitating the spastic components. The flow of the contrast medium was seen to be interrupted (Fig. 12.26 b). Interestingly, she experienced pain on dorsal extension of the wrist after the pressure was released.

The results of the small experiment become particularly significant when the following points are considered in relation to the development of the shoulder-hand syndrome in hemiplegia.

In the majority of cases the syndrome develops between the 1st and the 3rd month after onset of the hemiplegia. Davis et al. (1977) show a figure of 66% for that period. The patient has therefore reached the stage where he is no longer being so intensively nursed and observed as he was during the first weeks. A few hours may pass before his position in bed or sitting in the wheelchair is adjusted, or some nursing duty needs to be carried out. The patient's hand may therefore remain for a considerable time, undetected, in a position of relatively forced flexion.

The tone in the arm is still relatively low, even though some hypertonus may already be present in the wrist flexors and the flexor pattern at the shoulder. The wrist extensors, however, are almost certainly still hypotonic, and provide no protective resistance to the wrist flexion.

Many patients demonstrate neglect of their affected arm in the early stage of the illness and do not notice when it adopts an awkward position. Added to the neglect there can be an actual sensory loss: 91% of the patients examined by Davis et al. (1977) are reported as having either moderate or severe sensory loss.

Most of the venous lymphatic drainage of the hand is located in its dorsal aspect (Cailliet 1980). The oedema is predominantly on the dorsum of the patient's hand in the early stages of the syndrome.

The oedema is very localised and usually ends just proximal to the wrist joint. Throughout the day and night the patient's wrist is almost exclusively in some degree of flexion, particularly if he is not carefully positioned and supervised. The flexion is often more pronounced if he wears some form of sling, or sits with his hand in his lap.

It would seem that the mechanism of flexion of the wrist joint interfering with venous drainage is the commonest primary cause of the shoulder-hand syndrome in hemiplegia.

12.3.2.2 Overstretching of the Joints of the Hand May Produce an Inflammatory Reaction, with Oedema and Pain

The amount of movement possible in the numerous joints of the hand varies considerably from person to person. The therapist may unwittingly force the patient's hand into a range which is for him excessive, and so traumatise the joints or structures surrounding them.

This can easily occur, for example, when the patient is being encouraged to take weight through his extended arm. The hand is placed beside him on the plinth, and the therapist holds his elbow in extension. The patient is then asked to transfer his weight to that side as far as possible. The movement of his body sideways moves the wrist into more dorsiflexion, and if performed in a very enthusiastic or uncontrolled way, dorsiflexion could be forced beyond its normal range.

The same may occur during occupational therapy, where the patient is carrying out tasks with his sound hand while attempting to support himself on the affected arm. While concentrating on performing the task successfully he may not notice that dorsiflexion of the wrist is being forced (Fig. 12.27).

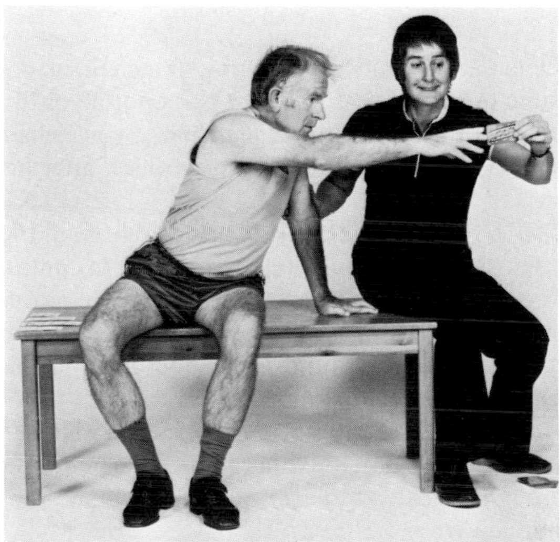

Fig. 12.27. Forced dorsiflexion of the wrist while the patient is concentrating on a task (left hemiplegia)

The same mechanism can occur in all situations where the patient's weight is taken through his extended arm while he is prone kneeling, standing or sitting. If the patient is asked to practise flexing and extending his elbow while weight-bearing, the wrist may inadvertently be forced too far into dorsiflexion. If passive movements are performed too vigorously the same may take place.

Patients whose oedema is triggered off in one of these ways are often those patients who experience a later onset of the syndrome, or who are more active in the early stages of their illness. A typical example is the patient who has little involvement in the lower limb and can walk and exercise at a level far in advance of his upper extremity function.

12.3.2.3 Fluid from an Infusion Escapes into the Tissues of the Hand

It is common practice to use the veins of the hand when repeated infusions are required. Understandably, the medical staff is loath to use the sound hand, as the patient would then be unable to help himself at all in bed. Should the infusion fluid escape into the hand a marked oedema occurs.

12.3.2.4 Minor Accidents to the Hand

The patient may suffer small injuries to his hand, particularly in the presence of sensory loss or inattention. He may sustain a fall towards the hemiplegic side and compromise his hand. He may burn the hand through inadvertent contact with a hot plate, a cigarette or a hot-water bottle. The hand may be caught in the wheel of his chair, and he pushes the chair forwards without noticing what has happened. As a result of such injuries the hand becomes oedematous.

12.3.3 Prevention and Treatment

12.3.3.1 Prevention

Prevention of the shoulder-hand syndrome aims at avoiding all the causes of oedema in the hand.

The patient is carefully positioned when in bed and when sitting in a chair, as described in Chap. 5. If he is not yet able to ensure that his wrist does not lie in full flexion or that his arm does not hang over the side of the wheelchair, a wheelchair table can prevent the danger until he has progressed sufficiently to look after his arm himself (Fig. 12.28).

Great care must be taken when activities which entail weight-bearing through the hemiplegic arm are being practised. The therapist should help the patient to control the movement when necessary. Before such activities or any form of passive movement are undertaken, the therapist carefully establishes the patient's individual range of movement by comparing it with that of the sound side. Should the patient complain of discomfort or pain during therapy, the therapist should change the position of the hand; for example, more outward rotation of the arm at the patient's side while he is sitting will reduce the amount of dorsiflexion required, as he moves his body sideways to take weight through the extended arm. If the pain is still produced, the activity should be discontinued.

Every effort should be made to avoid infusion into the veins of the hemiplegic hand. Using one of the subclavicular veins may offer an alternative.
All in the team, as well as the patient's relatives, must help to avoid the minor injuries to the hand. A hot-water bottle should not be used.

The patient's ability to take care of his own hand may easily be overestimated, especially if he has good motor activity or if he can talk well.

12.3.3.2 Treatment of the Established Syndrome

The best results are achieved if the treatment is started in the early stages of the condition, as soon as the oedema, pain or loss of range of movement is observed. The treatment can also be effective, however, even after a few months, if the hand is still inflamed and if there are acute pain and oedema. Once consolidation has occurred and the hand has returned to its normal size and colour, little if anything can be done to overcome the fixed contractures. The main aim of treatment is clearly to reduce the oedema as quickly as possible, and hence the pain and stiffness. The condition of the hand must be regarded as acute and inflammatory.

12.3.3.2.1 Positioning. In bed, the positions described in Chap. 5 are continued to prevent the shoulder from becoming involved. When the patient is sitting, his arm is positioned forward on a table at all times. A pillow can be placed beneath the arm for added elevation and comfort. It may be necessary to use a wheelchair table when the patient is moving around the hospital in his chair, or to ensure that the hand does not hang down unnoticed (see Fig. 12.28).

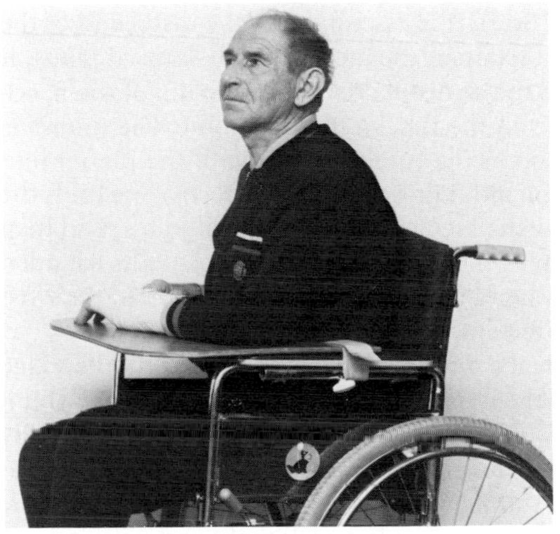

Fig. 12.28. A wheel chair table. The patient is wearing a wrist splint for his swollen hand (left hemiplegia)

It has been recommended that the patient's arm be mechanically suspended above cardiac level, both when he is lying and when he is sitting, but unfortunately the suspension is contra-indicated. The downward pull of the scapula against the abducted or elevated arm inevitably traumatises the shoulder, with severe pain as a result.

12.3.3.2.2 Avoiding Flexion at the Wrist. Maintenance of dorsal flexion of the wrist throughout the 24 hours is most important, to improve venous drainage and to prevent sustained extension of the metacarpophalangeal joints, which occurs mechanically if the hand lies in the patient's lap, and even when it is supported on a table or lies flat in bed (Fig. 12.29).

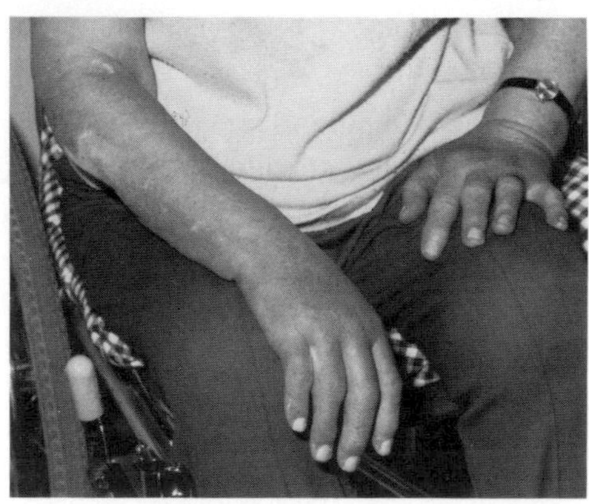

Fig. 12.29. Sustained extension of the metacarpophalangeal joints (right hemiplegia)

A small cock-up splint to support the wrist is made for the patient out of plaster of Paris, using eight to ten layers of an 8-cm plaster bandage:

The patient sits at a table with his arm supported forwards. An assistant stands next to him keeping his shoulder forward and supporting the wrist in a comfortable amount of dorsal flexion. The therapist stands in front of the patient and places the wet bandage carefully in place (Fig. 12.30 a). It is essential that the distal end of the splint when dry should not restrict the flexion of the metacarpophalangeal joints. It should therefore be moulded proximal to the distal crease in the palm of the hand, and slope appropriately downwards from the first to the fifth joint. The thumb is left free (Fig. 12.30 b). The assistant smooths the forearm portion of the plaster into place while the therapist concentrates on moulding the hand correctly. She folds the plaster back into the desired line below the metacarpal-phalangeal joints, and then uses her thumbs to press into the palm of the patient's hand to ensure its rounded form. Her fingers on the dorsum of his hand give counter-pressure to hold the wrist in dorsal flexion, in a slightly radial direction.

When the splint is dry it is bandaged firmly in place with a crêpe bandage (Fig. 12.30 c). Care must be taken that the wrist is correctly positioned in the splint and fixed in place. Even a few degrees of wrist flexion will push the splint distally and restrict the flexion of the metacarpophalangeal joints. The dorsum of the hand is well covered by the bandage, which starts over the knuckles and continues to the proximal end of the splint. The patient wears the splint both night and day, and it is only removed for skin checks, for washing and during therapy. Extension of the wrist is ensured at all times, no matter where the patient has his hand (Fig. 12.30 d).

The splint is worn continuously until the oedema and pain have disappeared and the colour of the hand is normal. Even while wearing the splint the patient is able to carry out the self-assisted activities which maintain full range of shoulder movement.

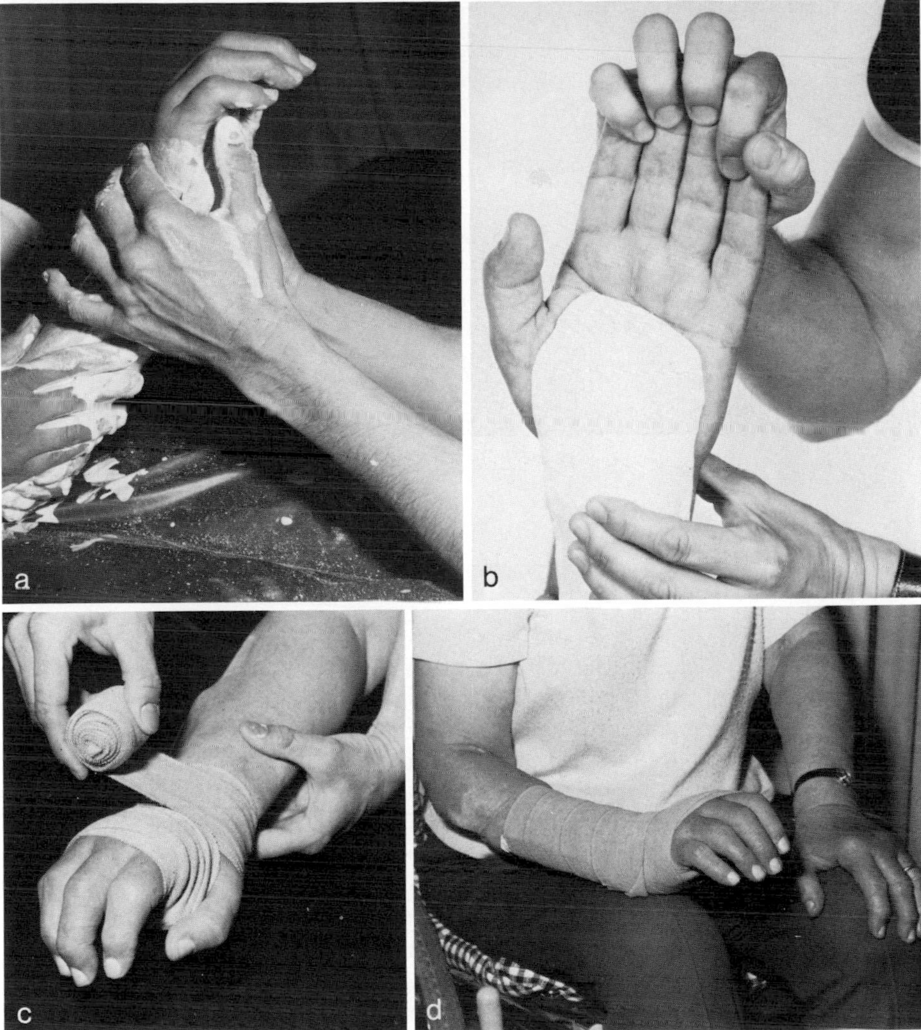

Fig. 12.30 a–d. A splint to support the wrist. **a** Placing the wet plaster of Paris bandage; **b** correct position of the splint; **c** bandaging in position; **d** flexion of the wrist prevented

12.3.3.2.3 Compressive Centripetal Wrapping. "Centripetal wrapping of digits or extremities has proved to be a simple, safe and dramatically effective treatment for reducing peripheral edema and its deleterious concomitants" (Cain and Liebgold 1967). Using a length of string of about 1–2 mm in diameter, the therapist wraps the thumb and then each finger from distal to proximal. She then proceeds to wrap the hand, and continues to just above the wrist joint. Wrapping commences with a small loop made in the region of the finger-nail in such a way that it does not press on the sensitive cuticle (Fig. 12.31 a). The therapist then wraps the finger firmly and

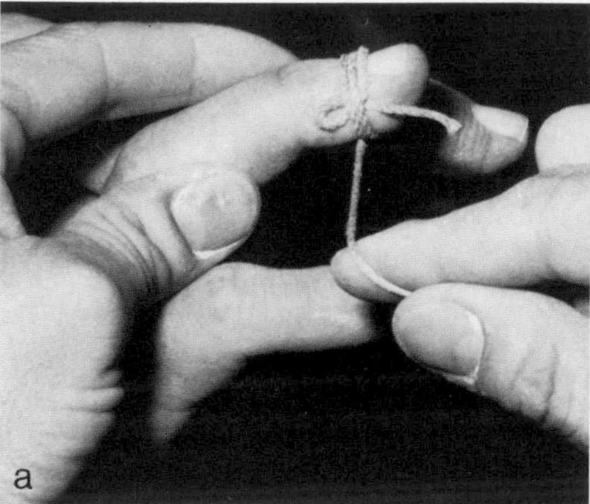

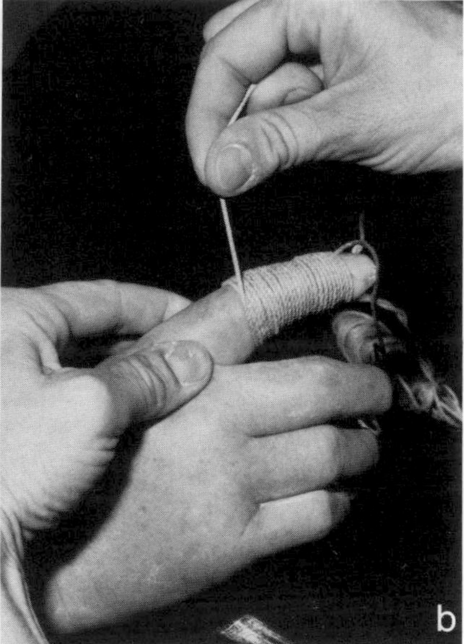

Fig. 12.31 a, b. Compressive centripetal wrapping

rapidly until she reaches the hand and can go no further (Fig. 12.31 b). She immediately removes the string by pulling on the free end of the loop.

When each finger and the thumb have been individually wrapped, the therapist proceeds to the hand itself. Once again she commences with a small loop and wraps the string over the metacarpophalangeal joints and proceeds proximally. On reaching the base of the thumb she adducts the thumb, so that its proximal joints are included in the wrapping. The last stage in the procedure includes the wrist joint, and the therapist starts wrapping there from where she ended the area of the hand.

The patient's relatives can soon be taught to carry out the procedure to save valuable time during therapy. The results are most gratifying and can be dramatic. "The amount of benefit has ranged from uncovering of trace motion in an apparently completely paralysed hand, to complete and lasting normal function in a hand previously swollen, painful and incapacitated" (Cain and Liebgold 1967). Certainly, the circulation is immediately improved by the reduction of the oedema, and other forms of therapy can proceed more effectively.

12.3.3.2.4 Ice. When crushed ice is available, the therapist immerses the patient's hand in a bucket containing a mixture of ice and water. The mixture consists ideally of approximately one-third water and two-thirds ice, so that the hand can be introduced easily, and additional cold is produced by the melting ice (Fig. 12.32). The therapist dips the patient's hand three times into the ice, with a brief pause between immersions. The sensation experienced by her own hand will guide her as to how long the cold can be tolerated.

12.3.3.2.5 Active Movements. Movements performed during therapy should be active whenever possible, rather than passive. Whatever active muscle function the patient has should be incorporated, even if the hand itself is completely paralysed.

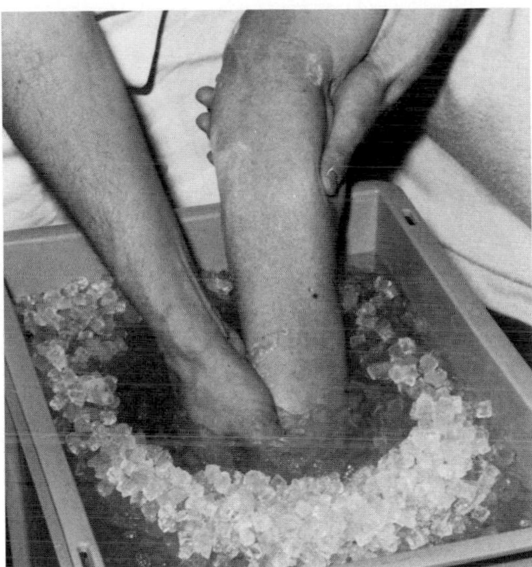

Fig. 12.32. Immersing the hand in ice

For example, it is usually possible to stimulate some activity in the elbow extensors with the patient lying supine and the arm held in elevation. Muscle contraction provides the best pumping action to reduce the oedema. The activities are carried out with the arm in elevation, after the scapula has been mobilised. Any activity which stimulates return of function in the hemiplegic arm can be used, particularly those activities where gripping is required, e.g. holding a towel and swinging it with the therapist's help, clasping a wooden pole and releasing it.

On no account should exercises involving weight-bearing through the extended arm be practised until all signs of pain and oedema have been eliminated. They may have been the precipitating cause of the syndrome and in any case will often cause pain and perpetuate the condition. In fact, any activity or position which elicits pain should be assiduously avoided. The same applies when passive range of movement is being carried out by the therapist.

12.3.3.2.6 Passive Movements. Careful passive range of movement prevents the shoulder from becoming painful, and passive movements to the hand and fingers are performed very gently indeed, so as not to produce any pain. The loss of supination which accompanies the problems in the wrist and carpal area should not be forgotten. The therapist includes the component in the therapy by easing the forearm into as full a range of supination as is possible without pain. All the movements can be carried out with the patient lying supine and the arm in elevation to increase venous drainage.

Because therapists dread contractures arising, they tend to be too vigorous when treating the swollen hand. In this condition too little rather than too much is infinitely preferable. When the oedema resolves and the pain decreases, range of movement is soon restored.

12.3.3.2.7 Oral Cortisone. Occasionally, despite the treatment regime having been strictly followed for a few weeks, the symptoms may remain marked. They may cause concern, particularly if the patient has some return of activity in the hand, and future function could be jeopardised. Persistent pain may be making the patient's life intolerable and interfering with his total rehabilitation. The treatment of the hand may be disproportionately time-consuming.

The administration of an oral cortisone preparation such as that described by Davis et al. (1977) is dramatically effective for these cases. The pain often disappears within a few days and the patient can once again participate fully in the rehabilitation programme. The medication is seldom required, but should be considered if treatment is not proving effective. The regime is continued in the same way as before, with the oral steroids being given in addition. In spite of the rapid relief of symptoms the medication should not be discontinued too soon. A 2–3 week period is generally necessary for lasting results.

12.4 Considerations

Distressingly painful conditions of the hemiplegic shoulder and hand are unfortunately all too common in many hospitals and rehabilitation centres. The patient suffers not only from the pain but also through being unable to benefit fully from the rehabilitation programme available to him. Some of the painful stiffness may lead to permanent deformity with limitation of function as a result. With careful supervision and treatment the painful complications can usually be avoided altogether, once the factors which cause them are understood. Should the problems arise despite the careful prophylactic measures, they can soon be overcome, particularly if detected in the early stages of their development. The whole team needs to be involved in the prevention or treatment of the painful shoulder and the swollen hand. The patient and his relatives are an integral part of the team and need to be carefully instructed and encouraged to participate in the necessary measures for preventing or overcoming the problems. Once the pain has diminished or disappeared, the patient is able to co-operate fully and his rapid physical progress and improved emotional state are most rewarding.

13 The Neglected Face

Many patients who have suffered a hemiplegia will have some disturbance of movement or feeling in the area of the face and mouth. No matter how slight the disorder, it will be most distressing for the patient himself. Our faces play an important role in our lives because, for each of us, it is as if we exist just behind our eyes. Unlike other parts of the body, the face is always on show, and cannot be concealed or disguised by clothing. When we meet someone new, we form our first impression from his face and its expression. We say that someone has "such a friendly smile", "an intelligent face", "an intent look". From the information we receive we decide whether we would like to know the person better, and it also influences how we speak to or behave towards that person.

With the fine richly innervated muscles of the face we are able to alter our expression by a wide variety of very small movements. Together with movement of the head, facial expression is a prime communicator, and we use both constantly to support what we are saying or to replace speech altogether at certain times. Through minute changes we can express pleasure, disbelief, love, disapproval etc.

Getting to know someone better entails talking, and we listen not only to what is said but also to the quality of the voice. We appreciate the sound of the voice with its melody, pitch and the way in which the words are pronounced, and while listening to someone talking we make further judgements about him.

When people meet and talk, usually they eat or drink something together. We eat and drink not only for nutrition but for enjoyment and as part of our social custom. We continue to form an opinion of the other person while he eats. Any abnormality or strangeness in facial expression, voice or eating habits is immediately obvious and disturbs communication and easy contact with others. Most of us have had the experience after a visit to the dentist which entailed an injection, or when a small pimple has assumed the imagined proportions of a carbuncle, of feeling that everyone was staring at us.

In the total rehabilitation programme, where learning to walk and self-care are in the foreground, the problems of the face and mouth are often overlooked and not included in the treatment. The persisting difficulties will detract from the patient's quality of life. He may no longer enjoy eating and drinking, either alone or with others. Other people may misjudge him or misinterpret his reactions due to inappropriate or reduced facial expression. If the patient cannot speak as he did before, he may have difficulty in establishing new relationships or in maintaining previous ones. Other people will react differently towards him, and may converse with him at an inappropriate level.

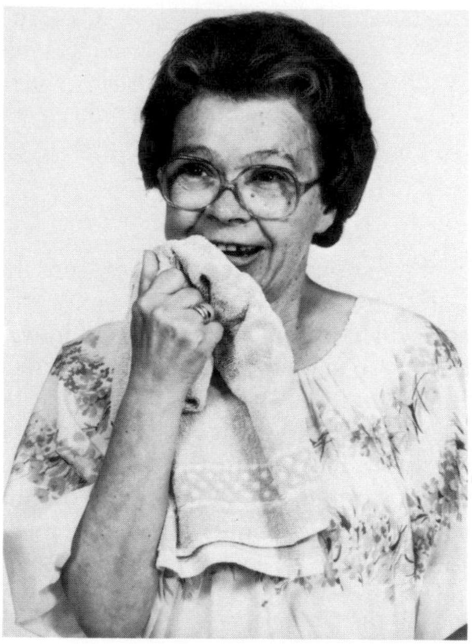

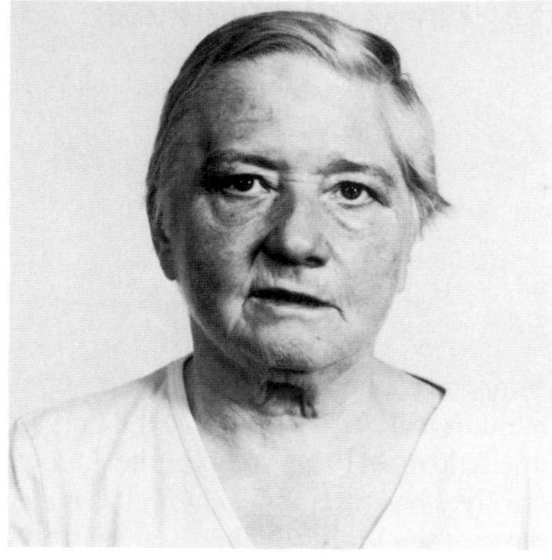

Fig. 13.2. Slight facial asymmetry (left hemiplegia)

◁ **Fig. 13.1.** A patient who is not able to eat or speak at all. The towel collects the saliva (right and left hemiplegia)

The degree and type of difficulty varies considerably, from a patient who is unable to eat at all (Fig. 13.1) to another whose face is not quite symmetrical (Fig. 13.2). When any difficulty is noticed, careful observation and investigation are necessary if the patient is to be helped to overcome the problems. Because the therapist usually meets the patient after his stroke, she may be unaware that the problems exist. The patient and his relatives may be better able to offer information as to any differences they have noticed, if carefully questioned.

13.1 Important Considerations for the Facilitation of the Movements of the Face and Mouth

Before she can observe, analyse and treat the problems experienced by hemiplegic patients in the area of the face and mouth, the therapist needs to understand the basic normal movements associated with communication and eating. Despite individual differences we all have similar patterns of movement which are partly reflex and partly learnt from earliest childhood, so that we can receive adequate nutrition and at the same time be accepted by the people around us.

13.1.1 Movements Associated with Communication

The postures and movements of the head can in themselves express a wide variety of signals and emotions. We certainly use them to reinforce what we are trying to express verbally. The slight bowing and nodding movements when we meet and greet someone, the nodding and shaking of the head to express agreement, disagreement or surprise, and the aloof nose-in-the-air position are but a few examples. We turn our heads to look at someone who is talking to us and adopt a listening posture, frequently moving our head to acknowledge or emphasise what the other is saying. Turning the head away is often a negative signal.

Commonly observed difficulties include the following:

The patient's head remains stiffly in one position, due to the exaggerated pull of certain muscle groups. He may hold his head in a fixed position in his attempt to remain erect or to compensate for inadequate balance reactions, and fails to make the customary gestures which others expect.

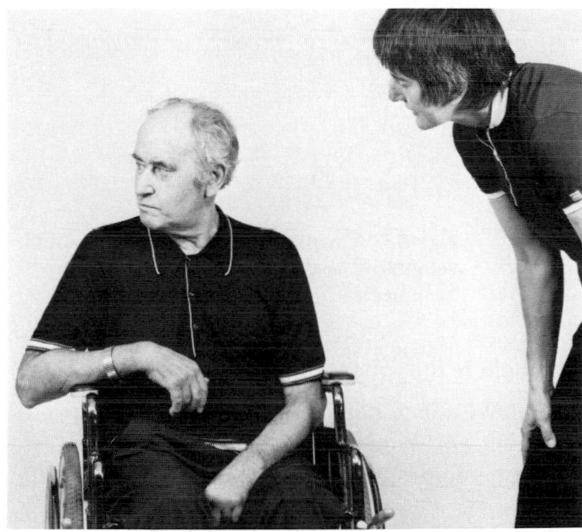

Fig. 13.3. The patient does not turn his head when someone addresses him (left hemiplegia)

Due to loss or reduction of the sensory modalities on his affected side, the patient fails to turn his head to look at someone who is addressing him, particularly if she does so from the affected side (Fig. 13.3). Patients frequently have difficulty in making eye contact with people who are on the affected side of their mid-line.

The face, with its wide variety of expressions, is a prime communicator in itself, as well as reinforcing or emphasising what we are saying. We can show someone else that we are listening to him. We frown and smile, we lower or narrow our eyes, and with hundreds of such tiny movements we can reveal what we are feeling or choose to disguise our real feelings. "The muscles of facial expression endow man with extremely subtle gradations of movement for non-verbal communication skills" (Moore 1980).

When we are communicating with other people our face is constantly moving, to a greater or lesser degree. We take for granted the customary movements of the face and head, but it is most disconcerting, for example, to be introduced to a person who neither moves his head nor smiles in greeting, or to talk to someone who fails to make eye contact and whose face remains totally immobile.

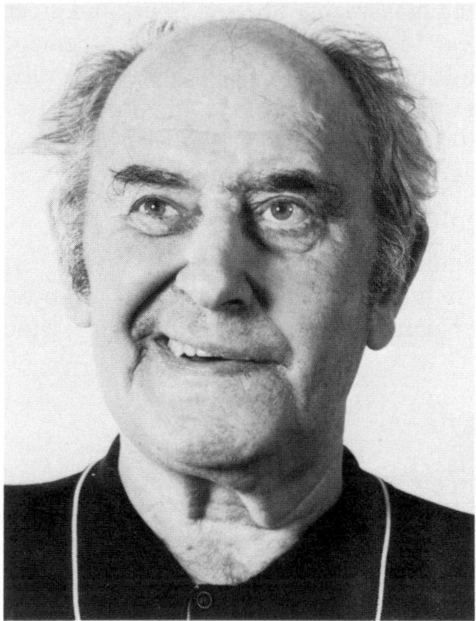

Fig. 13.4. Smiling emphasises the asymmetry (left hemiplegia)

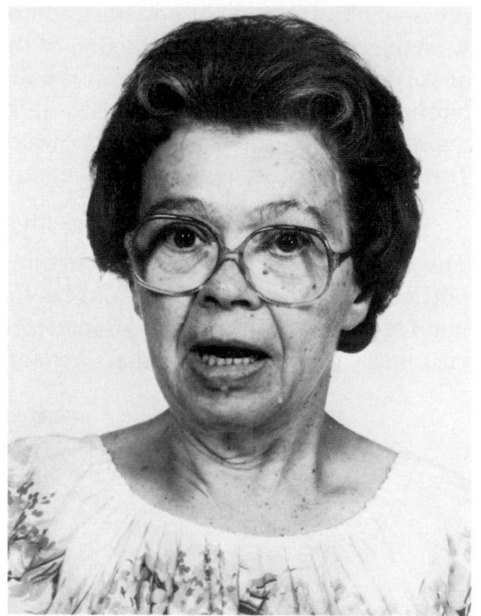

Fig. 13.5. The patient cannot close her mouth voluntarily, or prevent dribbling (bilateral hemiplegia)

Commonly observed difficulties include the following:

The affected side of the face does not move adequately and the asymmetry becomes more obvious when the patient is smiling, speaking or eating (Fig. 13.4).

The whole face may be completely expressionless and immobile or show very little change of expression.

There may be only a stereotyped change in expression, which occurs regardless of the patient's emotions at the time or the situation in which he finds himself. For example, a repetitive exaggerated smile appears.

The face assumes a constant abnormal posture perhaps with the mouth slightly open (Fig. 13.5), or with the lip drawn up over the teeth or held tightly down against the teeth.

The patient has difficulty in preventing dribbling, particularly when he is concentrating on something else, for example putting on his shoes. He dabs constantly at his lips with a handkerchief, just in case some saliva may have escaped. Because he can only use one of his hands, it is inconvenient to hold the handkerchief at the ready all the time, and the patient is permanently distracted from other tasks by the need to put the handkerchief somewhere or retrieve it again.

The ability to speak clearly and expressively is dependent upon many complex and co-ordinated movements. The tongue and lips are used to form the consonants, and clear articulation plays such a vital role in speaking that we are even able to understand when someone whispers, without producing voice. The movements of speech have developed from those originally designed for survival, i.e. the movements of eating and drinking. For speaking they are far more rapid and co-ordinated. Agile, selective movements of the tongue are necessary to produce consonants such as "t" and "d", when the tip of the tongue has to be placed accurately behind the front teeth, and "g" and "k", where the tip of the tongue is stabilised behind the lower teeth and the middle portion of the tongue has to elevate briskly. The tongue has to move without the jaw moving simultaneously in a primitive mass synergy. Quick, accurately graded movements of the lips produce the "p" and "b" sounds. We tend to associate slow, slurred speech with fatigue, illness, the influence of alcohol or even dim-wittedness.

Breath control is essential for voice production. Air passing through the vocal cords produces the sounds, and by altering the amount of air we change the volume of our voices. We speak more loudly or softly to emphasise, add interest or to express different emotions. In order to use sentences and phrases of an adequate length we need to be able to sustain a sound effortlessly for between 15 and 20 seconds. A trained singer could manage about 1 minute.

The larynx moves up or down as we change the pitch of our voice to add quality or to express emotion. The ability is under voluntary control and is dependent upon the normal tone of the muscles of the neck and throat, and of the vocal cords themselves. The sound of the voice is clear because of the co-ordinated tension in the vocal cords. Essential for the clarity and quality of the sound is the effective action of the soft palate, as it seals off the nasal cavity completely to prevent air from escaping through the nose during vocal sounds. The soft palate must also move downwards for the required nasal sounds. The movement has to be very rapid and co-ordinated, as the position of the soft palate changes repeatedly during a sentence, or even during one word. We alter the vowel sounds by changing the shape of our mouth, moving lips and jaw.

Commonly observed difficulties include the following:

The consonants are slurred or inaccurately produced and the speech may be difficult to understand as a result. The patient speaks slowly and carefully or even laboriously.

The patient speaks too softly and has difficulty in making himself heard. He uses short sentences and may need to rebreathe after saying only a few words. Very often he can only maintain a sustained sound for about 5 seconds.

The voice is monotonous, with little or no variation in pitch. It may be lower or higher than it was before.

The patient sounds hoarse, as if he constantly needs to clear his throat.

The voice may sound strained and effortful.

The patient speaks nasally or air may be heard escaping through his nose with certain sounds.

Saliva escapes while the patient is speaking.

13.1.2 Movements Associated with Eating and Drinking

We eat and drink in order to survive, but also for our pleasure. We are required to adhere to many learnt rules concerned with eating in order to be acceptable within our social group. Allowing for different habits and customs, the basic pattern of eating and drinking remains constant.

We sit in an upright position at the table to allow the head and neck to be in an optimal position for the act of eating. For this reason most societies have straight-backed dining-room chairs. In the erect position the mouth is horizontal to the food or liquid being presented, and within the mouth the movements of chewing and manipulation by the tongue are more easily carried out. The larynx can move up and down freely because the muscles surrounding it are not stretched and taut. The food is placed in the mouth from the front and in the middle, and the lips close to receive the mouthful. The swallowing programme begins with jaw closure in adults.

13.1.2.1 Solids

Chewing starts automatically, the food portion or bolus having been placed between the teeth by the tongue. It is kept in the correct place by the muscle tone of the cheeks laterally and the tongue action medially. The chewing action is an asymmetrical grinding movement, and the bolus is transported by the tongue from one side of the mouth to the other at intervals. The number of chewing movements is individual and continues until the bolus is sufficiently soft and moist to allow for a comfortable swallow. Intact sensory receptors allow the strength of mastication to be appropriate and to adjust automatically as the bolus becomes softer. During the chewing cycle small amounts of acceptably prepared food are selected by the tongue and swallowed. The whole bolus is therefore not usually swallowed in one piece.

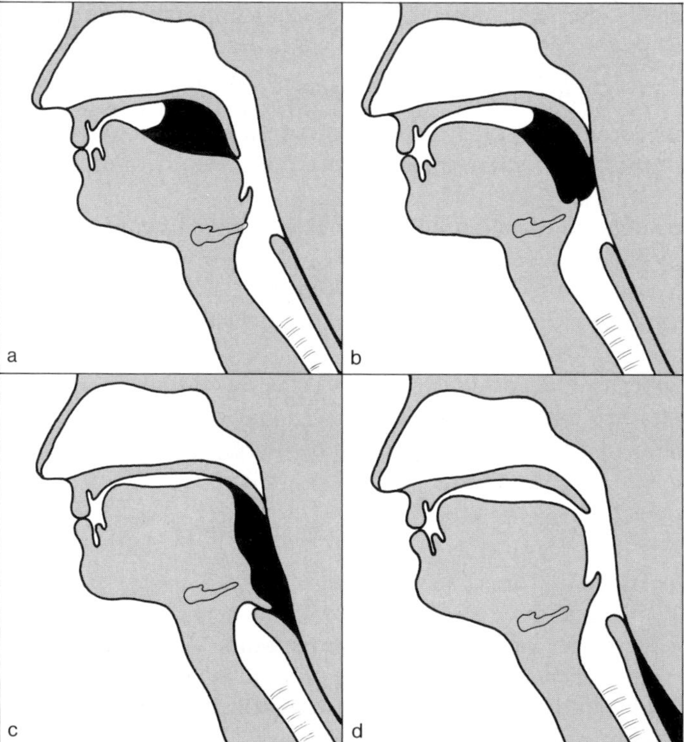

Fig. 13.6 a–d. Normal swallowing

The swallowing action starts with the bolus being placed centrally on the tongue, which makes a quick wave-like movement to push the portion back into the throat. The tip of the tongue elevates first and is followed by the middle and rear thirds, moving backwards as a piston (Fig. 13.6a). The soft palate elevates to seal off the nasopharynx, effectively preventing food from being pushed up into the nose (Fig. 13.6b). The bolus tips the epiglottis downwards and slides over its smooth convex surface to be guided into the oesophagus (Fig. 13.6c). The larynx, which has elevated, is sealed off by the epiglottis so that the airway is protected. The vocal cords themselves provide a second safety mechanism by snapping together to expel food particles, should any accidentally enter the laryngeal airway. When the bolus is safely in the oesophagus, the epiglottis returns to its original position and the soft palate relaxes so that normal breathing can be resumed (Fig. 13.6d). The swallow itself occurs reflexly.

13.1.2.2 Liquids

When drinking, the fluid is placed centrally on the tongue with an active suction to draw it from the cup or spoon which rests against the lower lip. The fluid is brought to the back of the mouth for swallowing by the same wave-like movement of the tongue used to swallow solids. Normally, one large swallowing movement takes place followed by one or two small additional swallows to clear the pharynx completely. In a relaxed situation the swallow is not audible to others, and is only possible for adults when the mouth is closed.

After eating or drinking, the teeth and mouth are cleaned most thoroughly by the tongue, and also by the movement of the lips and cheeks over the teeth. The saliva also washes the mouth clean. Eating and drinking with others is an enjoyable pastime. We take solids and fluids in rapid succession, and we can converse easily, even while food is held discreetly in the side of the mouth.

Commonly observed difficulties include the following:

The patient is unable to achieve an upright, symmetrical posture. With the trunk flexed he has to extend his neck at the back to eat and the muscles anteriorly are stretched. The movements of the tongue and larynx are more difficult as a result.
With the trunk and head flexed towards the hemiplegic side, the central presentation of the food is a problem, and within the mouth control becomes almost impossible. Food falls between the teeth and the cheek, or escapes from the corner of the mouth, the affected side being tilted downwards.
Pieces of food remain stuck in the mouth and may be observed long after the meal is finished. They may remain in the patient's cheek or on the roof of the mouth and can nearly always be seen on his teeth in front, or on his lips and chin. The patient often uses his finger to remove pieces of food that have become lodged within his mouth.
The patient chews only on the unaffected side and spasticity increases on the hemiplegic side. When the side is hypotonic with poor sensation, no activity is stimulated. The chewing is often more a "chomping" up and down action than the complex adult grinding motion and shows no alteration as the bolus becomes softer. The patient chews toast or crème caramel with the same amount of vigor.

Because chewing is slow and ineffective, the patient chews for a much longer period and often avoids hard food sorts altogether, or takes very small pieces. Due to reduced sensation or abnormal tone the patient often bites his cheek accidentally, and small painful ulcerations can be felt from the inside on examination.
Swallowing is audible and effortful, and the whole bolus is swallowed in one piece. The patient has to swallow several times before he succeeds in clearing the pharynx. The patient often chokes, particularly when drinking.
Eating and drinking become a slow and laborious chore, and the patient has to concentrate intently. He is unable to join in the conversation at table and often his food is cold and unappetising before he has finished.

13.2 Dentures

False teeth can be a problem for the patient when speaking or eating. A set of teeth that previously was held in place by normal muscle activity despite an imperfect fit slips down repeatedly when the patient has altered tone and sensation. The false teeth should be worn as soon as possible and held firmly in place by a dental fixative. When the patient has progressed sufficiently to visit the dentist, the necessary alteration can be made to ensure a good fit.

The dentures should be cleaned after each meal, as pieces of food tend to become lodged between the plate and the hard palate, and the patient can no longer retrieve them with his tongue.

13.3 Appropriate Treatment for the Common Difficulties

The problems that have been described are caused by:

Abnormal tone. The muscle tone of the face, mouth and neck is too high or too low.
Inadequate sensation. The patient is not able to feel the side of his face adequately, nor the inside of his mouth.
Selective movement is difficult or impossible for the patient. He is only able to move in stereotyped mass patterns.

Recognising the problems and including their treatment in the rehabilitation programme is the first important step. The area of the face and mouth tends otherwise to fall into a kind of "no-man's land" and is often neglected as a result. The nurse attends to the oral hygiene and ensures that the patient has sufficient intake. The occupational therapist enables the patient to prepare and eat the food with one hand, using aids if necessary. The physiotherapist deals with his ability to move about sufficiently to reach the dining-room table and sit correctly. In most cases the speech therapist is primarily concerned with language problems rather than with the nonverbal aspects of communication or with eating.

For more complex difficulties, specially qualified help will be necessary, but for the majority of patients the following treatment plan will be appropriate and helpful, and can be carried out by any of the therapists concerned with the patient. The emphasis of the treatment should be directed towards the specific difficulties which the patient has, although each difficulty will influence the other movements to a considerable extent.

When assessing or treating the face and mouth, two grips are particularly useful and can also be used when the patient is being helped to drink or clean his teeth.

1. Standing beside the patient, usually at his hemiplegic side, the therapist places one arm round the back of his head. With the crook of her elbow and her upper arm she keeps his head in the mid-line and elongates the back of his neck. She plantar flexes her wrist so that her thumb can rest against the tempcromandibular joint to feel any abnormal movement or muscle tone. The therapist holds the patient's chin between her index and middle fingers to guide jaw movements. With her index finger she assists lip closure and the middle finger can relax the tongue from below, or facilitate its movements (Fig. 13.7).
2. Sitting in front of the patient the therapist places her thumb on the patient's chin and her middle finger below in the space between the bases of the mandibles. Her index finger rests on the side of his face (Fig. 13.8). Her thumb assists mouth closure and her middle finger can influence the tongue musculature. The index finger provides information as to lateral movement of the jaw and the tone of the cheek. The grip is used when the patient has adequate head control and can inhibit the extension of his neck voluntarily. It is particularly useful when the patient has language difficulties, because he can see the therapist's face and follow what he is expected to do.

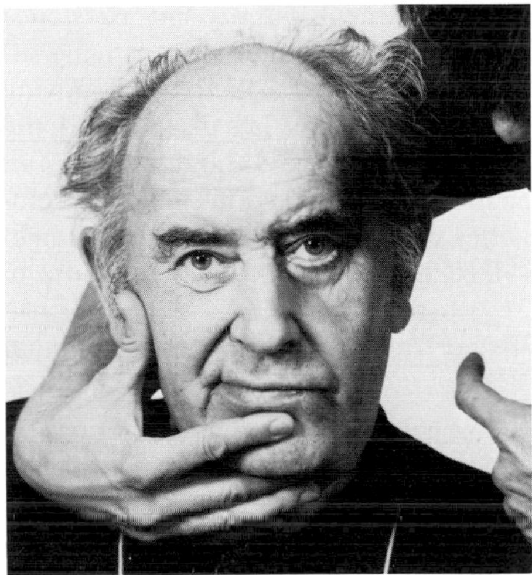

Fig. 13.7. Grip used when the patient cannot hold his head in the normal position (left hemiplegia)

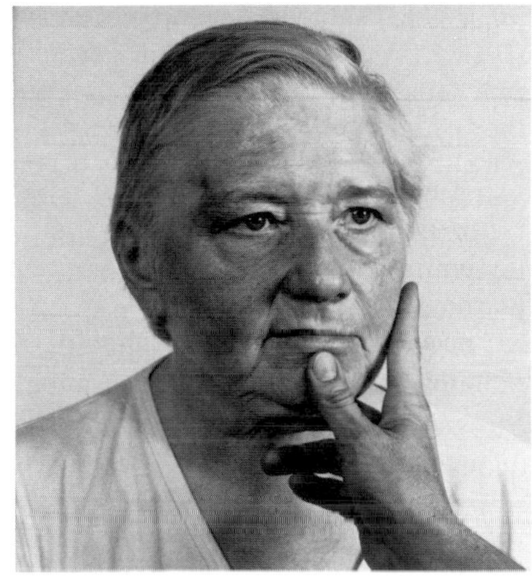

Fig. 13.8. Grip for patients who can maintain a correct head position (left hemiplegia)

When assisting the patient with eating or drinking the first grip is usually recommended. The patient can sit at the table in the normal way and see his food on the plate. Should the patient need help to bring the food or drinking utensil to his

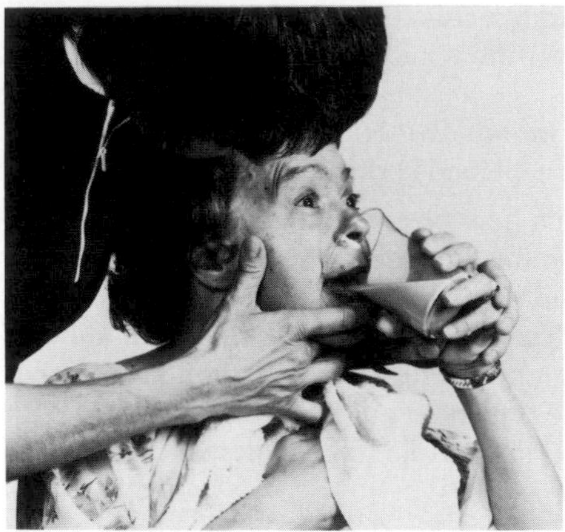

Fig. 13.9. Helping the patient with drinking (bilateral hemiplegia)

mouth, the therapist can guide his hand more easily, as the movement is the same one she would make herself (Fig. 13.9).

13.3.1 For Difficulties Associated with Non-verbal Communication

The neck should be kept fully mobile and the hypertonus or over-activity reduced. The therapist first moves the patient's head passively, emphasising the full range of movement, and the patient tries to allow the movement without any resistance (Fig. 13.10). It is often easier to regain full movement when the patient is lying supine. The therapist needs to fix the patient's shoulder with one hand when moving the head into full side flexion or rotation. Once the resistance has disappeared, the patient can be asked to move his head actively. All movements should also be full and free in sitting and standing positions, as these are the positions in which communication usually takes place. Group activities with music, balls or balloons help the patient to overcome the problem of a fixed head position and the failure to make eye contact with others.

Movements of the face should be facilitated from an early stage, to maintain mobility and to stimulate the sensation.

The therapist uses her fingertips to move the forehead into a frowning position, diagonally down towards the mid-line (Fig. 13.11). The movement is alternated with raising the eyebrows to produce a look of surprise, with an upward and outward action. The patient feels the activity and then helps actively, and the therapist assists less and less.

At first the movement may need to be a gross mass one, with the eyes closing tightly to reinforce frowning (Fig. 13.12) and opening wide when the eyebrows are raised. As the patient's ability increases the movements can become more selective and varied, until he can close his eyes without moving his forehead, close one eye or raise one eyebrow.

The therapist moves the patient's cheeks to normalise tone, from the outside and also from within the mouth. She rubs her little finger along the patient's gums

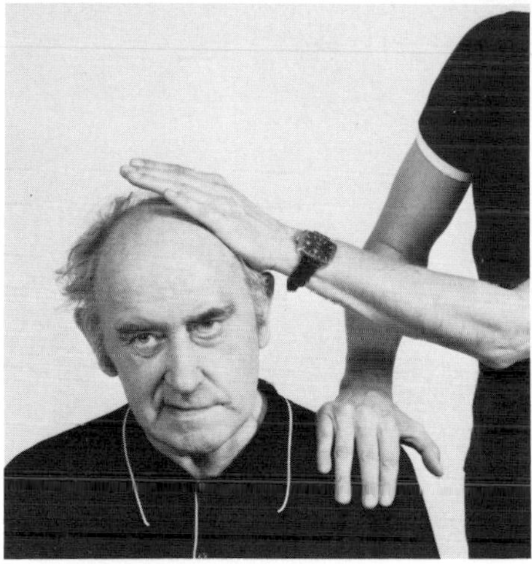
13.10

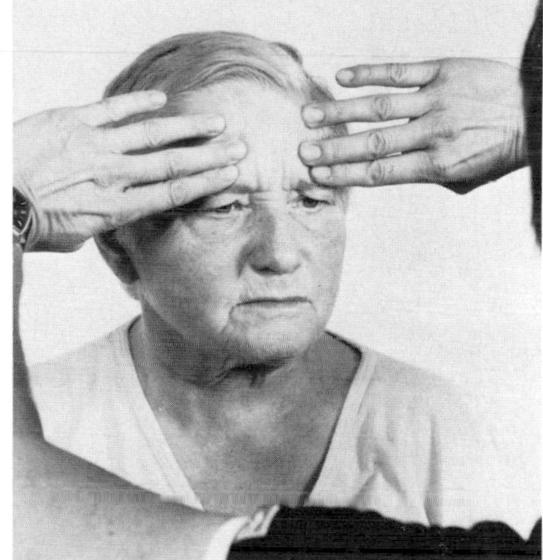
13.11

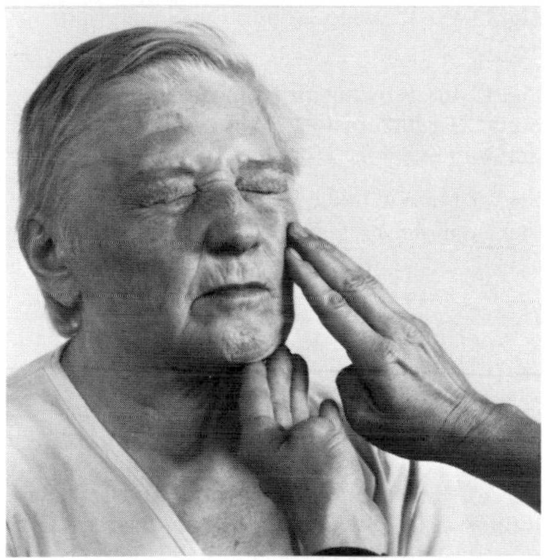
13.12

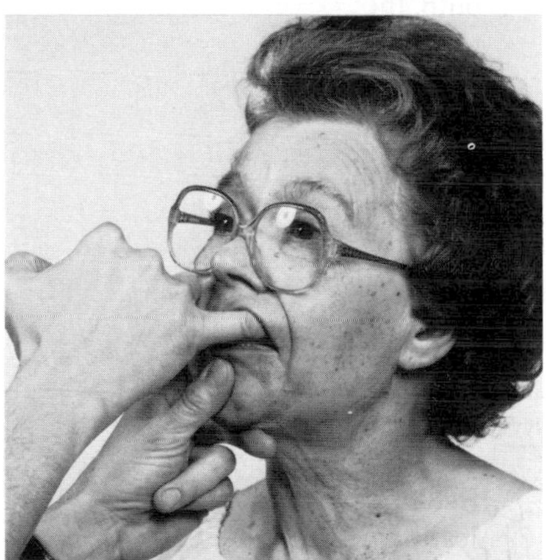
13.13

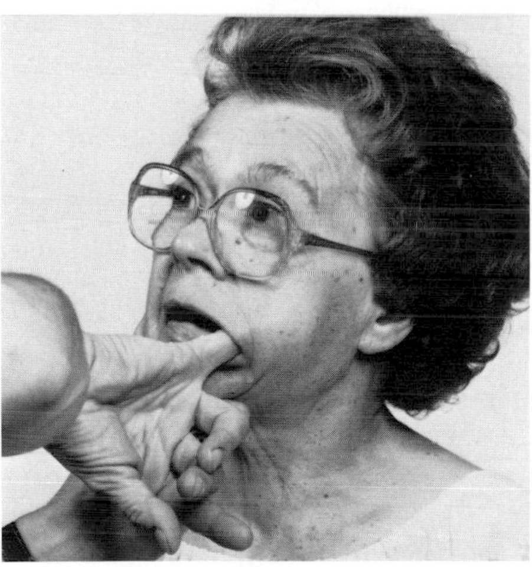
13.14

Fig. 13.10. Moving the head passively (left hemiplegia)

Fig. 13.11. Frowning (left hemiplegia)

Fig. 13.12. Closing the eyes tightly (left hemiplegia)

Fig. 13.13. Massaging the gums (bilateral hemiplegia)

Fig. 13.14. Releasing spasticity in the cheek (bilateral hemiplegia)

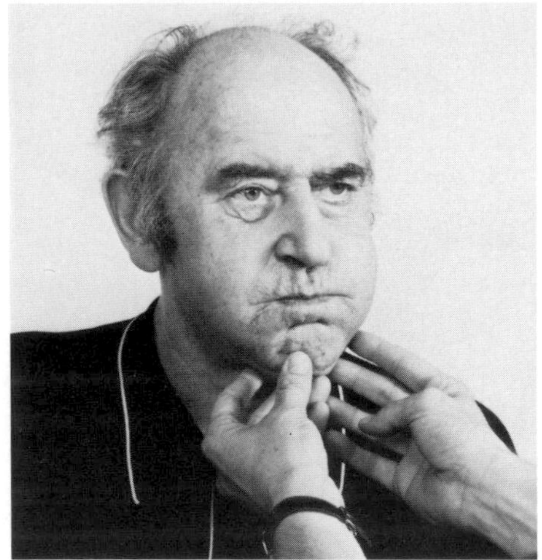

13.15

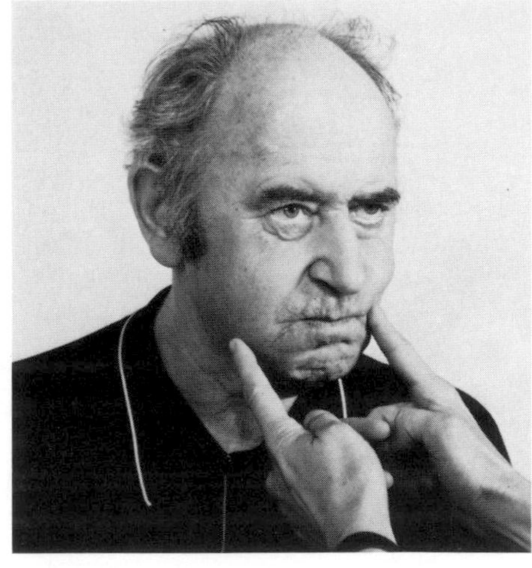

13.16

Fig. 13.15. Blowing air into the cheeks (left hemiplegia)

Fig. 13.16. Blowing air from one cheek to the other. The therapist assists the hemiplegic side (left hemiplegia)

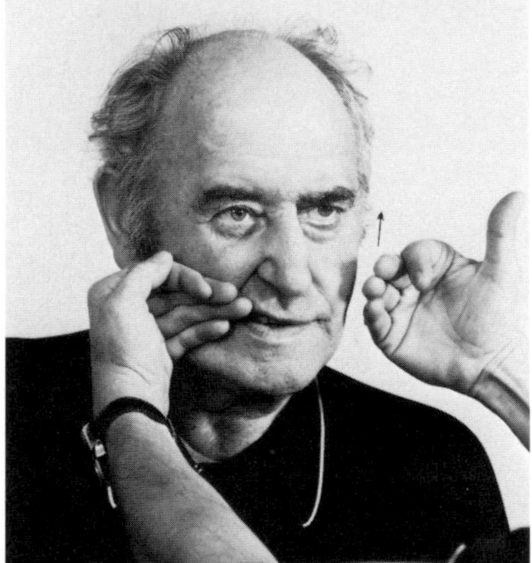

13.17

Fig. 13.17. Facilitating symmetrical smiling (left hemiplegia)

Fig. 13.18 a, b. Using the back of an electric tooth-brush (bilateral hemiplegia). **a** To normalize tone in the cheek; **b** to stimulate mouth closure

▽

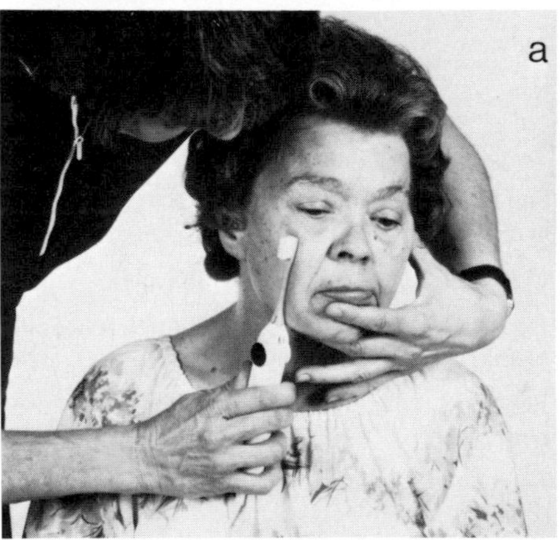

13.18

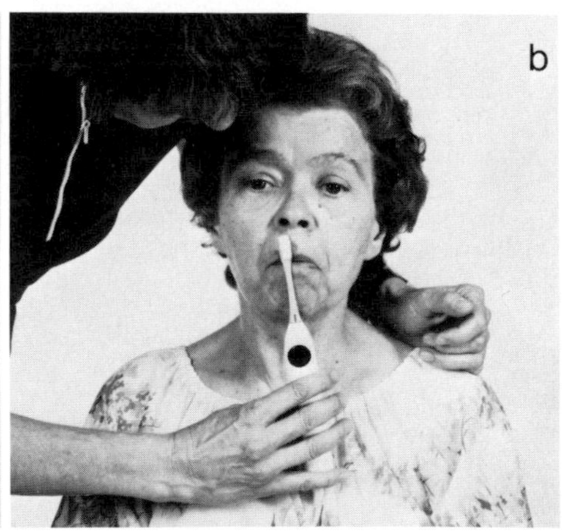

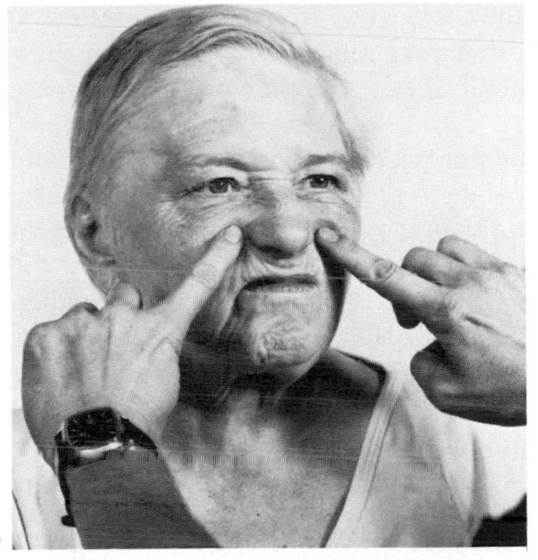

13.19

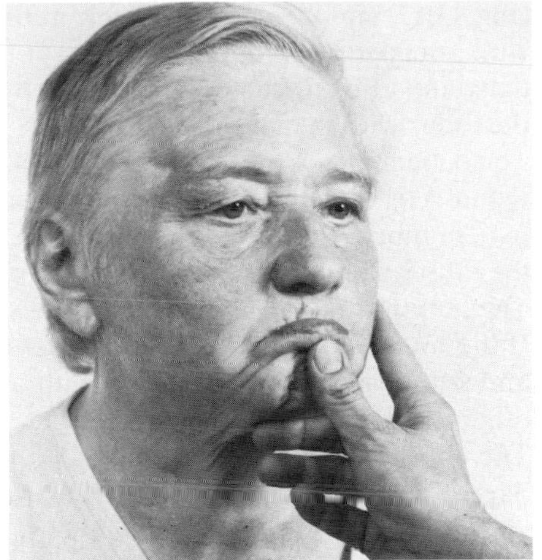

13.20

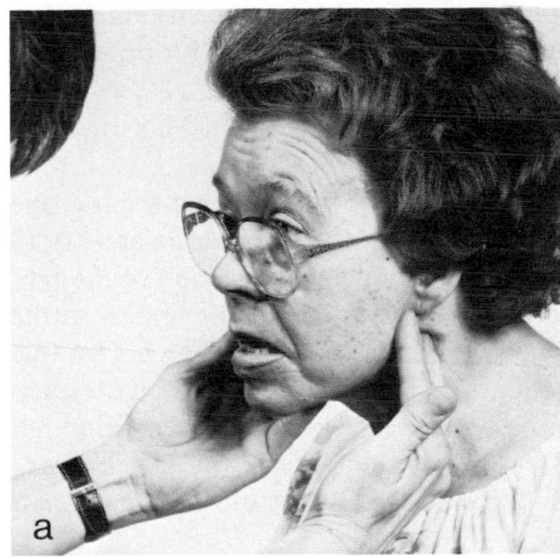

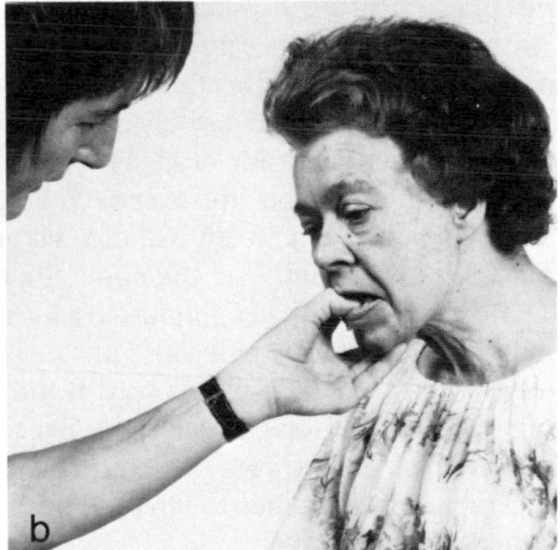

13.21

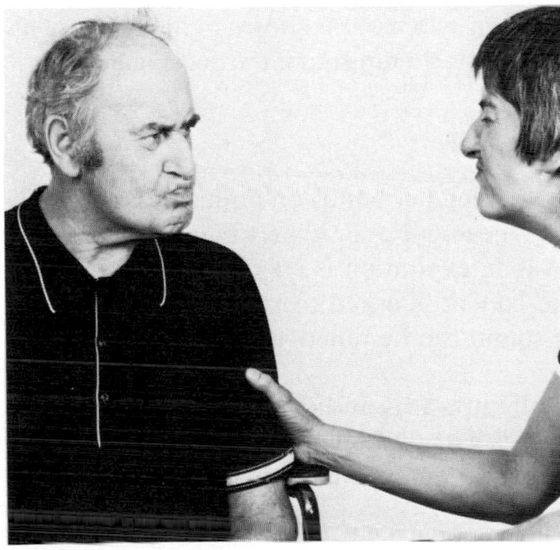

13.22

Fig. 13.19. Wrinkling the nose (left hemiplegia)

Fig. 13.20. Moving the bottom lip over the top one (left hemiplegia)

Fig. 13.21 a, b. Facilitating protraction of the jaw (bilateral hemiplegia). **a** From behind the angles of the mandible; **b** with the therapist's thumb hooked over the bottom teeth

Fig. 13.22. Copying facial expressions (left hemiplegia)

(Fig. 13.13) and then into his cheek, pulling the cheek away from his teeth at the side with a semicircular motion (Fig. 13.14). The stretching movement releases the spasticity and also stimulates activity in a hypotonic cheek. The therapist can compare the tonus with that of the other cheek.

The patient then blows air into his cheeks and holds it there (Fig. 13.15). The activity requires lip seal and movement of the soft palate to prevent air from escaping. The patient moves the air into first one cheek and then the other, stimulating activity in the muscles of the cheeks and the soft palate (Fig. 13.16).

The therapist facilitates a symmetrical smiling movement, followed by lip-pursing. If the sound side is too active, she uses the back of one hand to inhibit the activity, and stimulates the affected side with a quick upward brushing movement of her other hand (Fig. 13.17).

The cheek and lips can be stimulated by quick stroking with ice, or by using the back of an electric tooth-brush. The brush is moved from lateral to medial and the vibration increases sensation and helps to normalise tone (Fig. 13.18 a, b).

The patient is asked to wrinkle his nose, as if experiencing a bad smell. The therapist places her fingertips on either side of his nose to assist the movement (Fig. 13.19). As the patient becomes more skilled he tries to wrinkle his nose quickly and without moving other parts of his face at the same time.

The patient is asked to curl his lip upwards, as if to show the therapist his top teeth and the underneath side of his lip.

The patient moves his lips over each other, placing the bottom lip over the top one and vice versa (Fig. 13.20). He can also move his bottom jaw forwards and try to place his lower teeth over the upper lip, to combat the spastic retraction of the jaw. The therapist facilitates the movement using her fingers behind the angles of the mandible (Fig. 13.21 a). Because the area is sensitive to pressure, she may not be able to give sufficient help in this way. If the patient has considerable spasticity retracting his jaw, the therapist can place her thumb behind his lower front teeth and her index finger underneath his chin (Fig. 13.21 b). She then draws the jaw forward several times, and when the hypertonus has been reduced by the movement the patient takes over actively.

The therapist helps the patient to make different facial expressions, using her fingers to move his face. He can practise copying expressions shown to him, or vary his expression to express different emotions for the therapist to interpret (Fig. 13.22).

13.3.2 For Difficulties Associated with Speaking

Breathing is assisted, with the therapist placing her hands on both sides of the thorax to facilitate lateral costal breathing. Due to hypo- or hypertonus the hemiplegic side often fails to move adequately. A long expiration is encouraged by vibrating downwards over the sternum, and the patient is asked to produce a long sound without effort as he breathes out. The sound can be timed, and the patient tries to reach the necessary 15 s.

The larynx is moved passively, diagonally upwards and downwards to both sides (Fig. 13.23). The patient then makes sounds with a pitch change to move the larynx actively. The high and low sounds can also be practised using changing vowel sounds such as "ooh – aah" or "eeh – ooh".

13.23 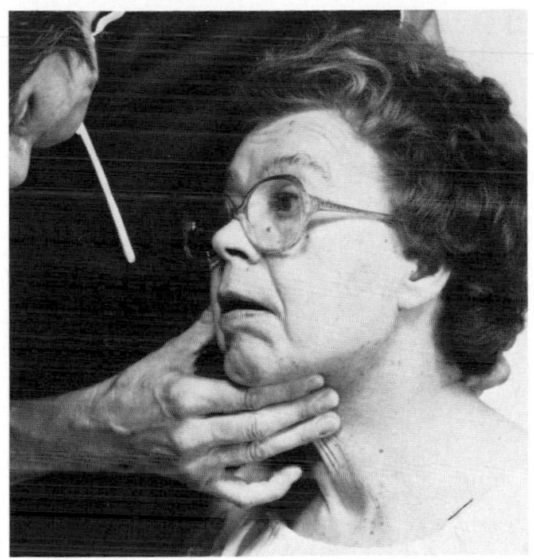

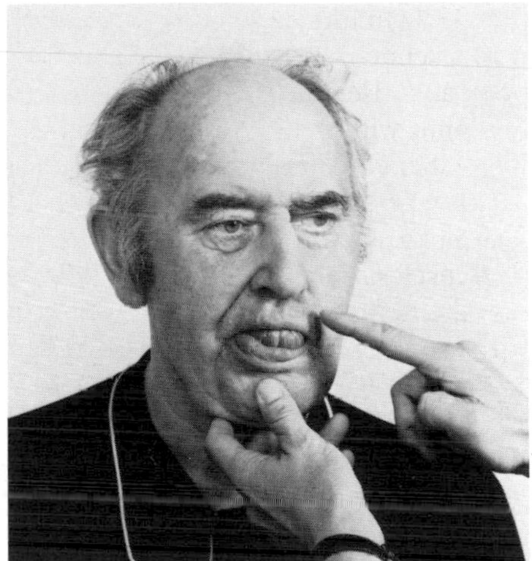 13.24

13.25 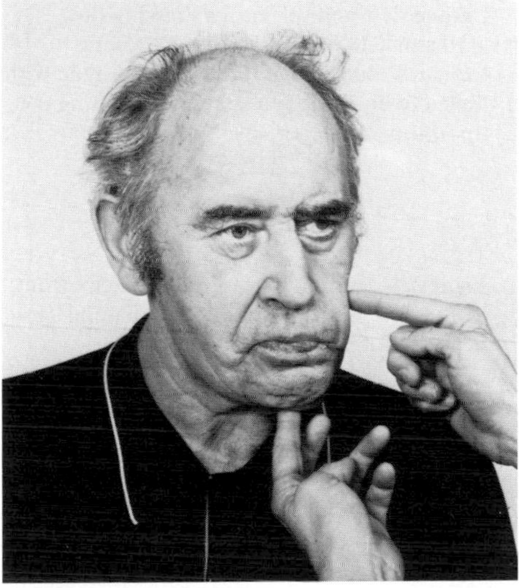

Fig. 13.23. Moving the larynx passively to normalise tone (bilateral hemiplegia)

Fig. 13.24. Licking the outside of the top teeth (left hemiplegia)

Fig. 13.25. Placing the tongue far back in the cheek (left hemiplegia)

The patient licks his lips moving his tongue right round the outside. He then moves his tongue around inside his lips, pushing them away from his teeth (Fig. 13.24). The therapist guides him to place his tongue far back in his cheeks to where her finger indicates (Fig. 13.25). He tries to stretch and massage his cheek with his tongue.

Should tongue movements be severely reduced the therapist needs to stimulate its movements more directly.

Placing her little finger in his mouth, she pushes down on the tongue and makes small steps towards the back (Fig. 13.26 a). Quick strokes forwards on the tongue can activate its intrinsic muscles (Fig. 13.26 b). Pushing against the lateral border of the tongue facilitates its movement sideways, and the patient tries to push his tongue against the finger.

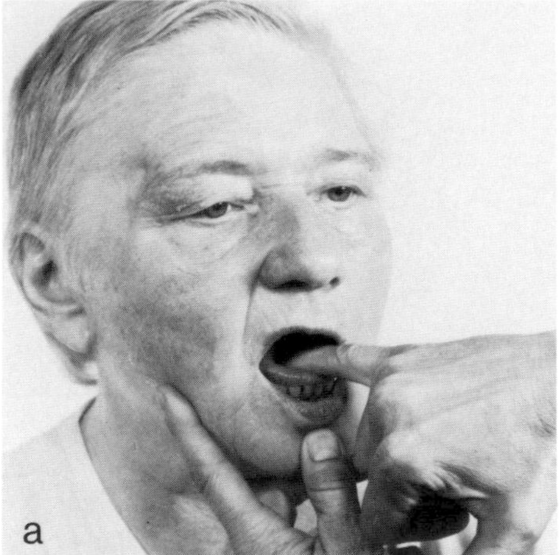

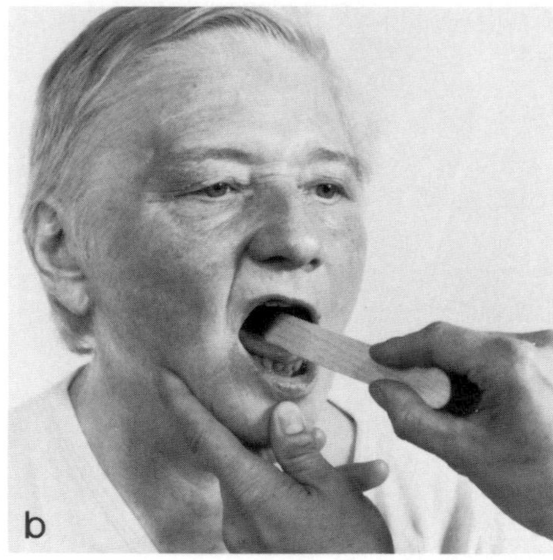

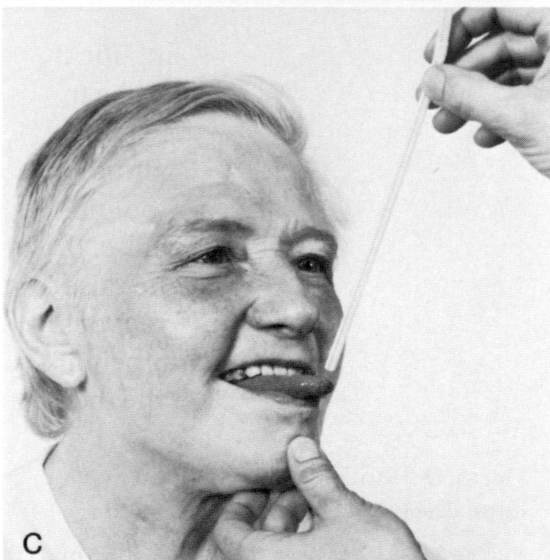

13.26

Fig. 13.26 a–c. Stimulating activity in the tongue (left hemiplegia). **a** Pressing down with small steps backwards; **b** stroking forwards along the middle of the tongue with the edge of a wooden spatula; **c** pushing the tip of the tongue against a drinking straw

Fig. 13.27. Inhibiting tongue spasticity from below and moving the tongue (bilateral hemiplegia)

Fig. 13.28. Facilitating movements of the tongue by holding it with a piece of damp gauze and moving it in different directions (left hemiplegia)

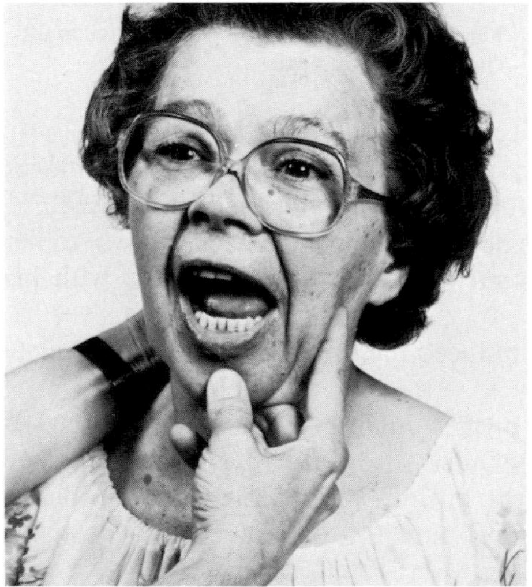

13.27

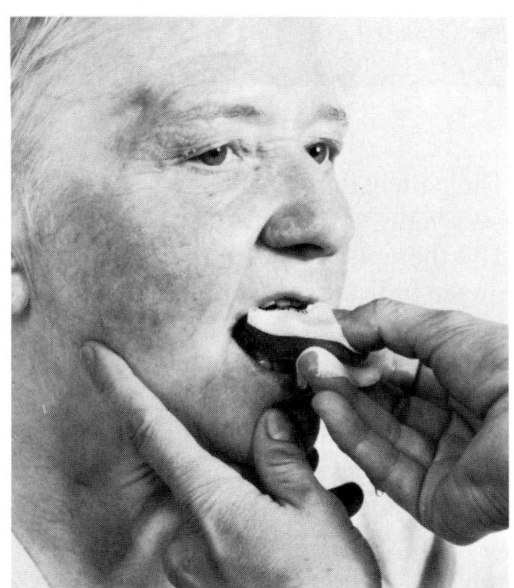

13.28

The therapist asks the patient to push his tongue against a spatula or drinking straw, and to follow its movements both inside and outside his mouth (Fig. 13.26c).
Before facilitating tongue movements the therapist should inhibit any hypertonus. She places her finger below the patient's jaw, in the area of soft tissue beneath the floor of the mouth. Using a semicircular movement she presses her finger upwards and forwards to influence the tone in the muscles of the tongue and to facilitate a forward movement (Fig. 13.27). To facilitate the wave-like movement necessary for swallowing, the therapist assists in the same way, only in this case her finger moves upwards and backwards in its semicircular motion.
For the patient who can hardly move his tongue at all, the therapist guides the movement completely at first. Placing a piece of damp gauze around his tongue, she is able to hold it between her finger and thumb and move it in the various directions required (Fig. 13.28). She draws his tongue forwards, taking care not to scrape it against the bottom teeth, lifts it upwards and moves it to either side. The therapist instructs the patient to feel the movement and to join in actively while she is assisting him.
The patient attempts to make the sounds "d" and "t" accurately, placing the tip of his tongue against the back of his front teeth. The speed is increased, and he tries to make the sounds without moving his lower jaw at the same time. The sounds "g" and "k" are practised, with the tip of the tongue forward against the bottom teeth. As the patient's ability increases he alternates between the „g" and "d" sounds.

The movements are those which are required for swallowing as well, i.e. the tip of the tongue first elevated for "d" or "t" and then the back of the tongue raised for "g" or "k". It may be necessary to guide the patient's tongue to the correct position at first, using a spatula to elevate the tip or point to the correct position behind the top teeth (Fig. 13.29). By pressing the spatula on the back of the tongue, the therapist can facilitate the upward movement required for "g".

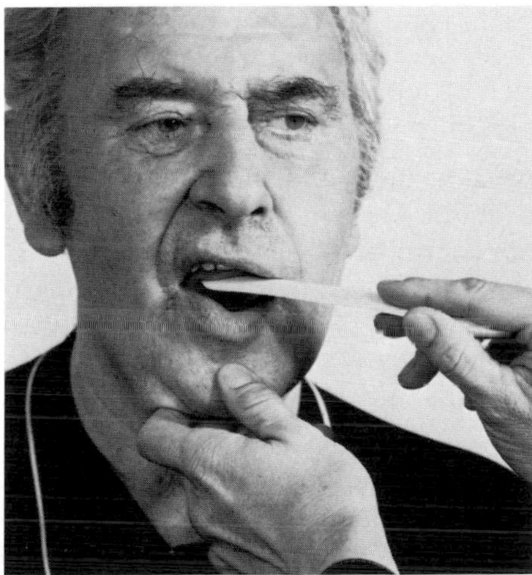

Fig. 13.29. Lifting the tip of the tongue with a spatula to touch behind the top teeth (left hemiplegia)

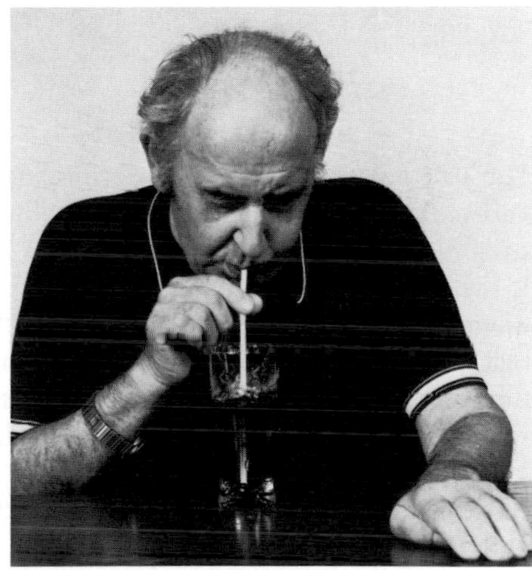

Fig. 13.30. Blowing through a straw (left hemiplegia)

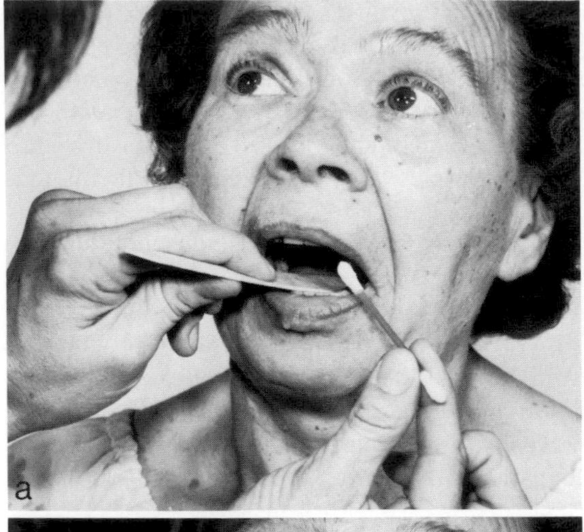

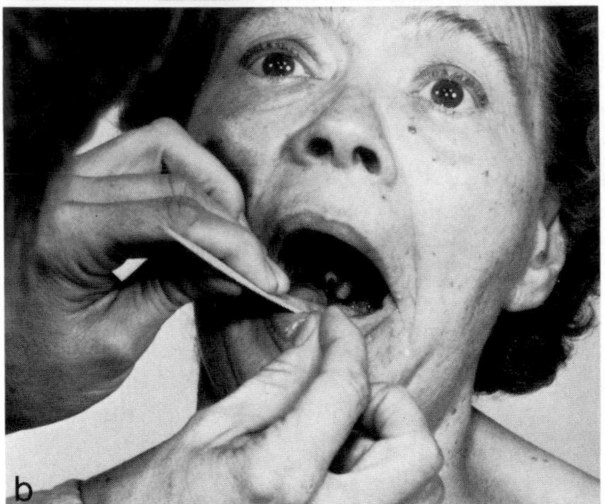

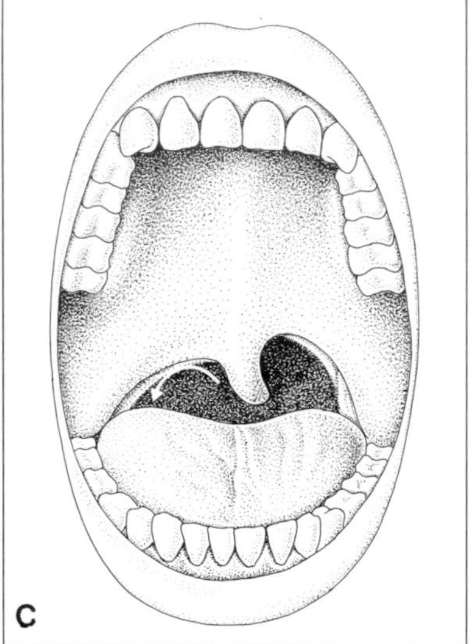

Fig. 13.31 a–c. Stimulating the soft palate with ice (bilateral hemiplegia). **a** Holding the tongue down with a spatula. **b** Stroking the soft palate with an iced cotton bud. **c** The direction of the stroking is upward and lateral

The soft palate activity can be stimulated by the patient blowing through a straw and making bubbles in a glass of coloured liquid. He tries to maintain a steady stream of bubbles, and will improve his breath control at the same time (Fig. 13.30). If the soft palate remains inactive, a wet cotton-bud placed in the freezer compartment of the refrigerator provides a useful means of stimulating with ice. The therapist holds the tongue down with a spatula and strokes the soft palate briskly with the iced cotton-bud (Fig. 13.31 a, b). After the icing, the patient makes some short, sharp "ah" sounds to elevate the soft palate.

To improve the melody and expression of the voice the patient is asked to say a short sentence in different ways, for example "What are you doing?" expressed with irritation, amazement, joy or rage.

13.3.3 For Difficulties Associated with Eating

The activities for improving speaking will all help to improve the patient's eating pattern. In the same way, correct eating movements will be beneficial for speaking. Even patients who are still being tube-fed should be treated, so that they can learn to take food by mouth again more quickly. They will benefit particularly from all movements and stimulation inside the mouth. Practising good clear phonation and changing pitch will ensure that the vocal cords and larynx are moving adequately, to prevent the patient from inhaling particles of food and choking.

Perhaps the most important factor of all is the patient's posture when eating. If he has any difficulties at all with eating and swallowing he should never attempt to eat or drink in bed. Even in a wheelchair the trunk tends to be flexed. The patient should sit on an upright chair at a table, and the therapist extends his trunk passively at first to enable a correct sitting position to be achieved. Placing the hemiplegic arm forwards on the table prevents the side from pulling down in flexion, and the position of the head can then be corrected.

Thick, slow-moving puree-type foods are the easiest to manage at first, but to stimulate chewing and sensation in the mouth the patient needs to be given crunchy food with more texture. Lightly cooked vegetables, biscuits and toast can be attempted. It is almost impossible for the therapist to facilitate chewing mechanically if the food in the patient's mouth does not require chewing.

The patient should be encouraged to chew on the hemiplegic side and place the food first to that side. If he only chews on the sound side the face becomes more asymmetrical, and the affected side is not stimulated into activity. If chewing is inadequate or there is a danger of the patient aspirating, the crispy food can be wrapped in a piece of gauze and placed between the patient's teeth on the hemiplegic side (Fig. 13.32). He can then chew on something and at the same time savour different tastes. The chewing action will also encourage movement of the tongue and lips.

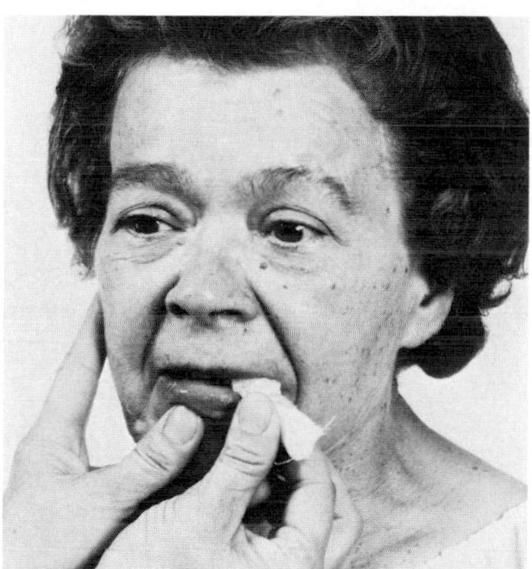

Fig. 13.32. Facilitating chewing with a piece of apple wrapped in gauze (bilateral hemiplegia)

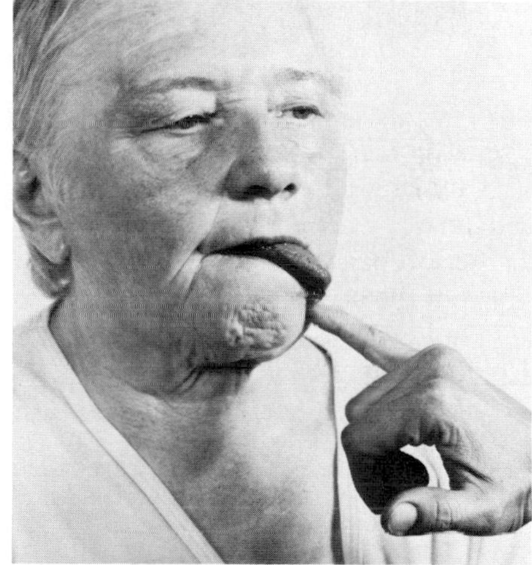

Fig. 13.33. The patient removes a piece of biscuit from her chin (left hemiplegia)

After eating, instead of dabbing at his mouth repeatedly with a napkin the patient is asked to reach for small pieces of food on his lips or chin with his tongue, or by moving one lip over the other (Fig. 13.33). He can also use his hand to wipe away small food particles or saliva, as we would do.

13.4 Oral Hygiene

When tongue movements are a problem or eating is restricted to soft foods, particular attention must be paid to oral hygiene. Food remains stuck to the patient's teeth and they deteriorate rapidly. The condition of the gums is often poor because the circulation is not stimulated by chewing solid foods and the tooth brushing is also inadequate. It is often assumed that because the patient can use one hand he will be able to brush his own teeth properly. With poor sensation and neglect of the hemiplegic side, he often fails to brush the teeth on that side adequately if at all. After each meal the teeth should be vigorously brushed, with the help of the therapist until the patient can manage alone (Fig. 13.34). An electric tooth-brush is a great help because its action compensates for the loss of the skilled manipulation required when using an ordinary tooth-brush. Its small brush is also more easily manipulated when the lips are paralysed or spastic, and the vibration stimulates feeling and movement within the mouth. Particular care should be taken to ensure that the inner side of the teeth is clean as well.

The patient learns a routine whereby he brushes first the top teeth from the very back on one side to the very back on the other side, both inside and outside. The lower teeth are then done in the same way. The therapist should guide the patient's

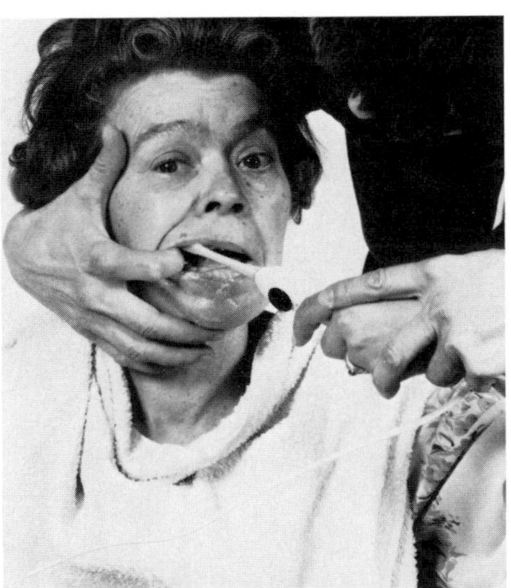

Fig. 13.34. Helping the patient to brush her teeth (bilateral hemiplegia)

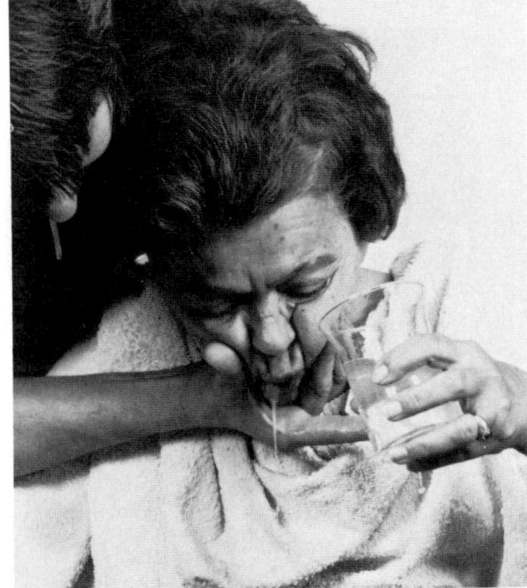

Fig. 13.35. Facilitation of spitting out the water after rinsing the mouth (bilateral hemiplegia)

sound hand so that he learns to carry out the movement routine by experiencing it. Many patients have difficulty in rinsing the mouth adequately and particularly in spitting out the water afterwards. The therapist may need to facilitate the necessary movement, using her thumb and fingers to draw the cheeks and lips forward into the correct position (Fig. 13.35).

If the condition of the gums is particularly poor, the therapist can massage them with her finger, or with a piece of gauze wrapped round her finger for added effect.

13.5 Considerations

The face is of such prime importance in our society, as the numerous advertisements for cosmetics repeatedly show us, that it seems strange that it has received so little attention in the rehabilitation literature and the various treatment programmes offered. Likewise, eating and drinking, which contribute so much to our quality of life, have seldom been emphasised apart from their nutritional aspects. Patients are most thankful for the help they receive through the treatment of their face and mouth. It would seem that certain inhibitions cause us to neglect this aspect of rehabilitation, but once these inhibitions have been overcome the results are most rewarding. The patient is more than willing to practise selected activities on his own.

The whole approach to the "neglected face" and the methods of assessment and treatment described in this chapter are based on the teaching of K. Coombes, (unpublished work).

14 Out of Line (The Pusher Syndrome)

Most studies concerning the rehabilitation of patients with hemiplegia have shown that the majority are able to achieve independent walking, irrespective of the quality of the gait pattern. Many patients learn to walk again even without formal rehabilitation. It is important to consider why the minority fail to learn to walk with conventional methods and how they could be helped to overcome their difficulties.

Various reasons have been offered for the failure in walking, such as old age, weakness, insufficient extensor tone, flexor spasticity in the leg and loss of sensation in the hemiplegic leg. Such hypotheses are obviously not valid, and tend to oversimplify the problem. Elderly patients with marked motor loss have learned to walk again. Polio victims, young and old, walk around despite marked weakness and loss of extensor tone in the leg. Spasticity bears no relation to achieving ambulatory independence, only to the pattern and quality of the gait. Patients with grossly diminished sensation in the lower limb can walk independently even without a stick.

The problem is far more complex, and observation of patients over many years has shown that those who have difficulty in achieving ambulatory independence will also demonstrate other difficulties in common. These difficulties are so uniform that they could be classified together as a syndrome, the *"pusher syndrome"*, the name deriving from the most striking of the symptoms. The patient pushes strongly towards his hemiplegic side in all positions and resists any attempt at passive correction of his posture, that is, correction which would bring his weight towards or over the mid-line of his body to the unaffected side.

In the acute phase after cerebrovascular accident, many patients pass through a transient phase of showing the symptoms. After a period, the more classic picture of hemiplegia develops, and the patient becomes independent. When the pusher syndrome is more pronounced and continues to be a problem, patients are often regarded as unsuitable for rehabilitation and are sent to nursing homes or other long-term institutions. Frequently, after many months in a wheelchair, the patient is sent to a rehabilitation centre, treatment in a general hospital situation having proved unsuccessful. It is often erroneously assumed that he was not sufficiently motivated.

14.1 The Typical Signs

Many more patients with left hemiplegia than right suffer from the pusher syndrome. However, when the symptoms are observed in a case of right hemiplegia of

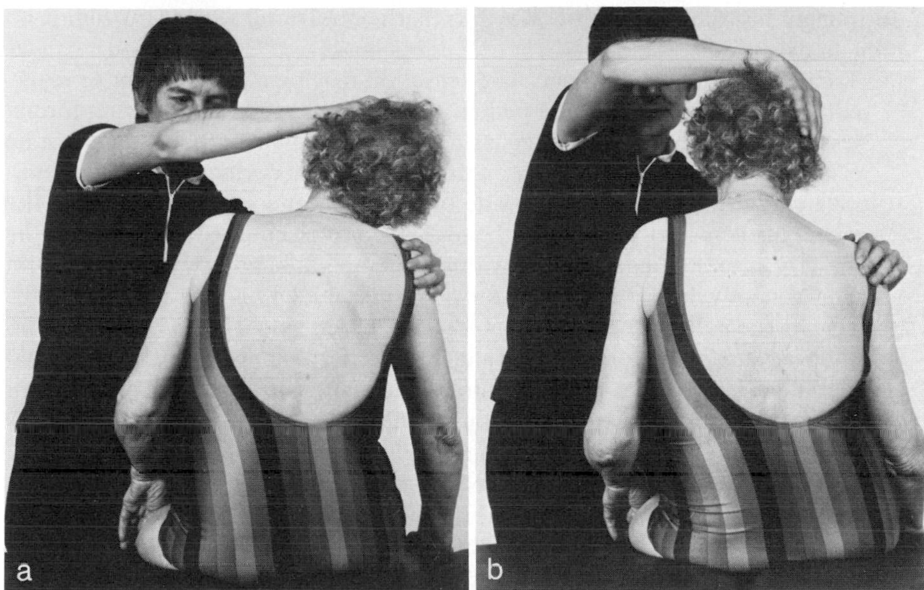

Fig. 14.1 a, b. Lateral flexion of the neck (left hemiplegia). **a** Free to the sound side; **b** limited to the hemiplegic side

long duration, the patient will either have a very severe aphasia or no problem with speech at all. The latter group may consist of those patients whose right cerebral hemisphere is dominant. The degree of difficulty will vary from patient to patient, and is not always directly related to a loss of active movement. Some patients may have selective movement in the hemiplegic hand and foot, despite marked manifestations of the syndrome. When the patient shows one or two of the symptoms, the others will usually be present as well, in varying degrees.

The syndrome in its most severe form, using a left hemiplegic patient as example, is characterised by the following problems:

1. The head is turned to the right and is at the same time shifted laterally towards the right, that is, the distance from the point of the right shoulder to the neck is markedly shortened. When the patient is sitting, he is unable to relax his muscles in order to allow the head to be side flexed towards the hemiplegic side, although it moves freely to the sound side (Fig. 14.1 a, b). When the hemiplegia is of some months' duration the neck may be so stiff that almost no movement is possible. When the patient is lying down the neck movements are noticeably freer, particularly if he is instructed verbally to give no resistance to the passive movements. The eyes are often turned to the right as well, and the patient has difficulty in bringing them to the left and then maintaining their position.
2. The patient's ability to perceive incoming stimuli from his left side is reduced in all the perceptual modalities. Mountcastle (1978), describing the profound contralateral neglect which he relates to parietal lobe lesions, writes: "Such a patient

no longer has the capacity to attend to that contralateral world: for him it no longer exists."

a) Tactile or tactile/kinaesthetic. The sensation may be almost absent or markedly reduced, but even if the patient appears to perform well during formal testing he neglects the hemiplegic side of his body when moving, or when he is not concentrating specifically on that side, as he is during testing. His hemiplegic arm may hang over the side of the chair, and even be caught in the wheel of the wheelchair. When being helped to clasp his hands together he may try to fold his sound hand with the therapist's hand, instead of his own. He frequently dresses or washes only the right side of his body.

b) Visual. The patient does not see objects on his left side. He may have a hemianopsia, and fails to turn his head slightly in order to compensate for the visual field defect. Even with no demonstrable hemianopsia he neglects the incoming visual stimuli, and frequently pushes his wheelchair against objects in his path. Because his head is turned to the right, any visual field loss is in front of him and his field of vision is severely curtailed.

c) Auditory. Because the patient does not hear when someone speaks to him from his left side he may be thought to be deaf. On formal testing, however, the hearing is found not to be diminished.

3. There is a general dearth of facial expression. The face is immobile and when activated is one-sided, with over-activity on the right.
4. The voice is monotonous, with poor breath control and little volume.
5. Lying supine on a plinth or in bed, the patient shows an elongation of his hemiplegic side from head to foot (Fig. 14.2). Particularly noticeable is the discrepancy between the left and right side of his trunk. The right side appears to be short-

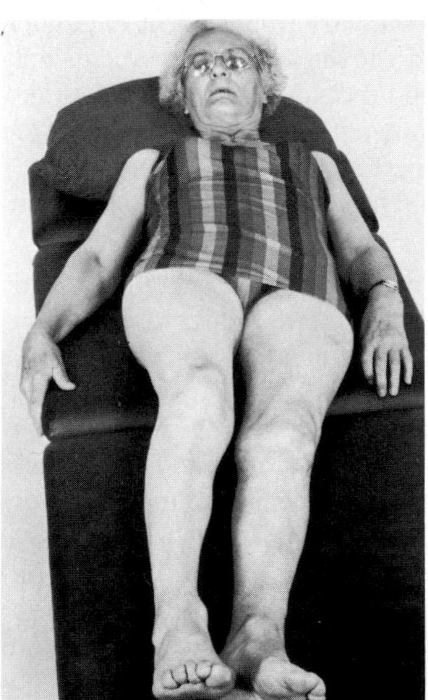

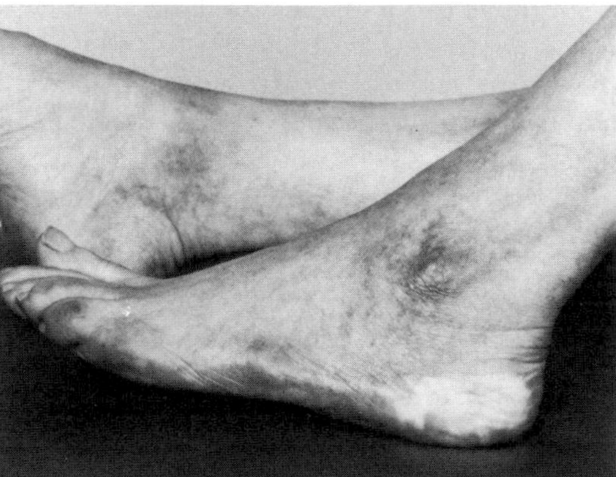

Fig. 14.3. Pressure mark after lying supine (left hemiplegia)

◁ **Fig. 14.2.** Elongation of the whole hemiplegic side in the supine lying position. The head is held off the pillow, the sound leg is actively flexed and the patient holds the side of the plinth (left hemiplegia)

ened. The right leg may be held actively flexed, the heel pushing against the supporting surface, and the therapist has to tell him to relax it and let it lie flat before she is able to place it on the plinth. The patient holds his head actively off the pillow until instructed to relax it.

The left side is at the same time retracted, the shoulder, thorax and pelvis lying below the level of their right equivalents. The left leg therefore lies laterally rotated, and if the patient has been nursed on his back, will frequently show pressure areas over the lateral malleolus and/or along the outside of the heel (Fig. 14.3).

6. When lying on the plinth the patient holds on to the edge with his sound hand and is anxious that he may fall over the side.
7. Placing does not automatically occur when the sound leg is moved, although when asked to hold that leg in a certain position the patient can do so easily (Fig. 14.4 a, b).

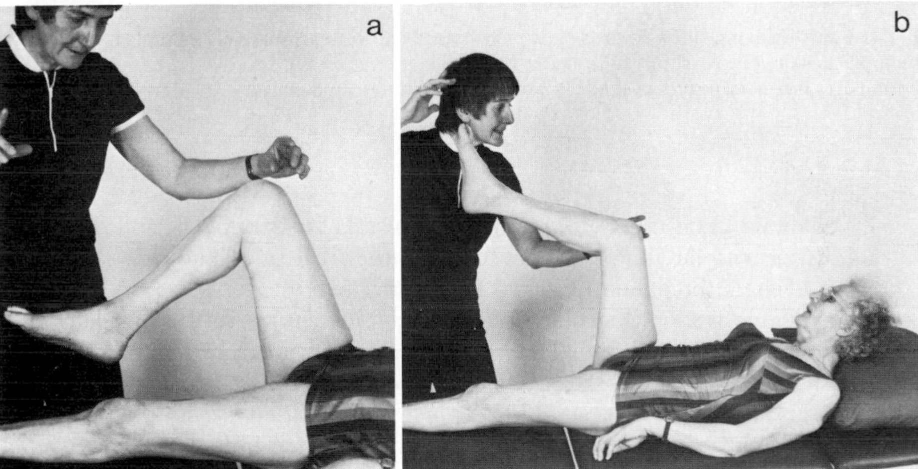

Fig. 14.4 a, b. Placing of the sound leg (left hemiplegia). **a** Fails without verbal command; **b** patient holds the position when verbal instruction is given

8. When both knees are flexed with the feet supported on the bed, they lean towards the left. A marked resistance is felt when trying to turn both knees to the right side, i. e. as if to lay them on the bed on that side. No resistance is met when rotating both knees to the hemiplegic side.
9. In sitting the difficulties become more obvious. The head is held stiffly to the right side and the right side of the trunk shortens markedly. The hemiplegic side is elongated and the navel is shifted towards the right, with hypotonus showing clearly in the muscles on the left side of the abdomen. The weight, however, remains over the left side. Resistance is encountered when an attempt is made to transfer the weight over the right side, with the patient pushing back with the help of his sound hand. He may protest, although no fear was expressed when he was overbalancing to the left.

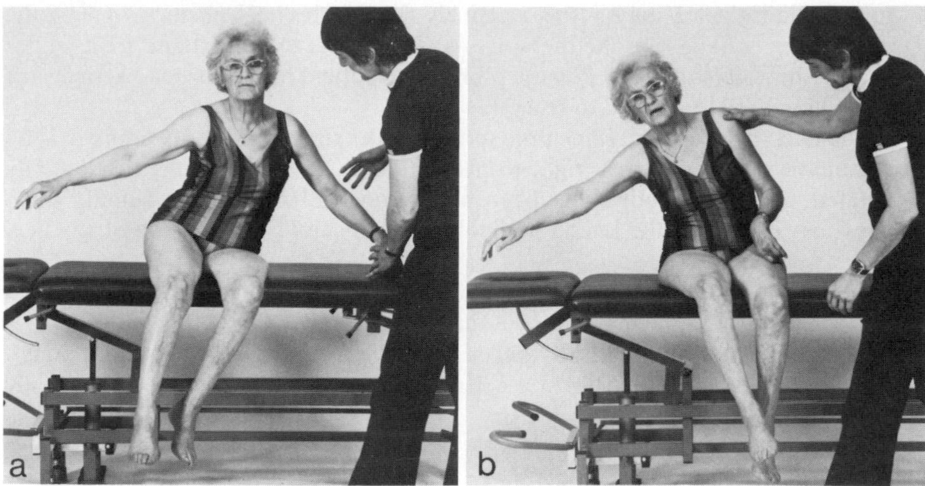

Fig. 14.5 a, b. Moving sideways in a sitting position: balance reactions (left hemiplegia). **a** To the hemiplegic side. The reactions of the head and trunk are almost normal. **b** To the sound side. The hemiplegic side does not react at all. The sound side shortens too actively

When weight is transferred to the left towards the hemiplegic side, the reactions appear to be almost normal, because the right side is already shortened (Fig. 14.5 a). If the patient is asked to take his weight over the sound side, no head-righting reaction occurs. The head remains fixedly to the right, and the side of the trunk fails to elongate, shortening actively instead (Fig. 14.5 b).

10. Transferring the patient into a chair presents difficulties, as he pushes backwards and away from the sound leg, which would otherwise support him. The transfer is particularly difficult if an attempt is made to move the patient to a chair placed on his sound side. His right hand and leg push strongly in the opposite direction to the movement.
11. Seated in the wheelchair the patient adopts a typical posture. His trunk is flexed, his head is turned to the right and his right arm maintains constant activity, pushing on the arm of the chair. He sits more towards the left of the chair, so that it may be difficult to replace the arm of the wheelchair on that side.
12. When leaning forwards in order to stand up or transfer into bed, the patient pushes towards the hemiplegic side, although his trunk is markedly shortened on the sound side (Fig. 14.6). His affected foot may slide back under the chair, or show no activity at all.
13. In standing, the patient's whole centre of gravity is to the left, so that a line drawn from his sound foot to his sternum would be diagonal to the floor. Perry (1969) has also described this symptom, and relates it to the patient who "with a distorted body image has lost awareness of the involved side of his body". The patient, however, remains surprisingly unperturbed, showing no fear, even though the therapist may be experiencing difficulty in holding him upright (Fig. 14.7 a).

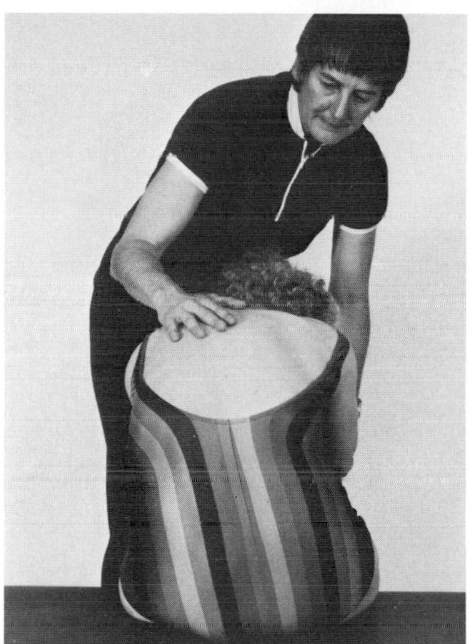

Fig. 14.6. When the patient leans forwards the hemiplegic side lengthens and there is no weight on the sound buttock (left hemiplegia)

As Perry writes, "he will make no attempt to support or otherwise accommodate for the weight of that side if the lesion is complete and thus falls toward the involved side without making an effort to protect himself". He only expresses alarm when the therapist tries to achieve a vertical posture for him. Remarkably, some patients actually pivot sideways with the sound foot to avoid being brought vertically over that leg. The legs are adducted, and the hemiplegic leg flexes and takes little if any weight. The flexion increases when the feet are apart (Fig. 14.7 b). As the patient stands up from sitting the leg may even flex up in the air, which it will certainly do if the therapist attempts to bring the patient's weight over the sound leg (Fig. 14.7 c).

Brunnstrom (1970) has observed this symptom and writes that in "rather unusual cases the flexor synergy dominates the motor behaviour of the lower limb", sometimes to the extent that the patient is unable to lower the limb to the floor in standing. During all standing attempts the sound leg is constantly held in exaggerated extension.

14. The patient either leans back against the therapist's supporting arm or flexes his trunk forwards from the hips and fails to come upright at all. The shortening of the sound side of the trunk becomes more marked in standing, through over-activity. The head is held fixedly, inclined towards the sound side (Fig. 14.8).
15. If it is possible to walk with the patient, the hemiplegic leg adducts so strongly that it may even cross over in front of the other leg as it is brought forward (Fig. 14.9 a). Brunnstrom (1970) describes how the affected limb assumes a "scissor" posture in front of the other limb when the weight is shifted towards the normal side. The patient has difficulty in taking a step with his affected leg because he is unable to transfer his weight over the sound side before doing so (Fig. 14.9 b). Taking a step with the sound leg is difficult due to the inadequate extensor support in the hemiplegic limb.

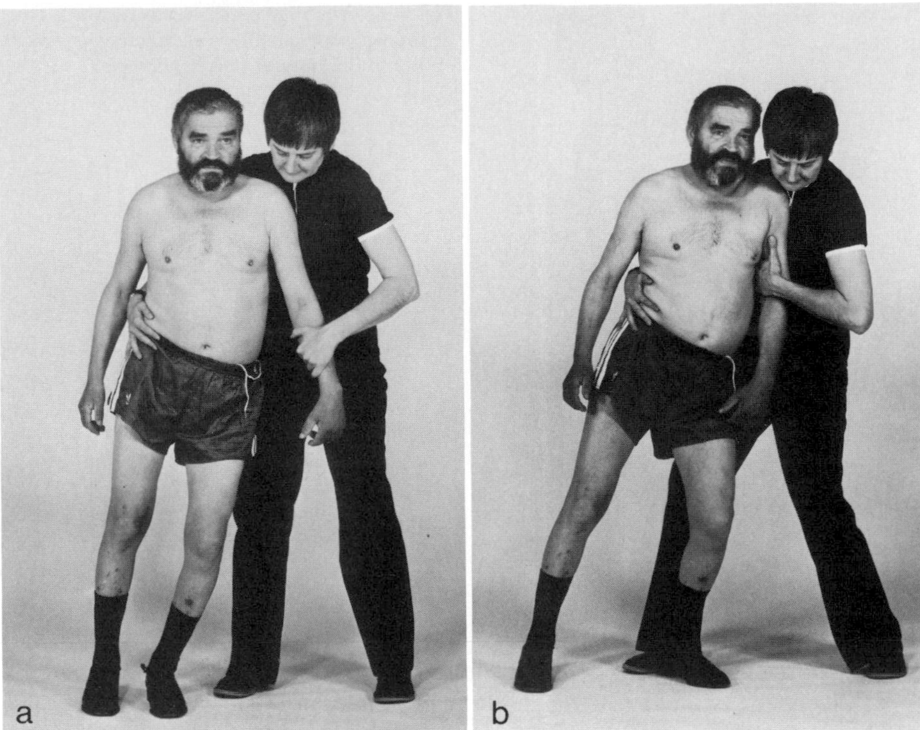

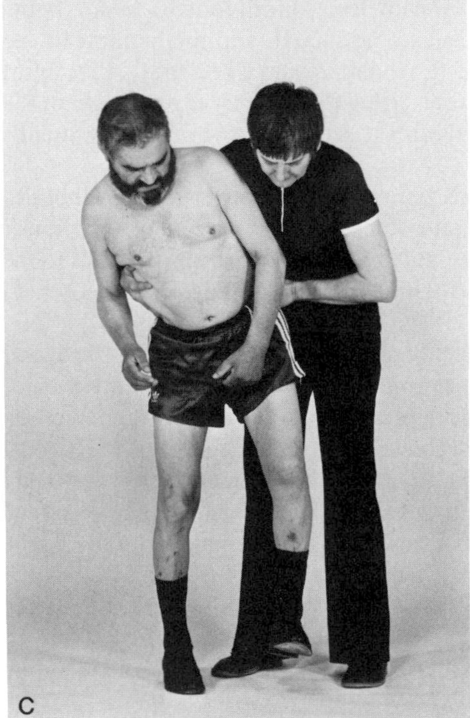

Fig. 14.7 a–c. Standing (left hemiplegia). **a** With feet together. **b** With legs abducted. **c** The therapist attempts to bring the patient's weight on to his sound leg. The hemiplegic leg flexes into the air

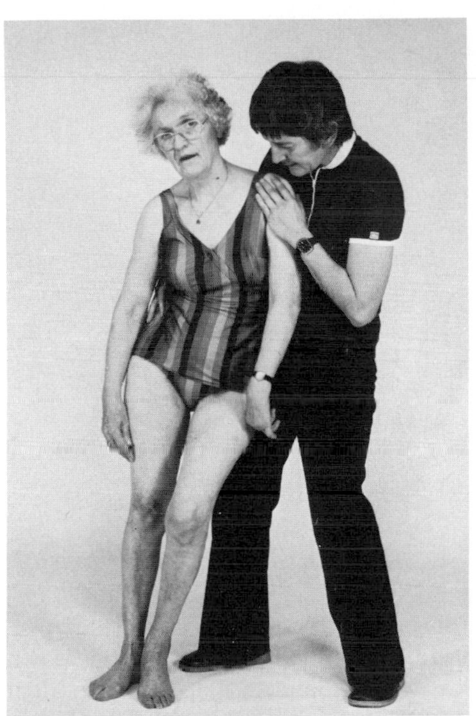

Fig. 14.8. Typical standing posture (left hemiplegia)

Fig. 14.9 a, b. Difficulties in walking (left hemiplegia)
▽

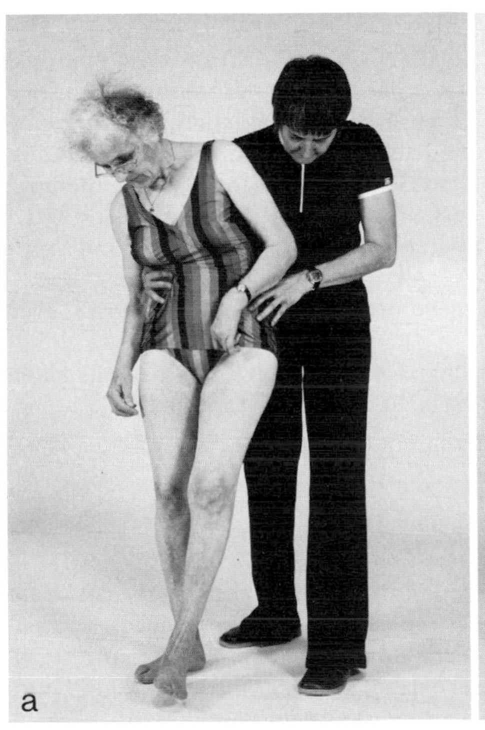

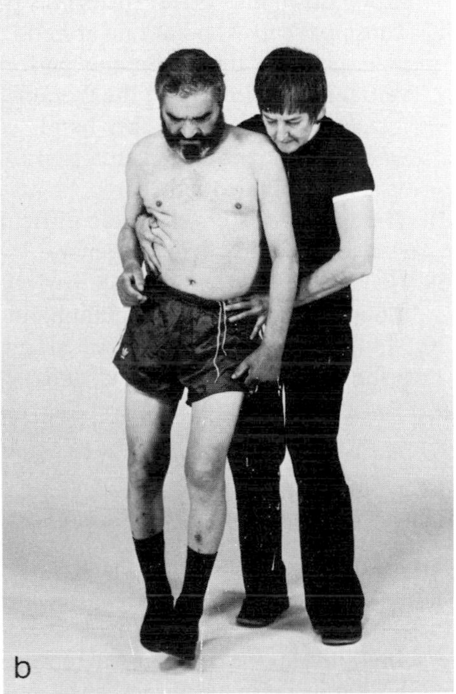

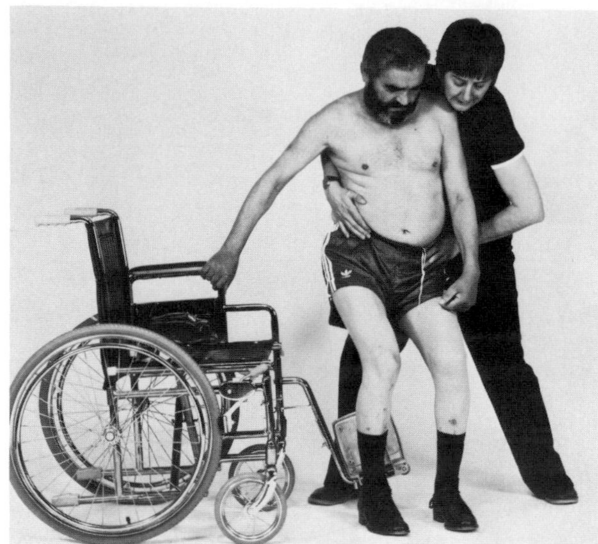

Fig. 14.10. Sitting down too soon (left hemiplegia)

16. As the patient walks towards his chair or the plinth, supported by the therapist, he sits down prematurely. He grasps the arm of the chair and starts sitting down when he is still inappropriately far away, and without turning round to align himself with his back to the chair (Fig. 14.10). The therapist has difficulty in supporting his weight, and the patient is often unable to interrupt the movement of sitting down in order to correct his position.
17. Those patients who have no aphasia tend to talk a great deal and offer many explanations for their failure in performance. The patient also requires constant verbal instructions from the therapist, even though the situation itself or the information provided by her hands would seem to be sufficient. For example, when the patient has taken a step forward with his right foot and the therapist asks him to take another step, he may ask which foot he should move.
18. The patient has considerable difficulty in learning to dress himself, and in the activities of daily living in general.
19. His sound hand appears clumsy when he tries to perform skilled tasks, even though it is often his dominant hand.
20. Many of the problems described in Chapt. 1 are experienced by patients manifesting the pusher syndrome, and will need to be treated accordingly.

14.2 Specific Treatment

All the activities which have been described in the preceeding chapters can be included in the treatment, when applicable to the patient's individual needs. Particularly important are those to enable the patient to bear weight on his hemiplegic leg, e.g. bridging, knee extension and retraining balance reactions in all positions. Guiding his hands during activities where a plan is required is most important.

The therapist needs to apply the principle of providing the patient with correct tactile/kinaesthetic input for his whole body during activity. She guides his whole body during the movement sequence if necessary. The patient's position in the wheelchair is particularly important, with a firm support to maintain extension of the trunk. He should sit with his weight inclined forward and his arms supported on a table in front of him, as the half-reclining posture seems to reinforce those symptoms which are seen when he is standing. The arm-rest on his unaffected side should be removed so that he does not constantly push on it during the day.

Attention is given to restoring facial expression and to improving the quality of the patient's voice and breathing. In addition, the following specific activities should be included in the treatment programme.

14.2.1 Restoring Movements of the Head

It is essential to free the head from its fixed position, particularly side flexion toward the hemiplegic side without resistance. The therapist maintains full passive range of movement of the neck, with the patient lying supine. There is far less resistance to the movements in this position, and she can ensure that no contractures develop. The movements are also carried out when the patient is sitting. The patient is better able to release the neck muscles when he is given tactile cues. The therapist places her hand against the side of his head and tries to move it sideways. When she feels a resistance she asks him to allow the movement, and to relieve the pressure against her hand. He moves his head so that the resistance against her hand decreases. She also facilitates the movement if she asks him to bring his head sideways to lean against her. The patient is then aware of achieving the correct movement when he feels his head against the therapist, to orientate him. When stretching the neck, the therapist will need to give counter-pressure against the shoulder on the opposite side to the direction of the lateral flexion.

Active movement is encouraged further by activities where the patient is required to move his head to look at an object, e.g. using a ball or balloon. Later the head movements also need to be achieved when the patient is standing. Correct rolling to both sides helps to re-establish head movement, and also to orientate the patient in space. As he rolls over he makes contact with the surface of the bed or mat, and the total resistance which he encounters informs him that he has completed the movement.

14.2.2 Stimulating Activity in the Hypotonic Trunk Side Flexors

Because of the hypotonus and inactivity of the hemiplegic side the patient has difficulty in transferring his weight towards the sound side (Fig. 14.11 a). For example, he cannot cross the hemiplegic leg over the other leg to put on a sock. When trying to walk he is unable to free the hemiplegic leg to take a step forward. The hemiplegic side lengthens instead of shortening, and the sound side shortens instead of lengthening.

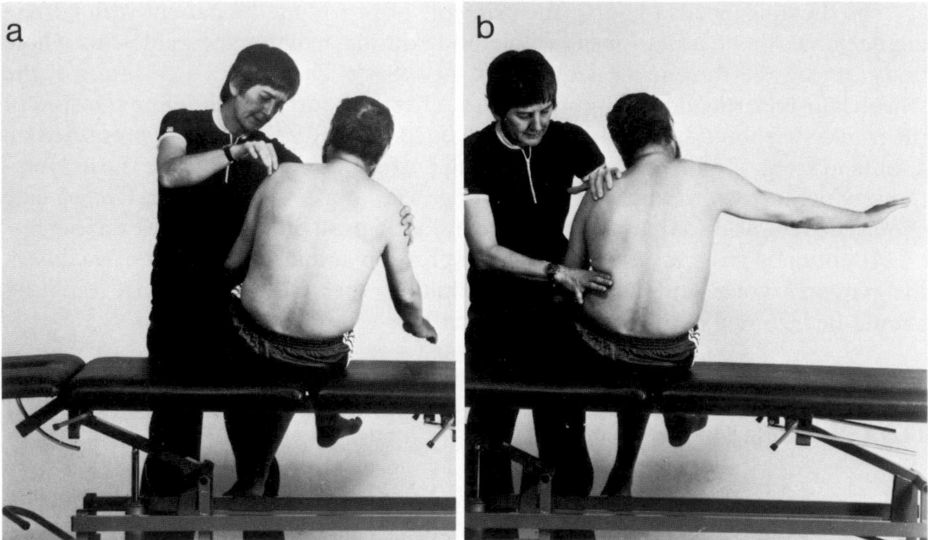

Fig. 14.11. **a** Transferring weight to the sound side when sitting with crossed legs is difficult due to inactivity of the side of the trunk. **b** The therapist stimulates activity in the hemiplegic side (left hemiplegia)

1. To facilitate shortening of the side of the trunk and head-righting to the left, the patient sits with his hemiplegic leg crossed over the other one. The therapist stands in front of him, keeping his legs in place with her legs. With her left hand round behind his shoulders and her right hand under his left buttock, she helps the patient to transfer his weight over the right side. When the head fails to come to the vertical, the therapist uses her left forearm to move it correctly, asking the patient not to push against her arm. He feels the pressure of his head against her arm and moves his head away to relieve the pressure, and the correct position is automatically achieved (see Fig. 7.3 b). He maintains the position as the therapist removes her supporting hands. The movement is repeated and the patient then tries to move into exactly the same position without the therapist's assistance.
2. Sitting or standing beside the patient, the therapist asks him to take his weight away from her. With one hand she presses the muscles of the side of his trunk firmly with the web between thumb and index finger to encourage their contraction. The pressure is applied intermittently. With her other hand she pushes down on the patient's shoulder to stimulate the correct righting reaction of the head, through stretch (Fig. 14.11 b).
3. The patient learns to lean towards the sound side, support himself on his elbow and then return to the upright position without pushing off with his arm. As he does so, the head rights automatically and the trunk side flexors are activated. The therapist facilitates the correct movement by placing one of her arms across the back of the patient's shoulders in such a way that she can control the speed of the movement and use her forearm to push down on his hemiplegic shoulder to stimulate head-righting to vertical (see Fig. 7.1 b). With her other hand she holds his sound hand lightly and reminds him not to use it to assist the movement. The

activity is progressed by asking the patient to lean slowly to the sound side and stop before his flexed elbow touches the plinth. He can also stop and start at various stages of the movement or change directions.

14.2.3 Regaining the Mid-line in Standing

The longer the patient remains seated in a wheelchair, the more the flexion in his leg and trunk increases. It is most important to start standing at an early stage. The lack of extensor activity in the leg makes the upright position difficult for the therapist to support. The more she holds the patient, the more he tends to lean or push towards her.

Using a back slab made of a firm material such as plaster of Paris (Fig. 14.12) to hold the patient's leg in extension changes the procedure amazingly. The back slab is bandaged firmly into place using 2 × 12 cm crêpe bandages and the patient is helped to stand up from a sitting position. It is difficult for him to come upright because of the extended knee, and so the therapist must help him adequately. Once he is standing, activities are immediately carried out which automatically elicit the desired posture and movement without the patient being dependent upon verbal instructions and feedback from the therapist.

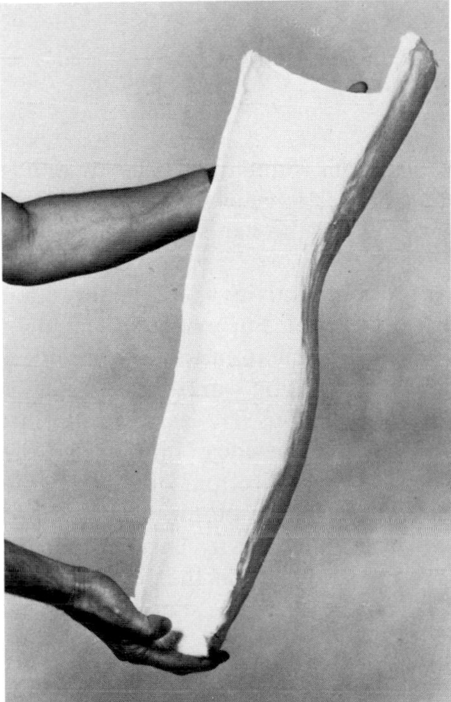

Fig. 14.12. Back slab (left leg)

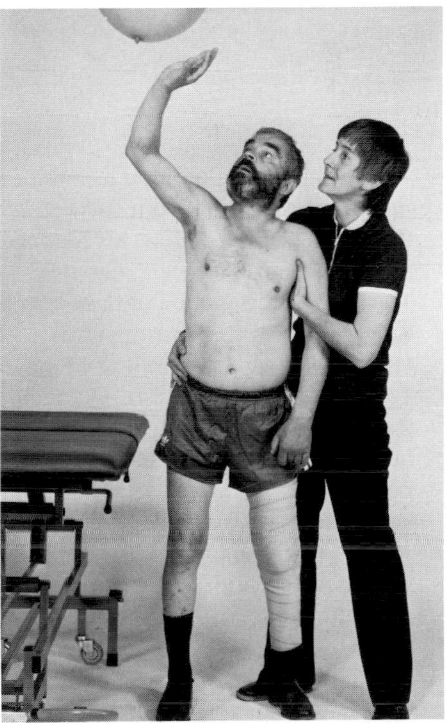

Fig. 14.13. Hitting a balloon with the sound hand elongates the side of the trunk (left hemiplegia)

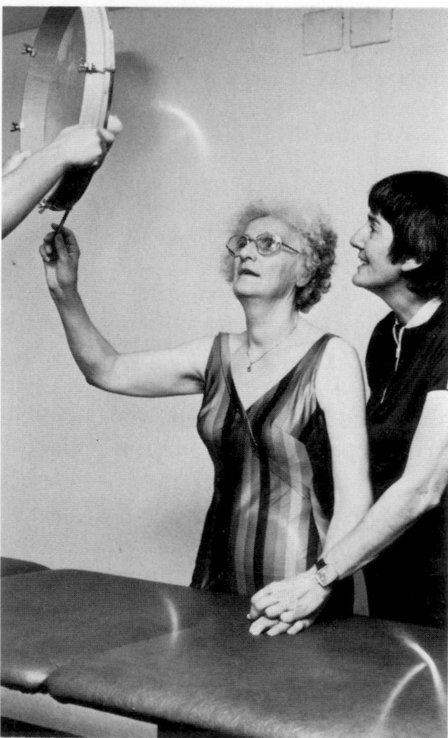

Fig. 14.14. Playing a tambourine prevents shortening of the sound side of the trunk (left hemiplegia)

1. The patient taps a balloon to a third person with his sound hand. The balloon is patted back to him high in the air so that he has to reach up to hit it back (Fig. 14.13). Immediately, his right side elongates and the standing posture is corrected.
2. The same effect can be obtained by any appropriate activity which requires that he reach forwards and upwards with his sound hand. For example, playing a tambourine with different rhythms or even beating time to music will provide a good stimulus (Fig. 14.14). The tambourine or the balloon can be placed so that the patient needs to turn his head in different directions. He learns to turn his head to the left and make eye contact with objects on that side of him. At first, the patient may feel more secure if a high plinth is placed in front of him, and he keeps his hips forward by maintaining contact with the plinth. The therapist stands on the patient's affected side and during the activity ensures that his weight is over both legs. She does not use verbal correction, as the patient is concentrating on performing the activity and will not hear her. She simply adjusts his pelvis to achieve the desired position.
3. Standing with his sound side to the plinth, the patient is asked to shift his weight until he feels his right hip touching it. At first he supports himself with his right hand on the plinth as he repeats the movement, moving his hip to the plinth and then away from it (Fig. 14.15 a). The therapist uses her hands to shorten the hemiplegic side of his trunk, one hand pushing down on his shoulder and the other

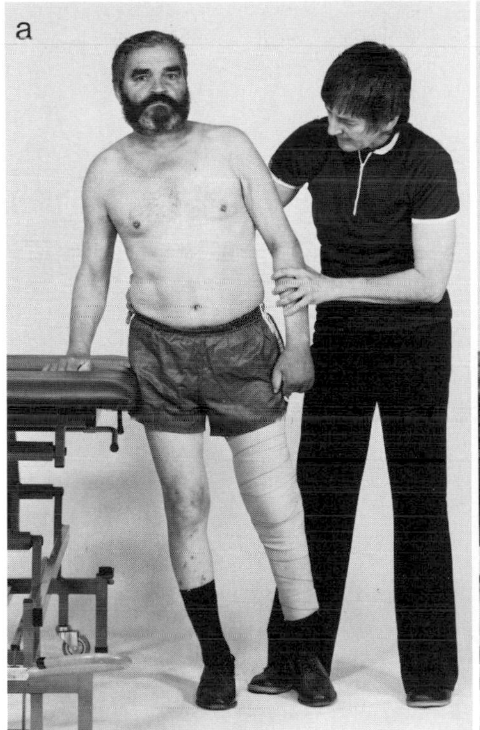

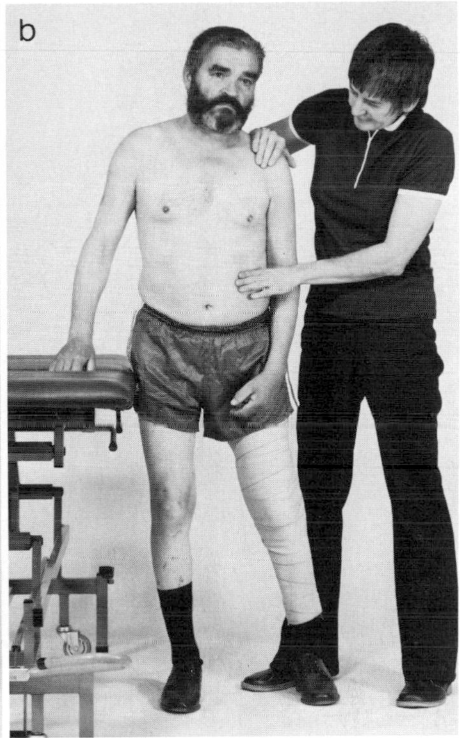

△

Fig. 14.15 a, b. Standing with the back slab, moving the weight sideways towards a plinth (left hemiplegia). **a** The patient leans too much on the plinth. **b** The therapist facilitates shortening of the hemiplegic side

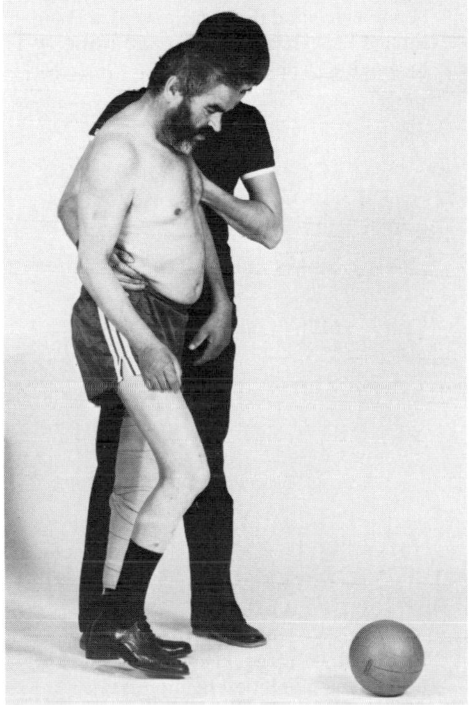

Fig. 14.16. Kicking a football with the sound foot (left hemiplegia)

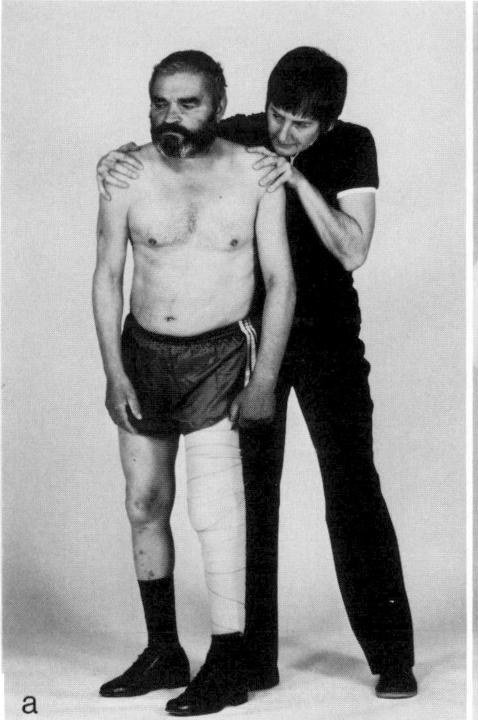

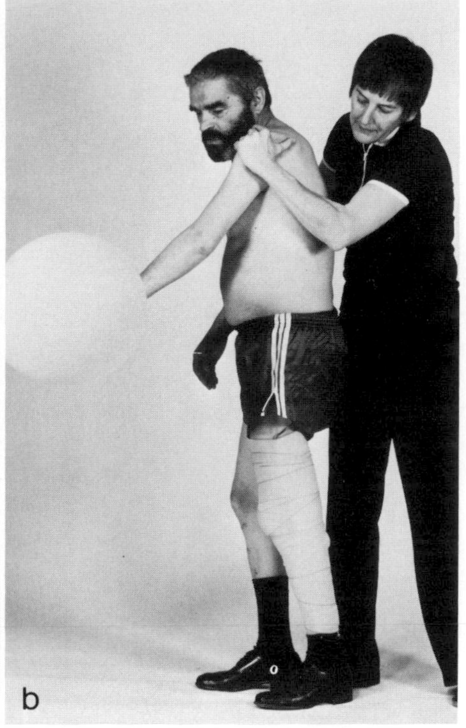

△

Fig. 14.17 a, b. Hitting a balloon with the hemiplegic hand (left hemiplegia). **a** Hand rotated back in readiness for the swing; **b** swinging to hit the balloon

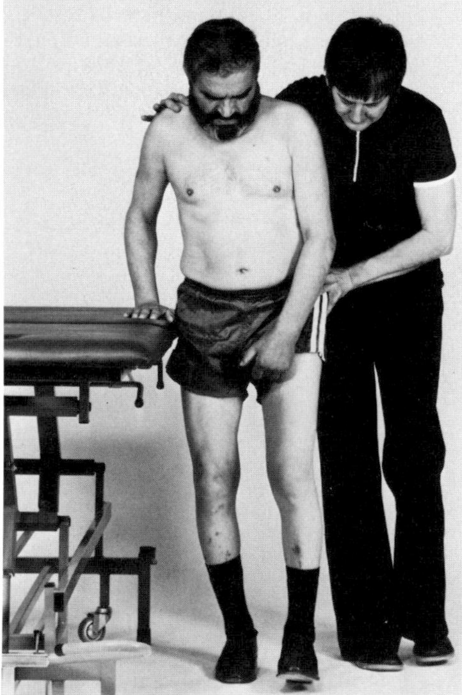

Fig. 14.18. Walking, keeping the sound hip against the plinth (left hemiplegia)

pressing into the trunk side flexors to stimulate activity (Fig. 14.15 b). The activity is performed with the patient standing with his legs more and more abducted.

4. The patient practises taking weight through the hemiplegic leg, and can be asked to kick a football with his sound foot (Fig. 14.16).
5. Because the hemiplegic side is rotated backwards, the patient needs to practise bringing his left shoulder forwards in order to improve his balance. The therapist helps him to bring the whole side forward and then he is asked to stay there, or to repeat the movement with less help. Swinging to hit a balloon with his hemiplegic arm often facilitates the correct movement. The therapist places her hands on the patient's shoulders and rotates the left shoulder back (Fig. 14.17 a). The balloon is thrown to the patient and the therapist helps him to swing the whole side forwards so that his hand hits the balloon (Fig. 14.17 b). Even if the arm has no active movement, the patient can hit the balloon away by swinging his hand forwards from the shoulder. He is instructed not to try to lift his arm but rather to swing it like a tennis racket.

Immediately following these activities the therapist removes the back slab, if possible with the patient still standing. He stands with his sound side against the plinth, and when the bandages have been removed attempts to maintain the extension actively. He is asked to walk around the plinth, trying to feel his hip against it all the time (Fig. 14.18). The plinth gives him the orientation he requires to remain in the mid-line position. After walking around the plinth he may be able to continue walk-

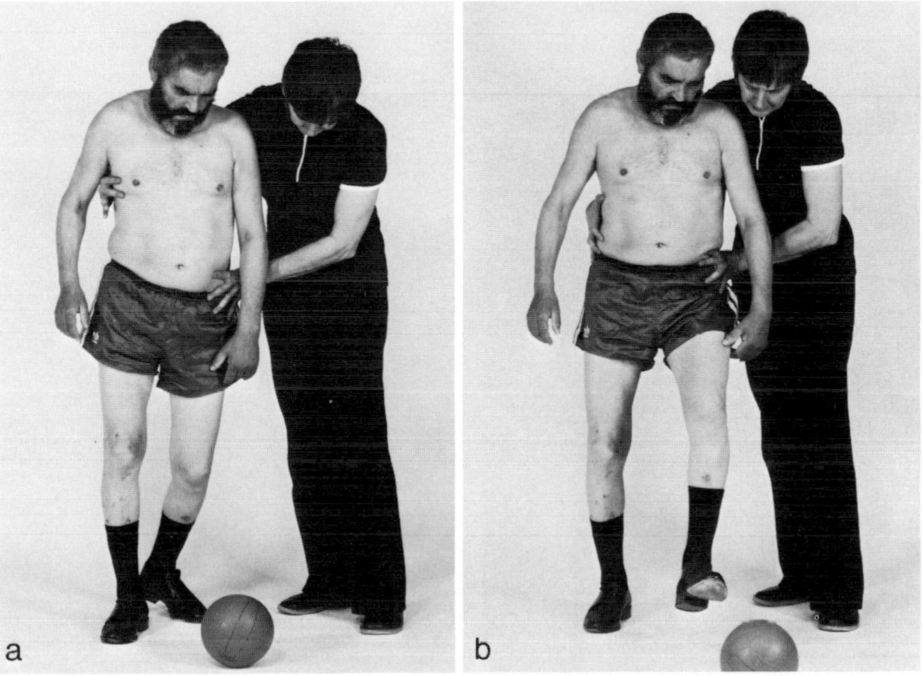

Fig. 14.19 a, b. Kicking a football with the hemiplegic foot (left hemiplegia). **a** Foot behind in preparation for the kick; **b** the kick

ing away from it, with the therapist supporting him from the pelvis. It is easier for him to walk to a set goal, for example to his wheelchair placed some way away.

Parallel bars are not used because the patient pulls himself towards the bar with his sound hand and does not learn the correct mechanism of transferring his weight over the sound side. Using the flat surface of the plinth or a table provides the correct stimulus for the activity.

When kicking a football with his hemiplegic foot the patient transfers his weight spontaneously over the sound leg. The therapist takes the patient's foot back to allow him to kick with a good swing, or he can take a step forward with his sound leg (Fig. 14.19 a, b). The ball is placed in the correct position for the kick until the patient is sufficiently advanced and can kick a moving ball. The action of kicking the ball also facilitates the swing phase of gait.

14.2.4 Climbing Stairs

Going up and down stairs provides the patient with an excellent stimulus. Even though he cannot balance while standing or walk without support, he can climb the stairs with facilitation from the therapist (Fig. 14.20). The flight of stairs offers him the information he requires to carry out the necessary movements. The therapist assists him in the way described in Chap. 7. It is often surprising how well the patient performs on the stairs, and how much better he can walk immediately afterwards.

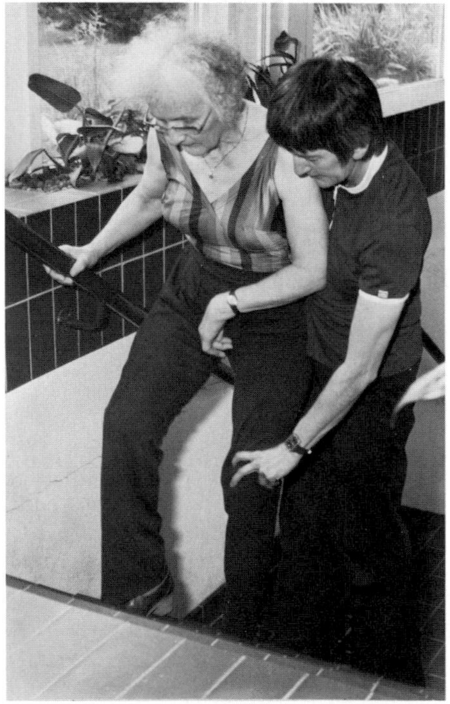

Fig. 14.20. Climbing stairs (compare Fig. 14.9 a) (left hemiplegia)

14.3 Considerations

Patients who cannot transfer weight towards the sound side have difficulty in learning to walk and regain independence. Giving the patient a stick does not help because he only uses it to push more strongly towards his affected side. Although the rehabilitation takes longer, it is well worth the effort, and the gait pattern is often surprisingly good in the end. The more the patient stands and walks, the sooner he learns to balance in the upright position. He should be helped to stand during those activities in his daily life which he normally performed in the standing position, for example combing his hair or shaving in the morning (Fig. 14.21).

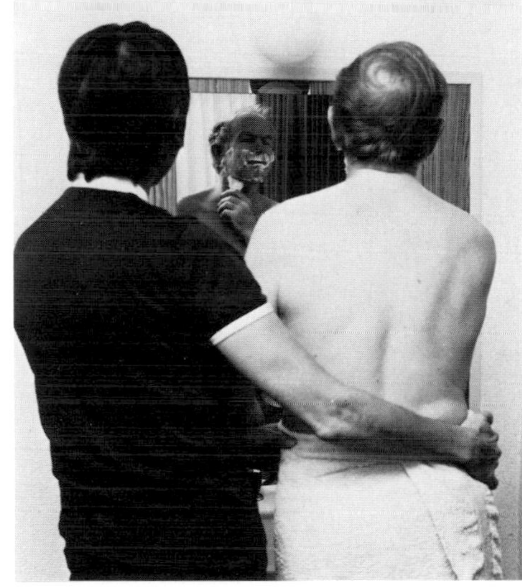

Fig. 14.21. Standing while shaving (left hemiplegia)

During therapy the patient should be given as much tactile information as possible from his environment, as his own internal feedback system is disturbed. He needs the information from his surroundings in order to orientate himself in space and to learn to move again. When the patient is leaning towards his hemiplegic side and he is told to move his weight to the other side, or to the right, he is entirely dependent on the information he receives from his own sensation. Very often he will be unable to respond correctly. In the same way he cannot react to the instruction from the therapist to "put your hip forward".

Placing a fixed resistance beside or in front of him will enable him to carry out the movement if he is asked to move his weight until he feels the table with his hip. The therapist can use her own body or her hand to provide the patient with a control point. She asks him to move his hip away from her hip or his head to or away from her hand. He feels the pressure or the resistance, and can then move so that he no longer feels it.

The principle is applied throughout the treatment and in the patient's daily life. When the patient is being assisted to transfer it helps if he puts his hands forward on to a stool placed in front of him, rather than just forward in space. As his ability to feel improves, the patient will require less and less information from his surroundings. He will have learnt the movements. Patients with the problems described respond far better to walking and climbing stairs than to trying to learn to stand. Standing balance improves as a result of walking and carrying out actual tasks while standing. Both the patient and the therapist become frustrated and resigned if standing is practised unsuccessfully in isolation, as a prerequisite for walking.

15 The Home Programme

Most important for the patient after being discharged from the hospital or rehabilitation centre is his 24-hour way of life, rather than having a long list of exercises which he has to perform each day. The activities of his daily life, when carried out correctly, will help him to maintain his mobility and will also encourage further improvement. He will have learnt how to lie in bed when he sleeps, how to dress himself without associated reactions, how to stand up symmetrically etc.

There are, however, certain movements which do not occur in his daily life, and he must therefore carry out specific exercises or activities to prevent muscle shortening or increased spasticity. There is no absolute prescription applicable to all patients, and special additional activities may sometimes be necessary. The following problems are most commonly seen when patients return for a check-up or a further period of intensive treatment, or are referred from another hospital:

1. The shoulder no longer has full range of motion and may have become painful.
2. The elbow flexors have shortened.
3. There is loss of full dorsal flexion of the wrist with full extension of the fingers.
4. Full supination of the arm is not possible, even passively.
5. The full range of abduction of the arm in outward rotation with elbow extension has not been maintained.
6. The knee is spastic in extension and the patient has trouble releasing the spasticity for functions such as crossing his legs to put on his shoe, walking or climbing the stairs.
7. The Achilles tendon has shortened – the patient cannot bear weight with his heel on the floor. Clonus may have developed.
8. The toes are flexed strongly and adducted, and sometimes corns have developed or painful areas on the pads of the toes from the pressure against the floor.

The patient must carry out specific activities each day to prevent these complications from arising. He must set aside an appropriate time each day to exercise, a time which fits in with his normal routine. First thing in the morning would suit a pensioner, but a patient who works might find a later time more appropriate. The following activities are suitable for the majority of patients and should be carefully taught from the beginning so that the patient can perform them easily and accurately before he goes home or stops having out-patient treatment. They must have absolute controls to enable him to carry them out correctly on his own, so that he does not waste time practising an incorrect or useless activity.

The number of activities included in the recommended home programme has been reduced to a minimum, as very few people would be prepared to practise a long list of exercises every day. Those which have been selected are considered essential for preventing the commonest complications. The activities are included regularly in the treatment sessions, so that the patient knows them well and can perform them independently. As a final test, the patient should be able to go right through the required activities without the therapist having to prompt him in any way or correct part of his performance.

There are several ways in which he can be assisted in remembering each activity and its key points, and the sequence in which to carry out the exercises. The therapist can write a list of the activities and describe how they are to be carried out, but the patient often finds the description confusing, particularly if he has a language problem. Drawings or diagrams can also be of help. The most useful aid would seem to be a Polaroid photograph of each activity with the most important features written on or next to it. For example, a picture showing the following activity would need the comment "The elbows must remain straight and the balls of the hands together. Continue with the exercise until your thumbs touch the floor beyond your head."

1. To prevent shoulder stiffness. The patient lies on his bed or on the floor and lifts his clasped hands above his head. He reaches with them towards his sound side to bring the scapula well into protraction, and then moves the arms until his hands touch the supporting surface, his elbows remaining extended (Fig. 15.1).

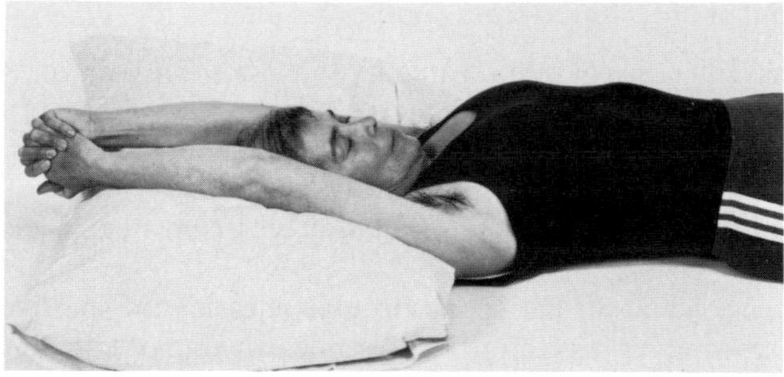

Fig. 15.1. Preventing pain or stiffness in the shoulder (right hemiplegia)

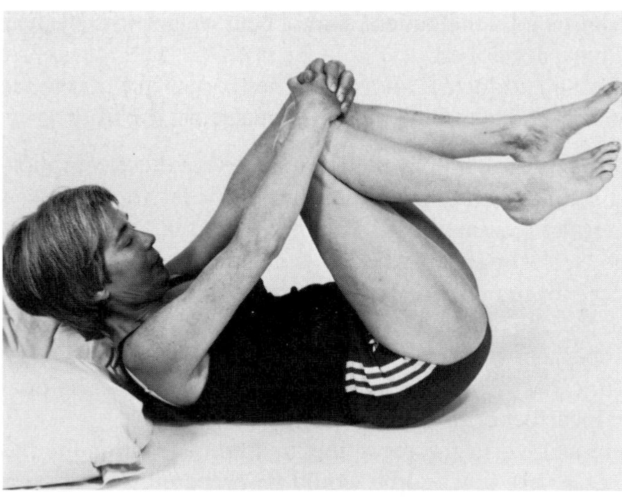

Fig. 15.2. Inhibiting extensor spasticity in the leg (right hemiplegia)

2. To inhibit extensor spasticity in the lower limb. Lying on his back the patient clasps his hands together and encircles his flexed knees with both arms. He draws his knees up to his chest and lifts his head at the same time. He then allows the hips to extend somewhat, until his elbows are straight and his shoulders have been drawn well forward in protraction. He then repeats the movement by flexing his legs again (Fig. 15.2). The activity can also be practised with only the hemiplegic leg being flexed, the other leg remaining flat on the bed.
3. To maintain supination of the forearm. The patient sits at a table with his hands clasped and his arms stretched out in front of him. He leans toward his hemiplegic side, pushing his affected arm into supination until the thumb is pressed on to the table (Fig. 15.3 a). Moving from side to side he releases the spasticity until he can place the sound hand flat on the other hand, holding the fingers in extension (Fig. 15.3 b).

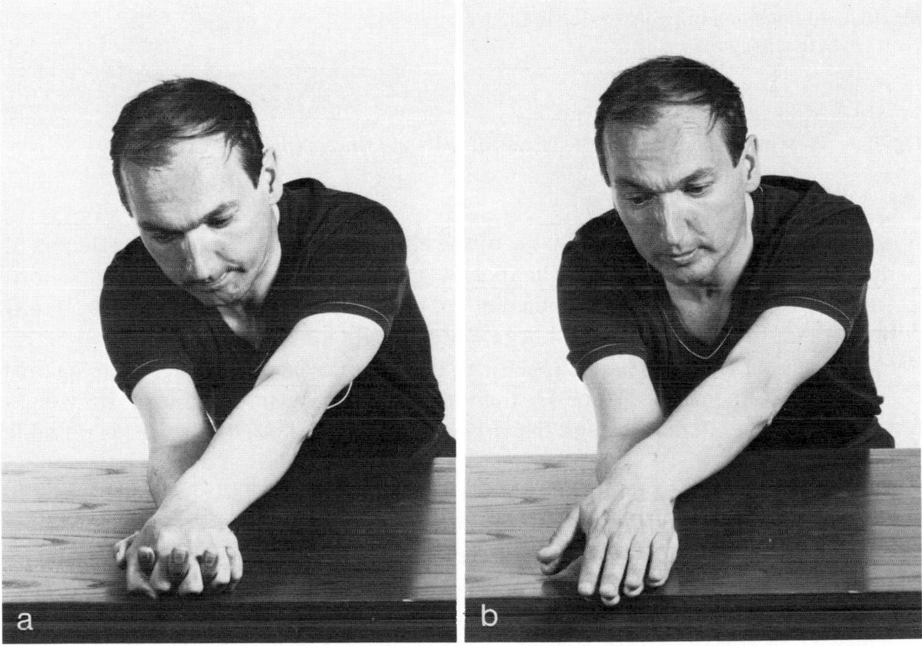

Fig. 15.3 a, b. Maintaining supination of the forearm (right hemiplegia)

4. To maintain full dorsal flexion of the wrist. The patient clasps his hands together, and with both elbows supported parallel on a table in front of him he brings his hands towards his face. Using his sound hand he dorsiflexes the hemiplegic wrist fully and then repeatedly moves the wrist into the corrected position. The activity can be repeated often during the day, and the position can be adapted when the patient is sitting talking or watching television (Fig. 15.4).

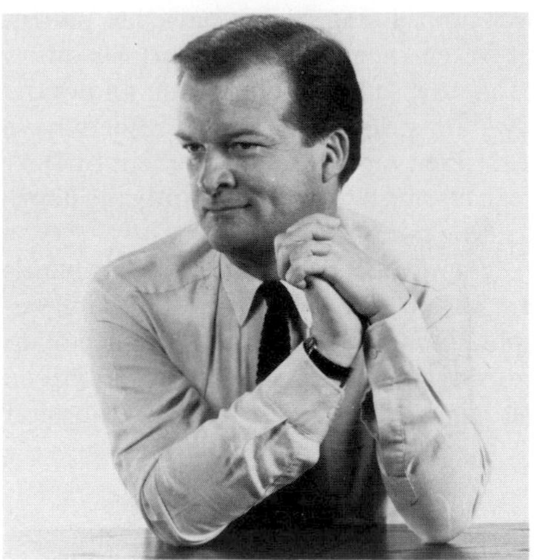

Fig. 15.4. Maintaining full dorsiflexion of the wrist (right hemiplegia)

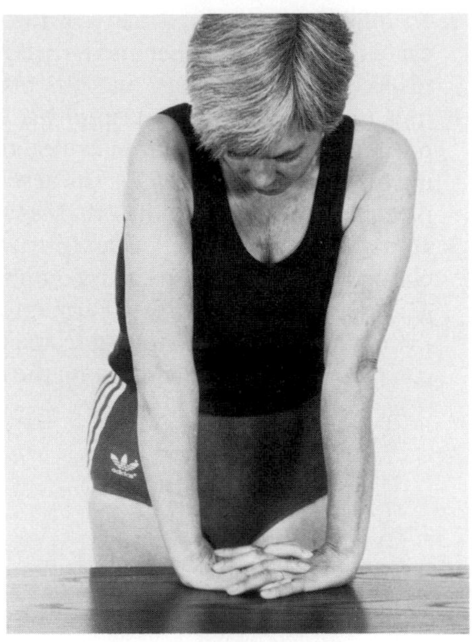

Fig. 15.5. Preventing shortening of the flexors of wrist and fingers (right hemiplegia)

5. To prevent shortening of the flexors of the elbow, wrist and fingers. The flexors of the fingers and wrist are often markedly spastic, and can easily become shortened. The patient must be taught a method of maintaining their full length. It may be difficult for him to achieve, but one of the following is essential.
   a) The patient claps his hands together, turns them over and pushes them against a table or other firm surface. He then straightens his arms and moves his weight over the extended arms until the wrists are in as full a dorsal flexion as possible (Fig. 15.5).
   b) The patient sits on a table, or on a chair with another placed alongside him. Using his sound hand he passively extends the fingers and wrist of his hemiplegic hand and then places it on the firm surface at his side. If the hand is very spastic he can use his sound leg to give counter-pressure against the dorsal aspect of the wrist while he opens the fingers passively (Fig. 15.6 a–c). With the sound hand he holds the affected elbow in full extension as he moves his body weight over the affected arm, taking care that the fingers do not flex as he does so (Fig. 15.6 d).
6. To prevent shortening of the Achilles tendon and toe flexors. The patient places a rolled bandage under his toes (Fig. 15.7 a) and then stands up. If necessary, he pushes on the affected knee with his sound hand to ensure that the heel maintains contact with the floor (Fig. 15.7 b). Standing upright, he brings his weight over the hemiplegic leg and lifts the other leg into the air. He can support himself lightly on the back of a chair, a chest of drawers or the wash-basin to maintain balance. The patient stands on the bandage and bends and straightens his knee, keeping his hips forward as he does so (Fig. 15.7 c).

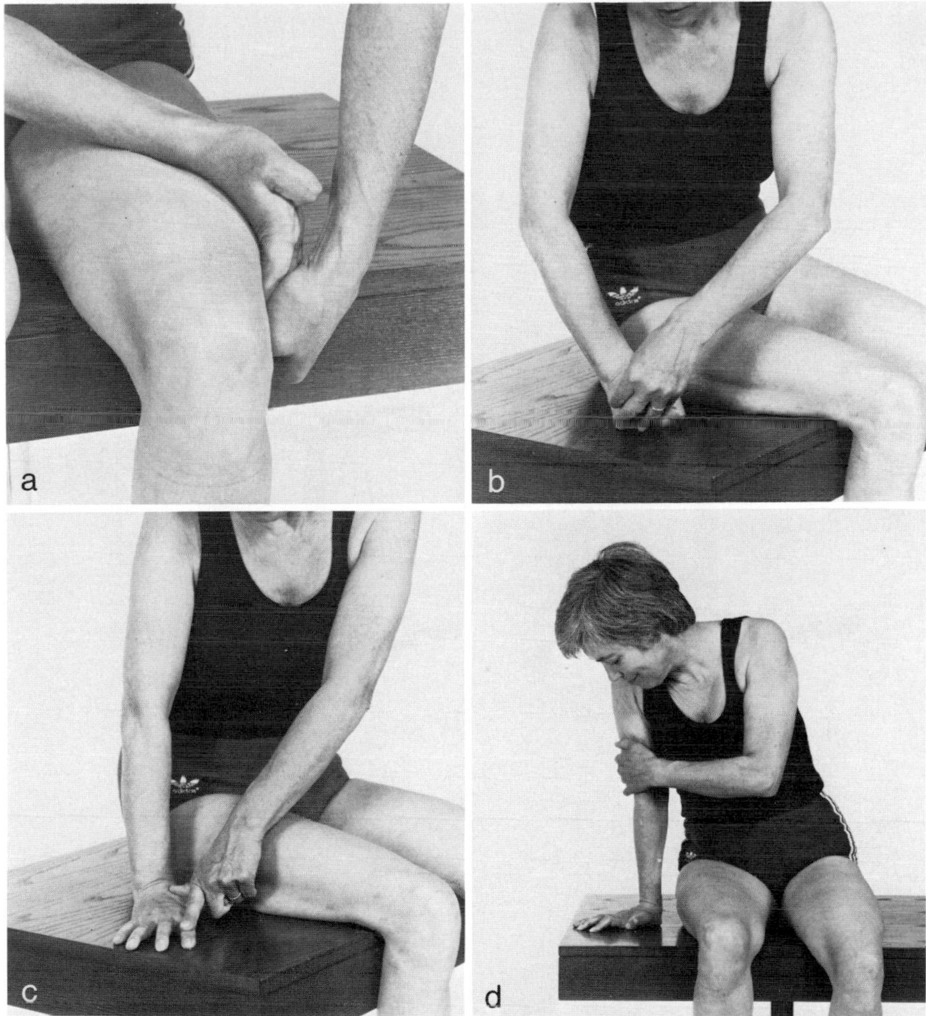

Fig. 15.6 a–d. Preventing shortening of the flexors of the elbow, wrist and fingers (right hemiplegia). **a** Passively extending the fingers with the sound hand, using the sound leg to provide counter-pressure; **b** placing the hemiplegic hand at the side with the fingers kept in extension; **c** bringing the flexed thumb into extension and abduction; **d** extending the elbow with the sound hand to maintain the extension while the weight is taken through the arm

7. To maintain the full range of horizontal abduction with the elbow extended. For full horizontal abduction with elbow extension, the patient usually requires the help of another person. It can be one of the family or a neighbour who has been taught the movement (Fig. 15.8). The patient first clasps his hands together and lifts them above his head. The helper then takes the hemiplegic arm and holding the elbow in extension moves it slowly sideways until it lies flat on the bed, with the palm of the hand facing upwards. The arm lies at an angle of 90° to the body.

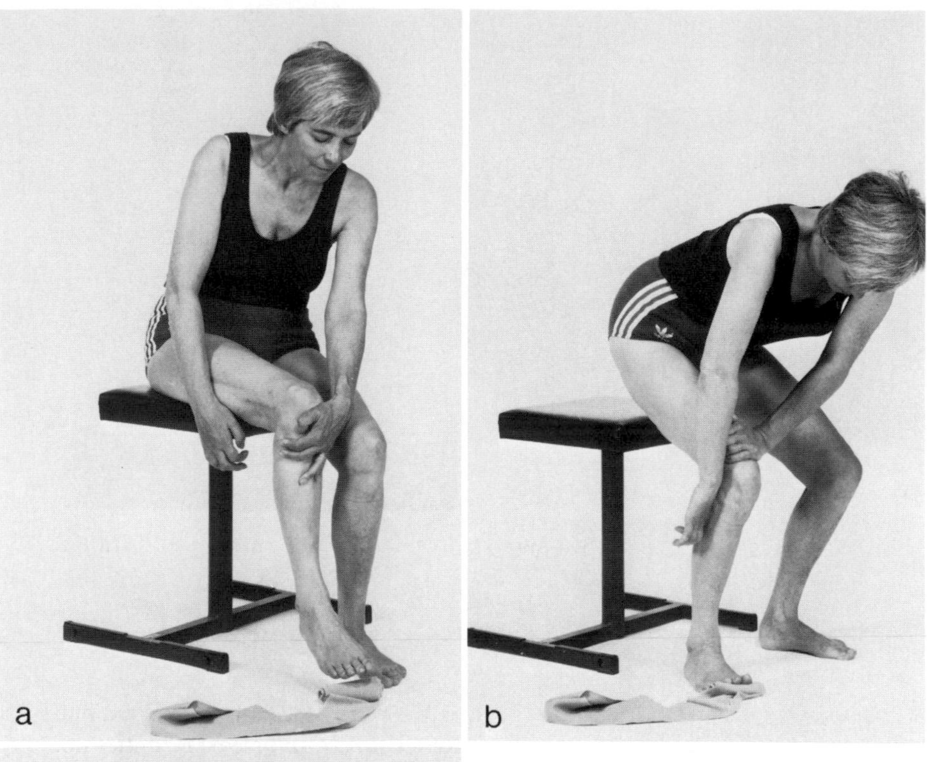

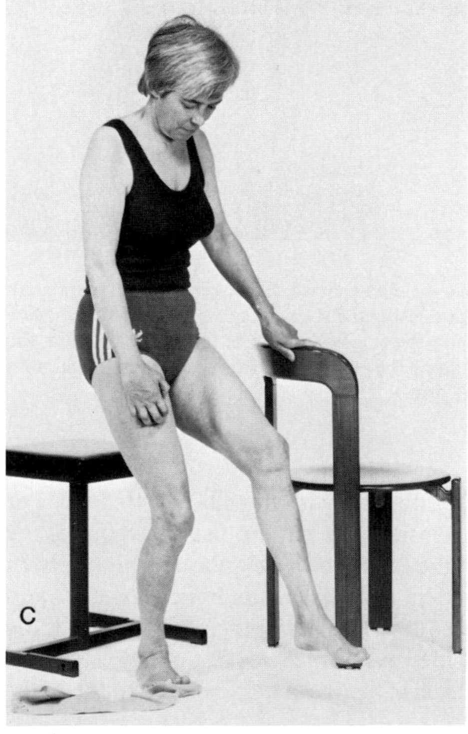

Fig. 15.7 a–c. Preventing shortening of the Achilles tendon and toe flexors (right hemiplegia). **a** The patient places her foot carefully on a rolled bandage, so that the bandage lies directly under all her toes. **b** She presses down on her knee until the heel is on the floor and then lifts her buttocks off the stool. **c** The patient stands, takes all her weight on the hemiplegic leg and then flexes and extends the knee. Her sound foot is held in the air and she holds lightly on to the back of a chair for safety

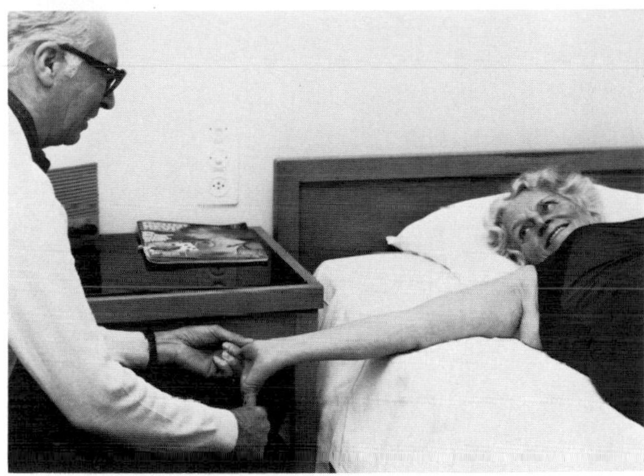

Fig. 15.8. Maintaining range of horizontal abduction with elbow extension (right hemiplegia)

The thumb is drawn out of the hand in extension and abduction, and with his other hand the helper extends all the fingers. The activity continues until the wrist, finger and thumb are fully extended. A pillow placed under the patient's chest during the activity will increase the effect, and will also maintain extension of the thoracic spine.

If the patient carries out these exercises regularly and correctly, he will maintain the full range of movement in the spastic muscles. The recommended activities not only prevent contractures but pave the way for any return of function in the future.

References

Adams GF, Hurwitz LJ (1963) Mental barriers to recovery from stroke. Lancet 14: 533–537

Adler MK, Brown CC, Acton P (1980) Stroke rehabilitation – is age a determinant? J Am Geriatr Soc XXVIII (11): 499–503

Affolter F (1981) Perceptual processes as prerequisites for complex human behaviour. Int Rehabil Med 3 (1): 3–9

Affolter F, Stricker E (eds) (1980) Perceptual processes as prerequisites for complex human behaviour. A theoretical model and its application to therapy. Huber, Bern

Andrews K, Brocklehurst JC, Richards B, Laycock PJ (1982) The recovery of the severely disabled stroke patient. Rheumatol Rehabil 21: 225–230

Atkinson HW (1979) Cash's textbook of neurology for physiotherapists, edited by PA Downie, chaps 2–4. Faber and Faber, London

Bach-y-Rita P (ed) (1980) Brain plasticity as a basis for therapeutic procedures. Recovery of function: theoretical considerations for brain injury rehabilitation. Huber, Bern

Bach-y-Rita P (1981 a) Central nervous system lesions: sprouting and unmasking in rehabilitation. Arch Phys Med Rehabil 62: 413–417

Bach-y-Rita P (1981 b) Brain plasticity as a basis of the development of rehabilitation procedures for hemiplegia. Scand J Rehabil Med 13: 73–83

Basmajian JV (1979) Muscles alive. Their functions revealed by electromyography, 4th edn. Williams and Wilkins, Baltimore

Basmajian JV (1981) Biofeed-back in rehabilitation: a review of principles and practices. Arch Phys Med Rehabil 62: 469–475

Bateman JE (1963) The diagnosis and treatment of ruptures of the rotator cuff. Surg Clin North Am 43: 1523–1530

Bobath B (ed) (1971) Abnormal postural reflex activity caused by brain lesions. Heinemann, London

Bobath B (ed) (1978) Adult hemiplegia: evaluation and treatment. Heinemann, London

Bobath K (1971) The normal postural reflex mechanism and its deviation in children with cerebral palsy. Campfield, St Albans (reprinted from Physiotherapy, november 1971, pp 1–11)

Bobath K (1974) The motor deficit in patients with cerebral palsy. Medical education and information unit of the spastics society. Heinemann Medical Books, London

Bobath K (1976–1982) Unpublished lectures given during courses on the treatment of adult hemiplegia. Postgraduate Study Centre Hermitage, Bad Ragaz

Bobath K (1980) Neurophysiology, part 1. Videofilm recorded at the Postgraduate Study Centre Hermitage, Bad Ragaz

Braun RM, West F, Mooney V, Nickel VL, Roper B, Caldwell C (1971) Surgical treatment of the painful shoulder contracture in the stroke patient. J Bone Joint Surg 53-A (7): 1307–1312

Brodal A (1973) Self-observations and neuro-anatomical considerations after a stroke. Brain 96: 675–694

Brunnstrom S (1970) Movement therapy in hemiplegia. A neurophysiological approach. Harper and Row, Hagerstown

Cailliet R (1980) The shoulder in hemiplegia. Davis, Philadelphia

Cain HD, Liebgold HB (1967) Compressive centripetal wrapping technic for reduction of edema. Arch Phys Med Rehabil 48: 420–423

Caldwell CB, Wilson DJ, Braun RM (1969) Evaluation and treatment of the upper extremity in the hemiplegic stroke patient. Clin Orthop 63: 69–93

Carr JH, Shepherd RB (1982) A motor relearning programme for stroke. Heinemann, London
Carslöö S (1966) The initiation of walking. Acta Anat 65: 1–9
Carterette EC, Friedman MP (eds) (1973) Handbook of perception, vol 3. Academic, New York
Codman EA (1934) The shoulder. Todd, Boston
Coombes K (1977–1983) Unpublished lectures and demonstrations given during courses on the rehabilitation of the face and oral tract. Postgraduate Study Centre Hermitage, Bad Ragaz
Coughlan AK, Humphrey M (1982) Presenile stroke: long-term outcome for patients and their families. Rheumatol Rehabil 21: 115–122

Davies PM (1980) Physiotherapeutische Maßnahmen im Umgang mit der Problematik der hemiplegischen Schulter. Der Physiotherapeut [Suppl] "Die Schulter" Nationaler Kongreß, pp 106–108
Davis SW, Petrillo CR, Eichberg RD, Chu DS (1977) Shoulder – hand syndrome in a hemiplegic population: a 5-year retrospective study. Arch Phys Med Rehabil 58: 353–356
Dewar R (1983) Personal communication
Dimitrijevic MR, Faganal J, Sherwood AM, McKay WB (1981) Activation of paralysed leg flexors and extensors during gait in patients after stroke. Scand J Rehabil Med 13: 109–115

Fiorentino MR (1981) A basis for sensorimotor development – normal and abnormal. Thomas, Springfield
Friedland F (1975) Physical therapy. In: Licht S (ed) Stroke and its rehabilitation. Williams and Williams, Baltimore, pp 246–248

Griffin J, Reddin G (1981) Shoulder pain in patients with hemiplegia. A literature review. Phys Ther 61 (7): 1041–1045

Houtz SJ, Fischer FJ (1961) Function of leg muscles acting on foot as modified by body movements. J Appl Physiol 16: 597–605
Hurd MM, Farrell KH, Waylonis GW (1974) Shoulder sling for hemiplegia: friend or foe? Arch Phys Med Rehabil 55: 519–522

Irwin-Carruthers S, Runnalls MJ (1980) Painful shoulder in hemiplegia – prevention and treatment. S Afr J Physiotherapy March: 18–23

Jeffrey DL (1981) Cognitive clarity: key to motivation in rehabilitation. J Rehabil 47: 33–35
Jimenez Y, Morgan P (1979) Predicting improvement in stroke patients referred for inpatient rehabilitation. Can Med Assoc J 121: 1481–1484
Johnstone M (1978) Restoration of motor function in the stroke patient. Livingstone, New York, pp 15–177

Klein-Vogelbach S (1976) Funktionelle Bewegungslehre. Rehabilitation und Prävention, vol 1, 1st ed. Springer, Berlin Heidelberg New York
Klein-Vogelbach S (1984) Funktionelle Bewegungslehre. Rehabilitation und Prävention, vol 1, 2nd ed. Springer, Berlin Heidelberg New York Tokyo
Knuttson E (1981) Gait control in hemiparesis. Scand J Rehabil Med 13: 101–108
Kottke FJ (1978) Coordination training. IRMA III Congress Lecture, Basle (unpublished)
Kottke FJ (1980) From reflex to skill: the training of coordination. Arch Phys Med Rehabil 61: 551–561

Lehmann JF, Delateur BJ, Fowler RS, Warren CG, Arnold R, Schertzer G, Hurka R, Whitmore JJ, Masock AJ, Chambers KH (1975) Stroke: does rehabilitation affect outcome? Arch Phys Med Rehabil 56: 375–382
Leviton-Rheingold N, Hotte EB, Mandel DR (1980) Learning to dress: a fundamental skill to independence for the disabled. Spec Articl Rehabil Lit 41 (3–4): 72–75

Maitland GD (1973) Peripheral manipulation, 2nd edn. Butterworths, London
Marquardsen J (1969) Natural history of acute cerebrovascular disease: retrospective study of 769 patients. Acta Neurol Scand 45 [Suppl 38]: 56–59
Mathiowetz V, Bolding DJ, Trombly CA (1983) Immediate effects of positioning devices on the normal and spastic hand measured by electromyography. Am J Occup Ther 37 (4): 247–254
Moore J (1980) Neuroanatomical considerations relating to recovery of function following brain in-

jury. In: Bach-y-Rita P (ed) Recovery of function: theoretical considerations for brain injury rehabilitation. Huber, Bern
Moskowitz E, Bishop HF, Pe H, Shibutani K (1958) Posthemiplegic reflex sympathetic dystrophy. JAMA 167: 836–838
Moskowitz E, Lightbody FE, Freitag S (1972) Long-term follow-up of poststroke patient. Arch Phys Med Rehabil 53: 167–172
Mossmann PL (1976) A problem-orientated approach to stroke rehabilitation. Thomas, Springfield
Mountcastle VB (1978) Brain mechanisms for directed attention. J R Soc Med 71: 14–28
Mulley G (1982) Associated reactions in the hemiplegic arm. Scand J Rehabil Med 14: 117–120

Najenson T, Pikielni SS (1965) Malalignment of the gleno-humeral joint following hemiplegia. A review of 500 cases. Ann Phys Med 8 (3): 96–99
Najenson T, Yacubovich E, Pikielni SS (1971) Rotator cuff injury in shoulder joints of hemiplegic patients. Scand J Rehabil Med 3: 131–137

Ofir R, Sell H (1980) Orthoses and ambulation in hemiplegia: a ten-year retrospective study. Arch Phys Med Rehabil 61: 216–220

Perry J (1969) The mechanics of walking in hemiplegia. Clin Orthop 63: 23–31
Pitt R (1976) Toward a comprehensive model of problem-solving: application to solutions of chemistry problems by highschool and college students. Dissertation, University of California, San Diego
Polya G (1973) How to solve it. A new aspect of mathematical method. Princeton University Press, Princeton

Riddoch G, Buzzard EF (1921) Reflex movements and postural reactions in quadriplegia and hemiplegia, with special reference to those of the upper limb. Brain 44: 397
Roper BA (1975) Surgical procedures in hemiplegia. Unpublished Lecture to the Hemiplegic Interest Group, London
Roper BA (1982) Rehabilitation after a stroke. J Bone Joint Surg 64-B (2): 156–163
Rosenzweig MR (1980) Animal models for effects of brain lesions and for rehabilitation. In: Bach-y-Rita P (ed) Recovery of function: theoretical considerations for brain injury rehabilitation. Huber, Bern
Ruskin AP (1982) Understanding stroke and its rehabilitation. Current concepts of cerebrovascular disease. Stroke XVII (6): 27–32
Russel WR, Dewar AJ (1975) Explaining the brain. Oxford University Press, London

Sagan C (1977) The dragons of eden. Speculations on the evolution of human intelligence. Ballantine, New York
Satterfield WT (1982) Hemiplegia – an 11-year summary. J Tenn Med Assoc 75 (8): 525–529
Semans S (1965) Treatment of neurological disorders, concept and systems. J Am Phys Ther Assoc 45 (1): 11–16
Seyffarth H, Denny-Brown D (1948) The grasp reflex and the instinctive grasp reaction. Brain 71 (2): 109–183
Skilbeck CE, Wade DT, Hewer RL (1983) Recovery after stroke. J Neurol, Neurosurg Psychiatry 46: 5–8
Smith RG, Cruikshank JG, Dunbar S, Akhtar AJ (1982) Malalignment of the shoulder after stroke. Br Med J 284: 1224–1226

Voss DE (1969) What's the answer? Phys Ther 49 (9): 1030

Wall JC, Ashburn A (1979) Assessment of gait disability in hemiplegics. Hemiplegic gait. Scand J Rehabil Med 11: 95–103
Walmsley RP (1977) Electromyographic study of the phasic activity of peroneus longus and brevis. Arch Phys Med Rehabil 58: 65–69
Walshe FMR (1923) On certain tonic or postural reflexes in hemiplegia with special reference to the so-called "associated movements". Brain 46: 1
Wyke B (1983) Clinical neurology of the spine, part 2. 7th international congress for manual medicine, Zürich, 9 September 1983

Zinn WM, Mason RM, Currey HLF (1973) Einführung in die Klinische Rheumatologie. Huber, Bern

Subject Index